Animal Hospice and Palliative Medicine for the House Call Veterinarian

Animal Hospice and Palliative Medicine for the House Call Veterinarian

Lynn Hendrix

Owner/Veterinarian,
Beloved Pet Mobile Vet, Davis, CA, United States

Former Board of Directors,
IAAHPC, Chicago, IL, United States

Consultant,
Hospice/Palliative Medicine/End of Life,
VIN, Davis, CA, United States

President/Founder,
World Veterinary Palliative Medicine Organization,
Davis, CA, United States

Owner/Consultant,
The Palliative Vet, Davis, CA, United States

ELSEVIER

Animal Hospice and Palliative Medicine for the House Call Veterinarian   ISBN: 978-0-323-56798-5

Notices

Practitioners and researchers must always rely on their own experience and knowledge in evaluating and using any information, methods, compounds or experiments described herein. Because of rapid advances in the medical sciences, in particular, independent verification of diagnoses and drug dosages should be made. To the fullest extent of the law, no responsibility is assumed by Elsevier, authors, editors or contributors for any injury and/or damage to persons or property as a matter of products liability, negligence or otherwise, or from any use or operation of any methods, products, instructions, or ideas contained in the material herein.

Publisher: Madelene Hyde
Acquisitions Editor: Jennifer Catando
Editorial Project Manager: Sam W. Young
Production Project Manager: Niranjan Bhaskaran
Cover Designer: TBC

3251 Riverport Lane
St. Louis, Missouri 63043

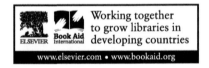

Working together
to grow libraries in
developing countries

www.elsevier.com • www.bookaid.org

Contents

CHAPTER 4   **Your first appointment** **51**

Lynn Hendrix, AA, BA, DVM, CHPV

CHAPTER 6 **Chronic pain management in the home setting......185**

Lynn Hendrix, AA, BA, DVM, CHPV and
Eve Harrison, VMD, CVA, CCFP

CHAPTER 9   **Supporting grief**.......................................**263**

Lynn Hendrix, AA, BA, DVM, CHPV

CHAPTER 10 Supporting a palliated death......279

Lynn Hendrix, AA, BA, DVM, CHPV

CHAPTER 11   **Providing a gentle death-Euthanasia**..................... **309**

Lynn Hendrix, AA, BA, DVM, CHPV and
Anthony J. Smith, BS, DVM, MBA, CHPV

Contributors

Eve Harrison, VMD, CVA, CCFP
Founder, The House Call Vet Academy, Los Angeles, CA, United States; Owner, Veterinarian, Marigold Veterinary, Los Angeles, CA, United States; Consultant, House Call and Mobile Practice, Ask Jan For Help LLC, Kansas City, MO, United States; Co-Founder, House Call and Mobile Vet Virtual Conference, Los Angeles, CA, United States

Lynn Hendrix, AA, BA, DVM, CHPV
Owner, Veterinarian, Beloved Pet Mobile Vet, Davis, CA, United States; Former Board of Directors, IAAHPC, Chicago, IL, United States; Consultant, Hospice, Palliative Medicine, End of Life, VIN, Davis, CA, United States; President, Founder, World Veterinary Palliative Medicine Organization, Davis, CA, United States; Co-Founder, House Call and Mobile Vet Virtual Conference, Los Angeles, CA, United States; Founder, Consultant, The Palliative Vet, Davis, CA, United States

Carolyn Naun, DVM, CHPV
Director, Medical Services, Arms of Aloha LLC, Kailua, HI, United States

Anthony J. Smith, BS, DVM, MBA, CHPV
Former Founding Board of Directors, President, IAAHPC, Chicago, IL, United States; Owner/Veterinarian, Rainbow Bridge Veterinary Services, Hercules, CA, United States

Mina Weakley, BSc
Veterinary Student, College of Veterinary Medicine, Western University of Health Sciences, Pomona, CA, United States; Office Manager, Beloved Pet Mobile Vet, Davis, CA, United States

Preface

In veterinary palliative medicine, all you need is love, human connection, and community.

In July 2018, I had a transformative experience at the first national lecture that I had done at the AVMA Conference on Veterinary Palliative Medicine. I am a veterinarian who does palliative medicine and end-of-life care for animals and their people and the AVMA provided me the platform to express why I do what I do. Veterinary palliative medicine is not just about the animals; I provide the service because I can often help them feel better at the end of their lives, but I also help provide comfort and support for the humans who love them. And to me, it warms my heart to give both more comfort and more support. The basis of what I do is rooted in human connections and the human—animal bond and the entire experience at the AVMA established how important these connections are through life.

My transformation began as I rode in my Lyft to the AVMA conference. I talked with the driver, and he chatted about his boys and the children of Africa that he helped go to school. He was from Africa originally, and he told me if the children in his country in Africa do not have money to pay a fee to go to school, then they do not go to school. His connection to these children, even being thousands of miles away, made my heart jump. Then, I arrived at the expansive convention center. Thousands of veterinarians and their families were milling about in the hallways. Music was playing in the background. As everyone bustled about, I saw a wonderful woman at the information desk. She was helping two preteen children, who appeared to be overwhelmed by the bigness of the conference center and the overwhelming number of humans there. She took the time to make a connection and quell their fears. When it was my turn, I kindly thanked her for it, and we made an authentic, if brief, connection.

Then, I saw Shiza Shahid, the keynote speaker at the 2018 AVMA conference, who had taught, Malala Yousafzai and then helped Malala create education for children worldwide. She currently works to lift women out of poverty and continues to make human connections to support the empowerment of people. She talked about the ripple effect that we have in the world; the connections we do not even know we have made. And as I was giving my lecture about Veterinary Palliative Medicine and making connections with my audience, I knew I had to write about the connections we form when I do what I do.

Palliative medicine vets who deal with death and dying every day hear from clients all the time. "This must be so hard. How do you do this day in and day out?" And in response, I connect what I do to what they do, I say that they have a much harder job because they are losing a beloved. The human—animal bond provides another human connection between us. The other question I often get from families is "Why do you do what you do?" And my answer is, this is not what I went to school for … however, when I connect with families and their beloved animals during a difficult time for them, and those connections, those bonds are why I am here, helping you and your beloved pet. I also find practicing palliative medicine to help those animals live better lives as they are going through their dying process personally satisfying. And though I euthanize most of my patients, even then, I help that beloved pet have a gentle death, sleeping on their bed, surrounded by their family.

In human connection, we all thrive, not from the superficial "Hi, how ya doin?" but from the deeper connections we form with one another. Building strong communities depends on deeper connections between people. And I see people during a challenging time in their lives and help them through to the other side of an emotional abyss. I often feel a part of the family, though I may only see them for an hour or two. We come together in grief and pain, and we bond over the very thing they are hurting over, the impending loss of their beloved friend. I spend more time learning about the family than I ever did when I was in the clinical setting, though I sometimes spent the same amount of time with people in the clinic. The intimate experience of death and dying brings people together unlike any other experience in life. Well, ok, maybe the birth of the child. But the birth of a child, if all goes well, is a joyful experience. While happy experiences are held in high regard, sad and painful experiences can move us through life and change us when we come out the other side and when there is human connection, are just as significant, if not more so.

I experienced profound complicated grief when my mother died in 1993. She was my best friend, my confidant, and my first experience with death, and I did not know how I could live without her presence in my life. It took me 6 months to smile again, and it took another 6 months for me to be able to function more normally. While friends and family were present for a brief time, the support that helped me through it was my hospice support group. We, in the group, had all recently experienced loss; one had lost her sister, another her soulmate of a husband, someone else a brother, and others still a father, and being able to talk, and laugh and cry and hug during our meetings, made our most human grief bearable and our most intimate moments normal. Blessed human connection and a deeper community.

When I sit with people and their pets in their homes, their intimate space, we laugh, we cry, we talk about the fun times they had with their beloved friend and the sad times come up too, we hug or shake hands or just a touch on the shoulder, and there is physical connection that melds with the emotional connection we are making. We express very core human emotions together, and we connect. We connect with their beloved animal who is dying. One bond is breaking, and one bond is forming to help bridge that emotional gap. That is why I do what I do and why we need to have a more human connection in each interaction we have. Human interaction can be a healing thing if done with love and empathy and vulnerability.

Making connections, looking people in the eyes when they need someone most, being present for them and their children, hearing their stories, sad or funny, and helping their beloved animal through a challenging, potentially painful, time in their lives, may bring you a fulfilling career if you so choose. Helping people in their homes may be an extraordinary heart connection for you. I hope this book enables you to find the kind of fulfillment that it has brought me. It may also bring sadness, frustration, learning about boundaries, and many other very human experiences in life.

My human connections in life that I am grateful for include my daughter Morgan and my husband Chris, for all their love and support and for helping me have the time to research and type and type and type. I am grateful for my dear sister Christine Craig. You came into my life when I needed it most and have been a tremendous support throughout the years.

I could not have written this book without the help of my friend and assistant, Mina Weakley. May you gather all the fruits of your labors. Thank you for showing up years ago and helping me build a business, an organization, a community, and being a connection for people and their pets. I am so grateful!

I am grateful for my UK "twin," Dr. Caroline Ficker, for it is your dear friendship from across the pond (and thank goodness for technology) and your challenge to me to be better that has taught me to be better and helped me write this book. And for walking this journey with me, though we live in far time zones.

I am grateful for Drs. Paul and Carla Pion. Paul, you, and VIN have taught me so much about veterinary medicine and human connection, and I believe when you learn, teach (thank you to Maya Angelou for all her inspiring words). Thank you for giving me the opportunity to do better, learn more, and teach more. And I am incredibly grateful for my dear friend Carla. Without your constant support, I do not know what I would do. I so appreciate your friendship every day. Thank you for always being there for me!

I am grateful for my friend Dr. Tobie Faith. Thank you, Tobie, for coming into my life. You are a joy, and I am glad of our connection! And thank you, thank you for helping me with this project!

I am grateful for Dr. Jessica Vogelsang, my dear classmate and friend. If you had not sought me out years ago and started me down this path, I would not be here today. May the synergy of the universe continue to expand our worlds.

I am grateful for my dear friend Dr. Cherie Buisson. You are an inspiration, not only to me but to all our many colleagues. You are a Rockstar!

Thank you to my fellow colleagues who contributed content, Dr. Anthony J. Smith, and Dr. Carolyn Naun. I appreciate you both and your contributions to veterinary palliative medicine and animal hospice.

To all the pioneers, Dr. Eric Clough, Dr. Amir Shanan, Dr. Alice Villalobos, Dr. Tina Ellenbogen, Dr. Kathy Cooney, Dr. Anthony J Smith, Dr. Page Yaxley, and Dr. Katherine Goldberg, thank you for leading the way. Special thanks to Dr. Amir Shanan for believing in me. I shall be forever grateful for your guidance. Thank you, too, to Dr. Cheryl Scott, Katherine Marocchino Ph.D., for getting me up in front of an audience and helping me up when I was a veterinary student and for providing the space on your Nikki Hospice board to starting me on the path to learn how boards work.

This is the most challenging, diverse profession that we have chosen all my beloved colleagues. Do not live a life that is not fulfilling. If you are unhappy, depressed, scared of what the future has in store, and work for someone who is not lifting you up, seek me out. Or seek out help somewhere. Living your best life is something we can all strive for. We do not have to stay in sorrow and misery. I was in that place once, more than once in my life, and my village helped me up and out. Find your village, find the loving human connection. Veterinary Palliative Medicine or Animal Hospice is one of many things you could be doing with your life. In spending time with dying people and dying animals, I have learned that life is too short and making human connections can be scary or fulfilling, purposeful, and more. May this book help you on your journey, wherever your journey may lead you. ♥

Addendum to this forward: This forward was originally written in 2018. It has taken me a long journey to get this book finished. I am grateful to my publishers for giving me time and space to do the work (5 years is a long while!).

I want to add a few more thank yous. To Dr. Eve Harrison, for helping me edit many of these chapters when my eyes had tired of looking at the manuscript. You made it even better! So grateful to have connected in the world. And to Dr. Shenandoah Diehl and Dr. Jill Pomrantz, my dear classmates who helped me with the symptom management chapter. They not only gave me many edits but also made the text better.

Things have changed a bit. I have met new friends, have lost others, have seen more pets and their people in the past few months than I had seen in a month's time in the past 10 years. Covid-19 changed our lives in 2020 in many profound ways. Many lost their human connections, resorting to Zoom and curbside veterinary services and minimizing contacts as we sorted through a pandemic that shut much of our world down. I am grateful to science for creating a vaccine that may help us move past this pandemic and back to more human connection.

In the adversity of a pandemic, our world also brought to our attention the challenges of facing other human failings, racism, sexism, poverty, and the loss of connection between individuals and the challenges faced that prevent us from seeing each other. I realized as I reread this and as I study how to be antiracist, how privileged my statement of living our best lives may sound with the adversity our fellow black, Asian, indigenous, and LGBTQ colleagues face. My perceptions changed with 2020, and I have a way to go, as do many people, to understand another's experience may not be your own and to stand up in the face of adversity, as tough as it is to do.

This book is a shift in paradigm, and I believe it has grown, with the changes in our world, and it is time for a major shift in paradigms, not only in veterinary medicine but in our way of embracing our differences as human beings and standing for each other. Ultimately, connection, whether it is our connections with our beloved pets or connections with our fellow colleagues or our fellow human beings, is what makes our lives rich at the end of our lives.

As we grow and become more educated and learn to be more inclusive people, be well and make connections with people and pets that help us create those bonds that matter.

Lynn Hendrix DVM, CHPV.

Introduction to animal hospice

Lynn Hendrix, AA, BA, DVM, CHPV [1,2,3,4]

[1]*Owner, Veterinarian, Beloved Pet Mobile Vet, Davis, CA, United States;* [2]*Former Board of Directors, IAAHPC, Chicago, IL, United States;* [3]*Consultant, Hospice, Palliative Medicine, End of Life, VIN, Davis, CA, United States;* [4]*President, Founder, World Veterinary Palliative Medicine Organization, Davis, CA, United States*

Animals of all shapes and sizes make up much of the life on our planet, from single-celled organisms to species that live around humans, from bug to elephant, veterinarians care for the multitude of animal species. The bond between animals and man has changed over time, from predators and prey to companions and animal workers. The relationship between animals changed from domestication to one of relation. Various species, including insects, arthropods, reptiles, fish and birds, and a multitude of mammals, may be considered part of the family. And as the relationship has changed, the medical care needs for our pets and other domesticated species have changed.

Veterinarians have accommodated their practices with the changing times. Once, animal doctors that helped with farm animals and working dogs and now veterinarians mimic human medicine, with specialists, and equipment, such as MRIs and CT scan machines. As veterinary medicine grows better at curative medicine, we have the opportunity to grow a potential gap in care. Veterinary palliative medicine and animal hospice can expand the opportunities for patients with life-limiting and chronic, progressive diseases. And as veterinary medicine hurtles toward corporate entities and large conglomerations, house call and mobile practices have increased value and connection to clients that those large entities have a harder time providing.

Animal hospice has recently become a hot topic in veterinary medicine. The history of animal hospice is relatively short when compared to the human model. Animal hospice and veterinary palliative medicine is a paradigm shift and it may take time for veterinarians and their team to be comfortable with shifting from clinical concepts and practice. This chapter will delve into the history of animal hospice and palliative care in animals. The following chapters will expand upon veterinary palliative medicine and how to become a house call practice devoted to animal hospice and palliative medicine.

Euthanasia (Eu—good, Thanos—death) has been the norm for the animal world for hundreds of years. The ancient Egyptians provided death for their animals, many animals went to the grave with them. The early models of animal control provide a more modern version of euthanasia, utilizing different methods of terminating life. Euthanasia has progressed to be the preferred way to deal with a terminal illness in our domestic, wildlife, and zoo species (Kleinfeldt, 2017). Euthanasia can be provided in various ways, from the use of a gun with larger animals and wildlife, to inhalant methods utilized in the past by animal control, to the current method of injectable medications for most domestic, zoo, lab animals. Euthanasia can be a source of profound emotions for both clients, and veterinarians. Education on euthanasia has been on the job training, with little direct education on how to perform euthanasia, what medications to use, how to guide and support the client. The AVMA came out with guidelines in best practices for euthanasia in 2013, and they were revised in 2020. There may be a gap in care between euthanasia and a terminal or life-limiting diagnosis. Animal hospice and palliative care was initiated by a few veterinarians when the gap between terminal diagnosis and euthanasia seemed too wide for either the veterinarian or the client.

Paradigm shift

The paradigm shift in human medicine adding human hospice began with Dame Cicely Saunders of the United Kingdom. Dame Saunders began her career as a registered nurse (RN) and then became an Osteopathic Doctor (OD) to help change the way people and their families have an end-of-life experience. She had already been helping terminally ill patients with their disease through death, adding palliative (comfort care) that included psychological, spiritual, and social support for the patient and family. Dr. Saunders saw a growing need for additional support for both the patient and family and developed the concept of hospice for human medicine. Early adopters of veterinary palliative care and animal hospice built on the concepts Dr. Saunders had developed.

Palliative medicine is symptom management to improve quality of life without trying to cure the patient (Doyle, 1993). Palliative medicine is at the forefront of the veterinarian's tools, allowing for the patient's comfort, and educating and empowering the family in their care. Palliative medicine may utilize standard pharmaceuticals, though dosing may vary from standard care. Hospice is the last stage of care with palliation.

Increasing awareness

Individual veterinarians in the latter half of the 1990s began changing how they practiced medicine. The earliest writings regarding animal hospice came from Dr. Eric Clough. Eric Clough, VMD, and his wife, Jane Clough, RN, BA, VNA, presented *"Helping Clients Say Good-bye: Hospice Care for Pets"* at the AVMA Convention in Baltimore, MD, in 1998 (Ann P. McClenaghan, 2011).

Dr. Alice Villalobos then picked up the torch and helped increase awareness of animal hospice concepts. Dr. Villalobos is a world-renowned veterinary oncologist who has provided palliative care and written many articles about Pawspice™ (her trademarked terminology for hospice) since 2000. She first became involved in animal hospice while studying oncology at UC Davis with her mentor, Dr. Gordon Theilen. In the 1970s, as they developed the field of clinical veterinary oncology, she felt it was a natural extension of her oncology practice and began writing articles for Oncology Outlook Columns and "The Bond and Beyond" in Veterinary Practice News. In 2004, she developed the first comprehensive Quality of Life Scale, the HHHHHMM scale, providing another tool for veterinarians to help further define for clients a way to consider euthanasia more objectively (Villalobos, 2017).

Dr. Villalobos has promoted the concept of home euthanasia as the best way for a hospice patient to transition (Villalobos, 2017). She has authored many articles and books on the subject of animal hospice, palliative care, and oncology. She feels passionate about end-of-life care, providing instruction on placing catheters with families, sedation before euthanasia to make the euthanasia experience a more respectful and symbolic process for the families (Villalobos, 2017).

Dr. Villalobos sees the future of veterinary palliative care encompassing certification and eventually becoming a specialty for providers to develop expertise in palliative medicine. Dr. Villalobos firmly favors veterinary-guided animal hospice including veterinary nurses and mental health professionals to provide support for both the caregivers and veterinarians. She also believes in a paradigm shift, thinking of our role as veterinarians in the euthanasia process as a "minister," helping animals on their transition for terminally ill patients. She believes that this change in our paradigm would help reduce the compassion and ethics fatigue that we so often find in veterinary medicine (Villalobos, 2017).

The earliest veterinary adopters of animal hospice who are still in practice include Dr. Amir Shanan, Dr. Tammy Shearer, Dr. Alice Villalobos, Dr. Anthony Smith, and Dr. Tina Ellenbogen. Other early adopters are Gail and Richard Pope with Brighthaven, Kathryn Marocchino with Nikki Hospice Foundation, and Dr. Ella Bittel with Spirits in Transition. They all have paved the way for the foundations of animal hospice.

Founding organizations

With the first writings occuring in 1998, the first organizations associated with animal hospice also began forming. Founded by Katherine Marochino, The Nikki Hospice Foundation was the first organization to recognize animal hospice and bring together veterinarians and others who were interested in providing this service. She felt one of her beloved kitties, Nikki, experienced a traumatic end-of-life experience and believed that veterinarians and owners needed more information and education (Marochino, 2008). In forming this organization, she brought together local veterinarians and mental health professionals to build a board of directors and added a UC Davis veterinary student (the author of this book) to the board meetings in 1999.

In 2008, The Nikki Hospice Foundation developed the first-ever Animal Hospice symposium at UC Davis. One hundred forty professionals interested in the concepts of animal hospice, from veterinarians to human hospice workers, attended. Difficult discussions ensued at this conference. The controversy arose between those who believed hospice meant little to no intervention letting the disease progress to "natural" death, or whether euthanasia should be provided for animals in a hospice program. This concept is still contentious today, though there is a shift amongst the current adoptors.

Dr. Amir Shanan saw a need for animal hospice in the early 1990s. He began offering in-home euthanasia in 1995 for his clients and began to see the need for other options besides euthanasia for end-of-life patients. Dr. Shanan was a member of the American Association of Human–Animal Bond Veterinarians at that time and listened to veterinarians talk about animal hospice with no forward movement. As late as 2007, and now a member of the International Veterinary Academy of Pain Management, Dr. Shanan once again heard talk regarding animal hospice but no plans for future integration (Shanan, 2017).

Dr. Amir Shanan was at the Nikki Hospice symposium in 2008 and recognized the need to meet on common ground to move the field forward. In addition to being an early adoptor and helping develop the animal hospice concept, Dr. Shanan wanted to have animal hospice recognized by mainstream veterinarians. He recognized the need for a vision and mission, to move the field. With that in mind, Dr. Shanan founded the IAAHPC, the International Association of Animal Hospice and Palliative Care, in 2009 (Shanan, 2017).

The original board of directors came from the Nikki Hospice symposium, Dr. Ella Bittel, Kathryn Marocchino Ph.D., Dr. Anthony Smith, and Dr. Tina Ellenbogen. In 2010, Dr. Kathy Cooney and Coleen Ellis joined Dr. Shanan, while Dr. Bittel and Ms. Marocchino left to pursue other avenues. In 2011, The IAAHPC, under the leadership of Dr. Shanan and Dr. Cooney, created the first Annual IAAHPC Animal Hospice Conference for veterinarians and other professionals in San Antonio, Texas. Dr. Cooney successfully ran the first annual conference and provided the support and the education for the following five annual conferences for the IAAHPC (Shanan, 2017). She has continued the education of veterinarians on euthanasia techniques with CAETA, the Companion Animal Euthanasia Training Academy.

The IAAHPC provided the first comprehensive guidelines for Animal Hospice and Palliative Care in 2013, and in 2016, the first Certification program was developed in Animal Hospice and Palliative Care. The first class of certified veterinarians and technicians graduated in 2017. The IAAHPC has become an umbrella organization, including veterinarians, veterinary technicians, and mental health professionals, and has paved the way for future animal hospice and palliative care field growth.

In 2013, two forward-thinking veterinarians, Katherine Goldberg DVM and Page Yaxley DVM, DACVECC, founded the first veterinary-only group, VSHPC, the Veterinary Society of Hospice and Palliative Care. They planned to further research and education in Animal Hospice and Palliative Medicine (Goldberg, 2017). As of 2021, the organization is no longer functional.

In 2018, Dr. Lynn Hendrix (Author of this book) and Dr. Caroline Ficker started the World Veterinary Palliative Medicine Organization. They began with a vision to improve the evidence base for veterinary palliative medicine, educate veterinarians in palliative medicine, and promote further research in palliative medicine. Dr. Hendrix and Dr. Ficker have a goal to be involved in the development of a specialty in veterinary palliative medicine.

Dr. Shanan sees slow progress. He hopes to see a greater demand for veterinary nurses to provide a more prominent role in animal hospice. The future will likely bring increased awareness of the field, providing more veterinary education on animal hospice and veterinary palliative medicine, adding animal hospice externships, research programs, more interest and education in veterinary technician schools and mental health programs, adding additional regulations and laws regarding animal hospice. Currently there is an organizing committee researching and working on a specialty in Animal Hospice and Palliative Medicine (Shanan, 2017).

Dr. Ellenbogen believes pet insurance will increase client's abilities to afford end-of-life care.

Similarities to human hospice and differences

Most of the animal hospice models started with an examination of the human hospice model. In 2013, a task force in the IAAHPC was made up of four veterinarians, a mental health professional, and an ethicist to develop the first- best animal hospice practices. A 50-page document came together over the year and is currently published online at www.IAAHPC.org. Several IAAHPC guidelines authors came together with AAHA and produced End-of-Life Guidelines for AAHA, published in 2016.

One of the similarities of animal hospice is the interdisciplinary team. It is also one of the differences. The current model for animal hospice providers recommends a team approach, including a veterinarian, a veterinary technician, and a mental health professional as the care provider team. However, as of this writing, most animal hospice practices are single practice veterinarians. Few practices employ one or more technicians and even fewer that employ a mental health professional. Those that do provide mental health providers, often do so as a referral and not as direct employment.

One of the most significant differences between human and animal end-of-life care is our ability to provide euthanasia for our patients. Veterinarians can perform euthanasia for animals in every state. As of this writing, in the United States, ten states currently allow physician-assisted death for human beings. There are four countries in Europe that allow for assisted death. The ability to provide assisted death is slowly changing in human medicine.

Euthanasia continues to be a controversial topic in veterinary medicine. Many veterinarians feel it is a gift to provide a peaceful death for their patients. However, stress levels are increased around the topic of euthanasia in the hospital setting (Newsome, 2019; Scotney, 2015). For the clients, it may be equally stressful to decide on euthanasia. In addition, providing euthanasia for some patients, or in large numbers daily can contribute to burnout among veterinarians and veterinary staff (Scotney, 2015).

The palliative philosophy offers support for the humans' caregiving their beloved animals at the end of their lives, and animal hospice affords support and comfort for the dying animals. Providing clients with adequate support and education. Meeting clients where they are, emotionally and physically, empathizing with client perception, understanding and being able to speak to a variety of educational background, listening to client goals and concerns, and educating clients on what to expect is included in the role of the palliative veterinarian.

Evidence-based medicine

Veterinary medicine is a science. The advances we make in medicine come from evidence-based science. Animal hospice and veterinary palliative medicine needs evidence-based science, and one of the challenges we currently have is little good research at the end of life for animals. The progress of increasing the research base has been slow to the date of this writing, but a few universities are starting to provide some research in this newly formed field. More research needs to be done to help provide the best care for animals.

In April 2016, The Veterinary Record, Dr. Katherine Goldberg published a comprehensive review of the literature published on Animal Hospice and Palliative Care (Goldberg, 2016). Bringing the literature up to date will continue to improve the knowledge base available to veterinarians and, hopefully, can start more evidence-based studies in the field (Goldberg, 2016).

Conclusion

Animal Hospice and Veterinary Palliative Medicine may have started with challenges but has skyrocketed into the consciousness of veterinarians worldwide in a short amount of time. Organizing has begun and created a foundation in animal hospice and palliative medicine in the veterinary field.

More veterinarians want to know more about veterinary palliative medicine every day. Growing the field of veterinary palliative medicine will produce a more solid end-of-life experience for both pet and loving family members. This overview of history is to provide context for future endeavors in education and research.

References

Doyle, D. D. (1993). *Palliative medicine - a time for definition? Palliative medicine*. Edinburgh, UK: Sage Publications.

Goldberg, K. (2016). Veterinary hospice and palliative care: A comprehensive review of the literature. *The Veterinary Record*, 369–374.

Goldberg, D. P. (2017). *Email discussion. (D. L. Hendrix, interviewer)*.

Kleinfeldt, A. (2017). *Detailed discussion of animal euthanasia*. Retrieved from Animal Legal & Historical Center https://www.animallaw.info/article/detailed-discussion-animal-euthanasia.

Marochino, D. K. (2008). *Interview with Katherine Marrochino. (D. L. Hendrix, interviewer)*.

McClenaghan, A. P. (August 01, 2011). *An introduction to the concept of veterinary hospice care (proceedings)*. Retrieved from DVM 360 http://veterinarycalendar.dvm360.com/introduction-concept-veterinary-hospice-care-proceedings.

Newsome, J. T.-H.-K. (2019). Compassion fatigue, euthanasia stress, and their management in laboratory animal research. *Journal of the American Association for Laboratory Animal Science*, 289—292.

Scotney, R. L. (2015). A systematic review of the effects of euthanasia and occupational stress in personnel working with animals in animal shelters, veterinary clinics, and biomedical research facilities. *Journal of the American Medical Association*, 1121—1130.

Shanan, D. A. (March 21, 2017). *Interview with Amir Shanan. (D. L. Hendrix, interviewer)*.

Villalobos, D. A. (May 8, 2017). *Interview with Alice Villalobos. (D. L. Hendrix, interviewer)*.

Further reading

Shearer, T. (2016). *The 5 Step hospice and palliative care plan*. Retrieved from IAAHPC https://www.iaahpc.org/images/Shearerprogramabstracts.docx.

Veterinary Palliative Medicine changes the paradigm of veterinary medicine

Lynn Hendrix, AA, BA, DVM, CHPV [1,2,3,4]

[1]*Owner, Veterinarian, Beloved Pet Mobile Vet, Davis, CA, United States;* [2]*Former Board of Directors, IAAHPC, Chicago, IL, United States;* [3]*Consultant, Hospice, Palliative Medicine, End of Life, VIN, Davis, CA, United States;* [4]*President, Founder, World Veterinary Palliative Medicine Organization, Davis, CA, United States*

Highlights

- Introduction to palliative medicine
  - What is palliative medicine?
  - The importance of palliative medicine
  - Defining veterinary palliative medicine
- Veterinary palliative medicine versus animal hospice
- Goals of veterinary palliative medicine and hospice
  - When to involve a palliative medicine veterinarian
  - The palliative care team
  - Communication tools to improve conversations about end-of-life care
- Challenges faced in starting veterinary palliative medicine or animal hospice
  - Myths/FAQ
- Conclusion
  - Veterinary palliative medicine as a specialty

Introduction to palliative medicine

Human palliative medicine developed as the need arose for medical doctors to have additional training in end-of-life medicine. Though palliative medicine can be found around the world, this chapter will focus on the development of palliative care and palliative medicine in the United Kingdom and the United States. Becoming a specialty in human medicine in 2006 in the United States (Ruder, 2015) and even earlier in 1986 in the United Kingdom (Doyle, 1993), human palliative medicine revolutionized the approach to patient care for life-limiting and chronic, progressive, advanced illness. Organized animal hospice and palliative care in veterinary medicine have been around for 23 years (as of this writing). The newest concept in end-of-life care, veterinary palliative medicine, has just started to organize and is looking to become a veterinary medicine specialty.

What is palliative medicine and hospice?

When human palliative medicine became a specialty in the United Kingdom, the Association of Palliative Medicine of Great Britain and Ireland defined on their homepage: "Palliative medicine provides clinical leadership, care, and support to prevent and relieve suffering for people with life-limiting and life-threatening illnesses. Its diagnostic and therapeutic priorities focus on meeting every individual patient's goals through shared decision-making and those important to them."

"It is practiced both as part of multidisciplinary palliative care teams and in partnership with other relevant specialties to deliver individualized, holistic care." It is a medical specialty recognized by the respective nations' Royal Colleges of Physicians.

Practitioners of palliative medicine specific expertise is in:

"Assessing and managing physical, psychological, and spiritual symptoms and mitigating distress. Clinical analysis of and decision-making in complex scenarios, such as when a patient's clinical needs, preferences, and interests are delicately balanced and may require the skilled application of relevant ethical and legal guidance. Expert communication about and coordination of care, especially at disease transitions and boundaries between care settings. Working with partners, colleagues, and organizations across multiple sectors to provide excellent multidisciplinary care for patients and those important to them. Care and support to those significant to the patient, including facilitating their bereavement care."

Home page for the Association of Palliative Medicine (n.d.)

The chart below provides the difference between veterinary general practitioners, specialists and palliative medicine practitioners (Fig. 2.1).

Human hospice provides comfort and support for patients and their families in the last phases of an incurable disease or at the natural end of life. Hospice incorporates palliative care and is defined as a philosophy, a specialized program of care, and in some instances, an actual building to support the dying.

Human hospice recognizes dying as a normal process resulting from end-stage disease and seeing the end-of-life as an opportunity for growth. Hospice exists so patients in the last phases of life get care so that they might live as fully and comfortably as possible. There is a saying in human palliative medicine, "They live each day until the day they die, so let us make their days good ones." Through appropriate care and a attentive community sensitive to their needs, patients and their families may be free to attain a degree of mental and spiritual preparation for death that is satisfactory to them.

In the U.S. human hospice organizations, services may be limited to patients who have decided not to undergo any further curative treatments and have a limited life

DIFFERENCES BETWEEN VETERINARY GENERAL PRACTITIONERS AND SPECIALISTS, AND VETERINARY PALLIATIVE MEDICINE

VETERINARY GENERAL PRACTITIONERS	VETERINARY SPECIALISTS	VETERINARY PALLIATIVE MEDICINE PRACTIONERS
Trained in multiple species, general medicine	GP trained in a specific field of care, i.e., Oncology, Internal Medicine	Currently a General Practitioner with additional training and focus on palliative medicine.
Trained in medical care from birth to death of patients	Board Certified in Specialty Field	Further training in complex, chronic palliative medicine cases.
Trained in basic palliative care.	Trained in complex medical care in their specific field.	Trained in advanced, refractory pain and symptom management
Trained in general discussions about end of life care.	Additional training in grief counseling	Further training in serious disease discussion and family conflict resolution and grief counseling
Performs euthanasia, training may be on the job	Performs euthanasia, training may be on the job	Additional training in providing euthanasia
Basic training in grief counseling	Trained in palliative care for their field, in addition to basic training.	Is a specialty in human medicine, may be a specialty in veterinary medicine in the future.

Based on human model described here: Quill, T. E., & Abernethy, A. P. (2013). Generalist plus specialist palliative care–creating a more sustainable model. The New England Journal of medicine, 368(13), 1173–1175. http://doi.org/10.1056/NEJMp1215620

FIGURE 2.1

The differences between veterinary practitioners. Based on the human hospice and palliative medicine models of care and modified to 2021 standards found in practice. Graphic created on Canva by Lynn Hendrix ©2021 (Kittelson, 2015; Quill & Abernathy, 2013).

prognosis of 6 months or less. The management of palliative care patients who have progressed such that death will likely occur within days to weeks describes the current state of animal hospice. Animal hospice and palliative medicine are not yet distinctly defined (Shanan et al., 2017).

The importance of palliative medicine for animals at the end of life

"Palliative care is the active total care of patients with a life-limiting illness that is not responsive to curative treatment. Control of pain, other symptoms, and psychological, social, and spiritual problems are paramount. The goal of palliative care is to achieve the best quality of life for patients and their families." (Palliative Care, 2020). Palliative care can go on as long as it is needed, for months and even for years which differs from hospice.

Starting palliative care early can make a significant impact on life. In 2010, Jennifer Temel MD et al. did a randomized study on human patients with small cell lung cancer. Half the patients did standard oncology care and were sent to palliative care late in their disease, which is commonly done. The other group added palliative care early to their oncology care. The conclusion was the patients had improvements in quality of life and mood. Surprisingly, they also lived longer up to 6 months longer (Temel, 2010).

In 2017, Dr. Temel et al. did another randomized study on patients with terminal lung cancer and GI cancer. They found differences in quality of life again, although longer out from their starting point. There were differences in end-of-life communication for patients in early palliative care. Patients were more likely to discuss what they wanted and needed when they had a palliative care physician involved early (Temel, 2017).

Another study done regarding the caregiver of terminal patients showed enrolling the caregiver in palliative care early improved the caregiver's quality of life and gave them more support to better care for their family member (El-Jawahri, 2017).

In 2016, the American Society of Clinical Oncology emphasized in their guidelines need for palliative care in advanced cancer (Nelson, 2017).

Palliative medicine and care in human medicine has been restructured since the landmark Temel study. Terminal patients are placed earlier into palliative care. Hospice has become late-stage support to end-of-life patients. Veterinary medicine can bridge the gap of care between terminal diagnosis and euthanasia if we institute early palliative medicine.

Defining veterinary palliative medicine

To move the field forward, we need a definition for veterinary palliative medicine. The author proposes this definition for veterinary palliative medicine: The medical model for veterinarians managing complex and refractory pain and other symptom management with complex comorbidites for animals with advanced, chronic, progressive or terminal disease. Veterinary palliative medicine embraces the end-of-life human-animal bond, and is supported by additional education in palliative medicine, advanced serious disease communication, and complex grief counseling. Veterinarians skilled in palliative medicine should be able to support people with multifaceted psychological distress or recognize it and know when to refer to a mental health provider.

Veterinary palliative medicine versus animal hospice

Establishing the differences between veterinary palliative medicine and animal hospice can help us define when we add palliative medicine to patient's treatment and when it may need to escalate to end-stage hospice (Fig. 2.2).

Human palliative medicine can be established with advanced, progressive, chronic disease, not just terminal illness, and can be ongoing supporting current medical treatments. On the other hand, hospice is utilized for terminal illness only, and often when people are no longer seeking medical care outside of palliative care. One significant difference is the timing involved in care. Hospice is generally defined as 6 months or less to live, where palliative care has no time limit. Insurance

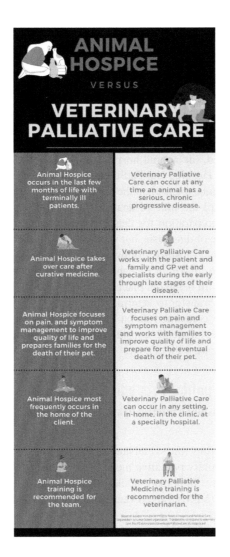

FIGURE 2.2

Animal hospice versus veterinary palliative care based on human differences between hospice and palliative care (NHPCO Staff, 2019). Graphic created on Canva by Lynn Hendrix © 2021.

companies have influenced the definition of hospice and palliative care in the US medical system. So how might that have influenced the veterinary field?

As discussed in the last chapter on the history of animal hospice, much of what the early adopters did was take the definitions in the human medical field of palliative care and hospice and adapted them to the veterinary field. Ideas like 6 months or less to establish animal hospice are considered the expected length of time for patients to be in "hospice." Other concepts regarding human definitions have influenced switching to not seeking curative treatment while providing hospice care for animals and only giving palliative care after discontinuing curative medicine. So, how can we improve care while using these concepts?

Goals of veterinary palliative medicine and hospice

As previously discussed, the animal hospice model is defined by the International Association of Animal Hospice and Palliative Care (IAAHPC) as follows: "Animal hospice is care for animals, focused on the patient's and family's needs; on living life as fully as possible until the time of death [with or without intervention]; and on attaining a degree of preparation for death" (Shanan et al., 2017). Palliative care should begin at the time of diagnosis, but when should hospice start? Since the early adoptors defined animal hospice following the guidelines of human hospice, 6 months or less to live, maybe it is a shorter time. In addition, hospice has some negative associations with being the place or the time in which people die in human medicine and this may transfer to veterinary medicine. Considering that an animal may suffer if they are concerned about the term hospice and then not likely to seek care, the author recommends considering using the term palliative care when discussing end-of-life care with clients.

When to refer to a palliative medicine veterinarian

Veterinarians could consider a referral to a veterinarian trained in palliative medicine when:

1. There is a life-limiting illness, advanced, progressive, chronic disease, or terminal illness. Veterinary palliative medicine is not separate from curative treatment, and studies in human medicine support early care. The veterinary palliative medicine (VPM) trained veterinarian would work in conjunction with the GP or specialist.
2. When there is a need for added support. Social, emotional, and spiritual support can be provided by hospice-trained or palliative-trained veterinarians, veterinary technicians, and mental health professionals. Medical support with palliative care increases over time and as the animal is declining and curative medicine intervention wanes. And if the house call veterinarian has established a relationship early, helping people through their postdeath grief benefits those who struggle with their grief.
3. Any time a client requests to take a pet home against medical advice. Palliative medicine can be a bridge for those animals who may not otherwise receive veterinary care because the owners are afraid, are not prepared to consider their death, or are in "denial." Palliative trained veterinarians, techs, and counselors can help people through this challenging time and can give the animal more comfort.

The palliative care team

The core team with human palliative care or hospice is the palliative medicine doctor, the nurse, and the mental health professional. The IAAHPC guidelines authors utilized the human hospice intradisciplinary core team model: having the veterinarian, the registered veterinary technician or nurse, and mental health professional. Each part of the team needs additional training either in human palliative care or with a conference. The most veterinary specific training (at the time of this writing) is the current IAAHPC conference or the certification program through the IAAHPC. More in-depth training can be found in human hospice and palliative care conferences but may need translation to veterinary medicine and research to support the use.

The medical director is the veterinarian and ideally, has supplementary training in palliative medicine, animal hospice, and end-of-life care. Veterinary technicians can also play an essential role in caring for the family and their pet. Technicians can also provide a link between the veterinarian and the other staff, carry out the veterinarian's medical care plan, and provide education, assistance, and respite for the families. Mental health professionals provide psychological care for the clients, and they can support team members and caregivers with topics like anticipatory grief, complicated grief, logistics of support, psychological support, and difficulties between family members. They can also facilitate a pet loss support group.

Who else may be on your team? Anyone who can provide palliative support to the family or the patient. Veterinarians do not need to hire specific individuals (though it may be a way to expand your business). Veterinarians can utilize other businesses in the area to help provide specialized services. Groomers, extended family members, pet sitters, general practice veterinarians, and their team, respite workers, churches, chaplains focused on animals and pet loss, human pharmacies, compounding pharmacists, and accredited pharmacists are preferred.

As of this writing, there may be many challenges to overcome to build a solid veterinary palliative medicine practice, much less a specialty. As more veterinarians embrace veterinary palliative medicine in their practices and enhancing what they currently do, with palliative care concepts, the team approach, and advanced planning, it is a significant step in supporting patients through end-of-life care.

Why are house calls important for hospice?

There are two standards in human medicine for hospice care. The first standard is care occuring in a building called a hospice, is the standard in Europe, and there are brick and mortar hospices in the United States. The second standard is in the United States, who has led in—home hospice care, sending nurses and other interdisciplinary team members into the terminally ill patient's homes. The palliative-trained doctor leads the interdisciplinary team, prescribing medicine and providing a medical plan for the team, consisting of registered nurses, paraprofessionals, and volunteers. The hospice team and family caregivers attend to the patient in comfort of their home. Both models are significant and needed, the brick and mortars can help care for people who need live-in care without moving them, the patient lives on site. However, we do not currently have a live-in model of care for animals in veterinary practices, and for them to live the remainder of their lives in a hospital would incur expense that many clients may not want. Thus in—home palliative practices become significant for end-of-life care.

In addition, for animals who stress going into the hospital, caring for them at home is often the least stressful way to support them especially when they have an advanced, progressive, chronic, or life-limiting disease. Veterinarians and their team can see the animal in their natural environment, watch them move around, and observe the obstacles in their environment which may challenge their mobility. The caregivers also feel more comfortable in their own home. Larger animals with mobility issues no longer have to get into vehicles to be transported to a brick and mortar, and cats can stay in an environment in which they feel more comfortable.

The challenges to at-home house call care may include difficulty testing, lack of imaging modalities, increased cost for owners with travel, and challenges with obtaining medications and timing of making appointments. Mobile practices, those with a van or motor home, can help provide some of these services for these patients. Small house call practices (one doctor or one doctor and technician) may get overwhelmed with patients, have challenges keeping up with the needs of multiple patients in palliative care, and be limited in the number of hours available. The IAAHPC guidelines suggests 24/7 care for hospice patients; however, it is not required (nor is it recommended for single-doctor practices) to provide 24/7 care for patients. Instead of being available 24/7, create a crisis plan and kit for the clients to support them for emergencies when the practice is not available. The better prepared the caregivers are, the more they are likely to have a great end-of-life experience.

Communication tools to improve conversations around end-of-life care

Effective, empathetic communication is essential to veterinary palliative medicine. Adjusting veterinary medicine's commonplace terminologies may support clients in various scenarios: from the diagnosis to a euthanasia decision. Advanced communication skills can improve the understanding of the disease process, the trajectory of care, quality of care, compliance, and the overall relationship between the family and the veterinary care team. The following points are regarded as common terminology used in current veterinary practice. The author suggests a different perspective on these terms to add to your lexicon.

Agonal breathing occurs when there is decreasing oxygen and increasing carbon dioxide levels and it stimulates the brain stem to generate a breath. This word, agonal, may make people think their beloved pet is in agony. Switching the term to brain stem or reflexive respiration and explaining the conscious brain has shut down, and therefore they are not in pain, may help people understand what is happening with their animal with this potentially scary-looking part of the dying process.

"Better a week too early than a day too late" … this is one of the most common things said to clients during euthanasia decision-making. However, this is a simplistic approach to a complicated and complex decision. Euthanasia can be a convoluted decision for people. Quality of life is not just about the physical but about the emotional and social aspects of the animal's life. The physical quality of life is often declining with the end-of-life patient, but the animal still may have a decent emotional and social quality of life. The client may also have complicating factors in their life that make this decision more difficult. Supporting clients by giving them tools to help them understand their animal's disease, comprehend clinical signs to monitor for, giving them specific instructions and specific medications in case of emergency or crisis. Understanding the difference between suffering and distress can also help them in decision-making. An advanced directive written for animals is far more helpful than a basic quality of life scale as it identifies what is important to the family, who will be making the decision. A checklist for planning, a list of clinical signs to watch for all can help this tough decision. Helping the client know more can help them identify the right day for the pet and for them.

"Call me when they are suffering." This comment comes from a perspective issue. The client does not always see what the veterinarian sees. The focus for the veterinarian may be the physical quality of life, while the client may be focused on the emotional quality of life. Here is an example. The animal comes in for diarrhea, not eating much, emaciated. From a veterinarian's perspective, it may be suffering from the physical aspects of its disease. From the client's perspective, this is their beloved 16-year-old dog, who has gotten them through their cancer and divorce, who is aging, but still eats a little and wags their tail when they walk through the door. They are also worried that the animal may be suffering and still see their beloved pet enjoying some aspects of life. The client may feel blindsided if talks about euthanasia commence and may balk at the suggestion and may leave against medical advice. Frustrated (in this example), the veterinarian might say … "call me when they are suffering."

Differentiating between each family member's and the veterinarian's perception and enhanced communication skills may help bridge the gap in perception. A person's definition of suffering is based on personal history and emotion. Utilizing the term distress instead of suffering may help. Distress can be objective, observable. You can help your clients know what specifically to watch for if you give them a list of clinical signs or distress points. Using this case as an example, talking about GI distress, clients can watch for vomiting, diarrhea, blood in either of those, abdominal pain, excessive gas, anorexia, nausea, and regurgitation. If you give your clients observable signs to watch for, then they feel supported, and now they know what specifically to observe and when to call you.

Quality of Life Scales. Quality of Life (Q of L) is an appropriate concept to discuss with clients; however, making a euthanasia decision for people is more significant than just the physical quality of life. There are numerous quality-of-life scales accessible on the internet. None of the current quality of life scales are validated in veterinary medicine, and most focus primarily on the physical quality of life of the pet. Some of the veterinary pain scales are validated and the author recommends using a validated pain scale vs an unvalidated Q of L scale. Neither address the emotional quality of life, the will to live, autonomy issues, and other clinical signs that may arise for the animal. They do not address the client's psychological and emotional suffering as a caregiver, the need for respite from caregiving. And finally a Q of L scale needs to address the expected trajectory of the specific disease, and the disease's progression.

A better Q of L scale including all of those aspects needs to be developed. It needs to be validated (making sure we are measuring what needs to be measured). Using advanced directives, validated pain scales, disease trajectories, death planners and specific targeted disease signs can more appropriately guide families through end-of-life discussions and determining goals for care.

"There is nothing more we can do ..." Whether a veterinarian or the client uses this phrase or the client perceives this to be true, it is often incorrect. When people are going through an end-of-life journey, they may need or want hope. They will start looking for other places or for alternatives that evidence-based medicine is not providing them where they can find hope. Hope may sound like denial, but it is not the same thing. Denial can be about fear; fear of the unknown, fear of not being able to do more, anxiety about cost. Client's may take their animal home against medical advice or euthanize prematurely for them and may carry guilt along with their decision, perhaps setting up complicated grief as a result. Clients may carry that guilt for years. A better way to phrase this is to say "There is nothing more we can do *to specfically treat the disease"*. However, palliative medicine can make the animal more comfortable and give the client time to process their emotions.

Challenges faced in starting veterinary palliative medicine or animal hospice

Understanding what palliative medicine or animal hospice is

Palliative care or hospice is not widely understood by the public. The terminology around death and dying can be complicated. The term, hospice gets associated with dying and death and attaching hospice to palliative care connects palliative care with death when it could be utilized to benefit other patients. Clients often believe that they are providing hospice or palliative care when they stop treatment and are given a single pain medication. Veterinary medicine could increase the awareness of the public to help resolve the understanding. However, veterinarians may not have a clear concept about what hospice or palliative medicine is either. Hospice is often confounded with euthanasia by both client and veterinarian. Additional education, could help resolve this challenge.

No veterinarian involved?

A veterinarian may not be involved in the care of a terminally ill pet. Currently, anyone can say that they provide animal hospice care. Look online, and one can find animal hospices that do not have veterinarians involved in the management of end-of-life animals. Articles are written about people feeding hamburgers and doing bucket lists for an end-of-life pet, and as endearing those articles are, those animals may be suffering from a lack of medical care. Laypeople can claim to be animal hospice specialists with no repercussion. As this chapter shows, there is no definition for veterinary palliative medicine. The IAAHPC has defined animal hospice. There are no laws or regulations in place that has defined the term Animal Hospice or Veterinary Palliative Medicine. Not having a veterinarian involved in the care of end-of-life pets puts animals at risk for pain and suffering and inadequate supervision. How do we protect the public and their pets from receiving inadequate care? The solution would be to institute laws and regulations to keep the public from harm.

Cost may be significant

The cost of adequate veterinary care in palliative care may be higher than people are anticipating. The cost of care in veterinary medicine is always a concern. Showing people the value of the service is key to understanding. Other considerations that veterinarians have employed include; having an "angel fund," Care Credit, or other ways to help provide funds will help more animals and their caregivers utilize your service. There may be charities and rescues that may provide funding for families as well.

Uncertain disease trajectory and progression

Sequelae and comorbidities may not be as easily predictable as we have few evidence-based veterinary medicine studies with end-stage disease. Looking at actual life spans in animals without euthanasia, establishing end-stage disease trajectories, and establishing other research in medications, pain, and symptom management for each species we treat will improve veterinary palliative medicine. For now, we utilize what we have provided in the one species we do not treat, humans.

The lack of evidence-based medicine in palliative medicine

Supporting veterinary palliative medicine will require an evidence base. Having evidence-based medicine is essential to providing the best care for our patients. Lack of studies will continue to make providing evidence-based medicine difficult, and the gold standard of palliative medicine should be evidence-based. More research must be done to improve our care.

More mental health support

Veterinarians may need additional training in the psychology of humans and communication of end-of-life care decision-making (McAteer, 2013). The lack of mental health professionals involved in veterinary palliative care limits our ability to support our clients. Most veterinarians are not trained in psychology or human behavior. More training in psychology and communication can help improve our understanding of client's perceptions and decision-making. Adding mental health providers to the team, who have been trained in pet loss, complicated grief, and other mental health challenges can help expand our abilities to support clients.

Myths and other FAQs

Do I not do hospice (palliative care or medicine)?

The common question veterinarians ask is, "Do I not do Hospice already? or Why do I need to send patients to a Palliative or Hospice Veterinarian?" Every veterinarian deals with animals at the end of life. So what makes a hospice or palliative veterinarian different from other veterinarians?

Hospice veterinarians are defined in the IAAHPC guidelines as veterinarians who have further training in human or veterinary hospice (Shanan et al., 2017). As of this writing, the training can be via the IAAHPC conferences, human hospice programs, or the IAAHPC certification program. AAHA has a short course on animal hospice to get the basics of hospice care. Hospice for animals involves a multimodal approach with palliative medicine and pain and symptom management. Hospice veterinarians may also have additional training in communication, pet loss, and grief support. They may have other certifications in pain management or pet loss. Currently, hospice veterinarians (as of this writing) are house-call general practitioners who have expanded upon their skills. A specialty in hospice and palliative medicine is in the early stages of planning as of this book's writing.

Palliative medicine veterinarians can provide pain and other symptom management for animals with chronic, progressive disease and terminal illness. Palliative medicine MD's work in many different fields, alongside internal medicine specialists, oncologists, emergency doctors, sports medicine, and more. Every veterinarian does take a palliative approach to medicine. However, veterinary palliative medicine will advance the field of end-of-life care, with additional training being developed.

Is euthanasia and hospice the same thing?

This is another common question from veterinarians and clients alike. Although euthanasia is part of what hospice or palliative care veterinarian provide, euthanasia is not the only service they provide. Palliative medicine is a philosophy that involves support and comfort for the animal with advanced, progressive chronic or life-limiting or terminal disease and the clients in a physical, social, psychological, and spiritual way. Veterinarians currently practicing palliative medicine or hospice support euthanasia as the family decides by educating them in the disease trajectory, imminent death, pain management, and symptom management and more.

Are you torturing the animal by making it live longer?

Another common question is this question in some form. Human palliative care has a saying, "They live each day until the day they die, so let us make each day a good day." Living better is the philosophy of veterinary palliative medicine. VPM is about making the animal comfortable and giving them a good quality of life for as long as we can provide for pain, distress, and other clinical signs with medical management and a good quality death, either in the form of euthanasia or a palliated death. VPM includes education and support for the families involved, increasing compliance, and providing personal care for animals who are not quite close to their end. Yet, their disease limits them, we improve their life through pain management and symptom control.

Are you just doing this for the people?

Another common comment is that the animal is suffering just for the human who cannot let go. Animals can and do suffer, but it is often due to lack of education or fear that prevents people from either seeking help or providing care. Clients may not feel supported in their decisions by their veterinarian. They may feel they have two choices: medical care or euthanasia. Supporting and understanding the client perspective as well as the medical management of the patient helps support the patient. Supporting the client alleviates fear and improves compliance. Keeping the animal comfortable with palliative medicine can help the pet live its best day until the day it dies, regardless of whether that is euthanasia or from its disease. Supporting the client helps support the pet.

Conclusion
Veterinary palliative medicine as a specialty

Veterinary palliative medicine is not yet a specialty in veterinary medicine. However, there is an organizing committee working on developing a specialty in the United States. The U.S. palliative medical model is a subspecialty, falling under 1 of 11 other specialties: anesthesia, emergency medicine, family medicine, internal medicine, obstetrics and gynecology, pediatrics, physical medicine and rehab, neurology, surgery, and radiology. In the United Kingdom, it is a specialty outright (Doyle, 2007−2008, pp. 77−88).

The organizing committee has discussed both avenues for veterinarians: becoming a subspecialty-though it would mean that veterinarians would have to become specialists in another field as the MDs do in the United States—or be our own standing specialty. The goal for the current organizing committee is to be a standing specialty.

Before developing a specialty though, we need to start with some basics. We need to define palliative medicine, how and when to use veterinary palliative medicine, and add it to our current medical training. As palliative medicine arose in human medicine, strategic planning went into place (Moses, 2019). Understanding and defining veterinary palliative medicine and animal hospice will be a significant step in moving the field forward.

Early-onset palliative medicine will help your patients live longer and have better-quality lives. House call practitioners who choose to develop a palliative medicine practice can work with your referring veterinarians and provide lunch and learns, giving them a better understanding of what you can do to help improve their patients' lives. Palliative veterinarians can give pets potentially longer and happier lives until the clients choose euthanasia or a palliated death. The path forward will build on using validated tools and improving the end-of-life standards of medicine. Embracing evidence-based palliative medicine will encourage your referring veterinarians to refer more patients to you and give your clients and their beloved pets a more substantial end-of-life experience.

References

Doyle, D. (1993). *Palliative medicine - a time for a definition. Palliative Medicine*. Edinburgh, UK: Sage Publications.

Doyle, D. (2007−2008). *Palliative medicine in Britain*. Westport: Omega.

El-Jawahri, A. E. (September 11, 2017). Effects of early integrated palliative care on caregivers of patients with lung and gastrointestinal cancer: A randomized clinical trial. *The Oncologist, 227.*

Home page for the Association of Palliative Medicine. (n.d.). Retrieved from Association of Palliative Medicine https://apmonline.org/.

Kittelson, S. M. (July−September, 2015). *Palliative care: A specialty that has come into its own*. Retrieved from Risk RX http://flbog.sip.ufl.edu/risk-rx-article/palliative-care-a-specialty-that-has-come-into-its-own/.

McAteer, R. M. (2013). Palliative care: Benefits, barriers, and best practices. *American Family Physician*, 807−813.

Moses, L. (2019). *Veterinary clinics/small animal practice/advances in palliative medicine*. Philadelphia: Elsiever.

Nelson, R. B. (September 22, 2017). *Palliative care curbs depression and trauma in HSCT patients*. Retrieved from Medscape https://www.medscape.com/viewarticle/886063.

NHPCO Staff. (2019). Palliative Care or Hospice? *Publication from NHPCO*, 1−2.

Palliative Care. (2020). https://www.who.int/news-room/fact-sheets/detail/palliative-care. (Accessed 17 November 2021).

Quill, T. E., & Abernathy, A. P. (2013). Generalist plus specialist palliative care—Creating a more sustainable model. *New England Journal of Medicine*, 1173−1175.

Ruder, D. B. (March-April). *From specialty to shortage*. Retrieved from Harvard Magazine https://harvardmagazine.com/2015/03/from-specialty-to-shortage.

Shanan, A., Hendrix, L., Cooney, K., Mader, B., Pierce, J., & August, K. (2017). Animal hospice and palliative care practice guidelines. *IAAHPC Website*, 1−50. https://iaahpc.org/wp-content/uploads/2020/10/IAAHPC-AHPC-GUIDELINESpdf.pdf.

Temel, J. E. (2010). Early palliative care for patients with metastatic non-small cell lung cancer. *New England Journal of Medicine*, 733−742.

Temel, J. E. (2017). Effects of early integrated palliative care in patients with lung and GI cancer: A randomized clinical trial. *Journal of Clinical Oncology*, 834−841.

Further reading

Linda Ganzini, M. M. (2008). Why Oregon patients request assisted death: Family members' views. *Journal of General Internal Medicine*, 154−157.

Tammie, E., & Quest, M. C. (2009). Hospice and palliative medicine: New subspecialty, new opportunities. *Annals of Emergency Medicine*, 94−102.

House call business basics

Lynn Hendrix, AA, BA, DVM, CHPV [1,2,3,4], **Mina Weakley, BSc** [5]

[1]*Owner, Veterinarian, Beloved Pet Mobile Vet, Davis, CA, United States;* [2]*Former Board of Directors, IAAHPC, Chicago, IL, United States;* [3]*Consultant, Hospice, Palliative Medicine, End of Life, VIN, Davis, CA, United States;* [4]*President, Founder, World Veterinary Palliative Medicine Organization, Davis, CA, United States;* [5]*Veterinary Student, College of Veterinary Medicine, Western University of Health Sciences, Pomona, CA, United States*

Setting up a housecall practice

Ok, so you are ready to jump into setting up a house call business in Animal Hospice and Palliative Medicine. Where do you start? What equipment do you need? How do you get licenses, the market for your new business, what insurance do you need? Marketing, social media, where to start? This chapter is for you!

First steps

The first thing to start with is your due diligence. Due diligence helps you assess the market you are starting up in. Understanding what the market can bear, what competition is in the community, what expenses one might have, what cremation services are currently available, regulations one might encounter.

Define your market area. Find out if there is a niche in your market area. Are there competitors? What is the population of your area you are going to drive? How far are you willing to drive? Are you going to provide emergency hours, is there an emergency clinic nearby to help if you are not available? What hours are you going to be available? It is good idea to start defining your boundaries at this stage of practice.

What cremation services are available in your area, what are their hours, will it fit with your hours, and type of practice? How do they care for the body? Do they allow witnessed cremation? Do they do single private cremations? Do they do partitioned private cremations? Do you know the difference? Have you visited each of them? Do you feel comfortable with their practices? What type of urns do they carry? How do they present themselves?

Defining your specific needs and what your expenses might be, is the next step, the business plan.

Business plan

The very next thing to do to make a successful business is to have a plan. One does not need a business plan to set up a house call practice, however, it can help you organize your business and help you clarify essentials. Writing a detailed business plan helps the veterinarian focus on what they need to prepare financially for setting up a housecall practice. It enables them to define costs and marketing plans. Business gurus will tell you that it takes at least 2 years for most businesses to establish themselves and be profitable. Veterinarians may need to have a backup income while they are building their business. Think about keeping your current job, at least part-time or working relief, to initially maintain some regular income. Other things to think about when beginning a business and starting a business plan are:

1. Can you take a pay cut? Do you have savings in case things are slow? How much are your monthly expenses? How much do you need past your monthly expenses?

2. What should you charge to make turn a profit? What will the market bear?

3. What should your business name be? You will want to see if there is an internet domain you can buy that will go with the name you choose, evaluate whether another business has that name or something similar, are you setting up a sole proprietorship or a corporation? Each has different rules for business names. Check your state database for "doing business as" or DBA names.

4. How do you plan to market? Are you going to buy ads? Think about what is the most effective return on your investment, often written as ROI. The most effective return on investment (ROI) is where you want to spend your ad dollars (as of this writing-Google Ads was most effective for the author, but consider Facebook, Twitter, Yelp, etc.) It may take some time to figure out what worked best. Another inexpensive way to get into the market is to go to your local practices and do lunch and learns or bring them a treat, and some cards, for some free advertising.

5. What do you need for compensation on a weekly, monthly, yearly basis? The author used a calculation for what was needed to clear bills for the week and then broke it down by what they needed to bring in, in a day. For example, if the author needed 2100 for the week (7 days), they would need to bring in at least one client a day at 300 dollars a day. 300 a day was above what they needed to pay for before medications and travel. So, the author would have charged maybe 350 to clear that. In the beginning, the author did not see one client a day. It took almost 2 years before the business was averaging one client a day, or seven in a week (some days I saw 4, other days, 0). The author suspects this has probably changed over the years and increased since more people seek out this service since covid changed the world.

6. What do you need to buy? Equipment, medications, car? Insurance? Are you going to start with one or more team members? Then you need to include payroll. Are you going to work out of a home office or get a small office somewhere? Can you write off that expense? Check with your CPA.

7. One formula to figuring out the cost of your product/services is this:

  a. Know your customer (back to due diligence). Are you going to see several in a day? How long will each appointment take? How much can your average client afford?

  b. Know all your expenses. Your expenses may be hard to know at first. Hopefully, this chapter helps. Make a spreadsheet so you can track them.

  c. Figure out your labor, marketing, website and domain cost to create and upkeep. You may choose to hire a company to build a website for you, or you may choose to do it yourself.

  d. Your other operating expenses. For a minimal house call practice, Office supplies (pens, paper, etc.), safe, car (even if you already own in, it should be factored in), operating car expenses, like gas and insurance, blankets, pee pads, medications, and medical supplies, tourniquet, bag for supplies, office equipment, either file folders, printer, printer paper (for medical records) or laptop, iPad, or computer, online medical record-keeping.

  e. Loan and loan cost (if you are taking out a loan to help you start)

  f. Your salary as the business owner, other employees, compensation if you start with tech or another doctor.

  g. Factor in your costs for setting up and add that to the total expenses so that you can be reimbursed.

  h. Set aside money to pay for emergencies, breakdown of equipment. Keep this as part of your expenses.

  i. Figure out your revenue target.

  j. Know the market, what others are charging, but do not use their price solely as a target. You might offer different things, different experiences. You do not want to be accused of price-fixing. You can see what the market may bear, but don't copy prices, show how you arrived at them.

A few references on setting prices:

Pricing guide webinar: https://www.score.org/event/power-pricing?
gclid=Cj0KCQjwvYSEBhDjARIsAJMn0licWM0AnI0DRrC00jLwTp_suxd-
rmPGrnwcf8B5iF42R5jOs1Et7ZgaAhWBEALw_wcB
The Art of Pricing: How to Find Hidden Profits to Grow Your Business
By Rafi Mohammed www.rafimo.com
How to Sell at Margins Higher Than Your Competitors: Winning Every Sale at
Full Price
by Lawrence L. Steinmetz, and William T. Brooks
National Federation of Independent Business
US Small Business Administration
This website has an excellent template for a business plan. https://www.score.
org/resource/business-plan-template-startup-business

Types of business plans

A traditional business plan should include (SBA, 2018):

1. An executive summary will consist of a mission statement, perhaps a vision statement, and a values statement, including information about the company, the team, location, and financial information. A mission statement is the present mission of your business, what is driving you to have this business? A vision statement is what you are going to do in the future, where do you plan to go with your business? What additional services might you provide? And a values statement evaluates your values for the business, develops your "elevator" speech.

2. A company description. It should include an overview of the products you are considering carrying, the services you plan to provide, the type of customers you plan to provide services to (who is your target audience). Think about your niche, what makes you different than other businesses in your area, how or what do you plan on providing that is different? What are your competitive advantages? What are some disadvantages? Do a SWOT analysis. This stands for S-Strengths, W-Weaknesses, O-Opportunities, T-Threat (Schooley, 2021).

3. Market analysis. Provide the research you have done here. Understanding what the market is currently doing and what it can bear can help you be successful.

4. Organization and management. How is the business going to be organized? If you are a sole proprietor, you may feel you don't need to do this step but planning for those changes can be very useful if you have employees in the future. This section should also include your legal structure for the business.

5. Service or Products you plan to provide. This section goes into more detail about the services available and products you are going to carry. This section is also an excellent place to provide a plan for research and development. If you provide products, then include a section on sales tax, you need to contact your state for information on sales tax, and calculate that tax.

6. Marketing and Sales. Understanding what will provide you with the most significant ROI will help you maximize your dollar spent on marketing. Planning for marketing in this section will help you not spend your hard-earned dollars on minimal return. Discussing what worked for others in the field is also an excellent place to start, and remember, this section may need changing over time as technology grows and markets shift.

7. Funding requests. If you need to take out a loan to start your business, understanding what you need and why you need it will be a necessary inclusion. You will need to provide the bank your assets and debts. Have a detailed description of what you will need the money for, whether it will be used to buy equipment or pay bills, or salaries and projections of future expected income, and how you plan to pay off debt as income increases.

8. Financial projections. This section should include what you need to charge to make your daily minimum, your project's needs for equipment, overhead, and salaries. You can include graphs and charts to help a bank see the progression and the plan.

9. Appendix. This section can include forms for a bank to examine that will support your claim that you can provide a business. Resumes, credit history, permits, legal documents, letters of reference, product pictures (if you are going to carry products that you want to sell)
10. Though not necessarily included in a traditional business plan, the author also had a section of equipment needed, licensing needed, organizations desirable to contact

A lean business plan may be utilized for a sole proprietorship or very small business.

Lean business plans can include (SBA, 2018):

1. Key Partnerships. These are the essential businesses you will work with to help run your business. For a housecall practice, these will include your referral hospitals, universities, specialists, crematoriums, medication and equipment suppliers, education providers, compounding pharmacies, (manufacturers [of a product]-less likely).
2. Key Activities. This section is like the section in the more traditional plan of what services and products you will provide.
3. Key Resources. This section is a resource plan to help you provide your business. The Small Business Association, VIN, the Veterinarian Palliative Medicine group on Facebook, the World Veterinary Palliative Medicine Organization, and the IAAHPC business circles groups are good resources for a Hospice/Palliative Medicine Housecall practice.
4. Value Proposition. This section includes your mission statement. The why of your practice, what are you bringing to the community.
5. Customer relationships. This section is to think about how you will treat your customer from start to finish with their experience with you. What are you going to do to exceed their expectations?
6. Customer segments. This section is to describe who your target audience will be. You will want to include your referral veterinarians, specialists, and the community in which you live. Please do your due diligence, get market analysis, and enter it in this section.
7. Channels. How are you going to reach out to your target audience? Through referrals, through a website, or word of mouth, or marketing through social media. Think about your marketing strategy here.
8. Cost structure. See the above information on figuring out pricing and place it in this section.
9. Revenue streams. Include in this section all the products and services from which you will generate revenue. Include time for driving, consultations, euthanasia, medications utilized, whether you will carry a small pharmacy with you or have an online pharmacy that you can attach to your website. Products that you might consider carrying are harnesses, wheelchairs, oxygen concentrators that you can rent out, prosthetic kits, orthopedic products, like braces, beds, and simple things like e-collars, bandaging material, pain patches, injectable medications.

Both business plan structures came from the SBA (Small Business Association), and you can find sample business plans there and other resources in an internet search. The author strongly recommends writing out a business plan, as it will help you think through what you need and minimize the cost of building a business.

Additional resources:

US Small Business Administration
This website has an excellent template for a business plan.
https://www.score.org/resource/business-plan-template-startup-business

For-profit or nonprofit?

Deciding on making your business for-profit or nonprofit may be the next step in creating a hospice and palliative care business. There have been some hospice businesses set up as nonprofit. The question is, why should you choose one over the other. According to the Harvard Business Review, the substantial difference is where you can source your capital (Chen, 2013). For-profit businesses can source from private investors, and a return on investment is expected. Nonprofit companies can receive donations from individuals, corporations, or foundations and expect a "social benefit or return." The IRS would look at these definitions. There may be additional rules for for-profit versus nonprofit debate (please check with your tax regulatory board).

Another reason to consider a nonprofit is the social benefit. The nonprofit has a mission that benefits society in some way, and an argument may be made that an animal hospice benefit society. Non-profits can have public ownership. One individual should not be the owner, and profits are not distributed to the owners (usually a board of directors) but to return to the mission of the nonprofit (Chen, 2013).

The work staff of a nonprofit is made up of primarily volunteers with few paid staff. In a for-profit business, the working staff is paid, depending on your state, may or may not have any volunteers.

The main advantage of setting up a nonprofit is the tax exemption for the nonprofit and a tax deduction for the donors. Other benefits include being eligible for grants, formal structure, limited liability. Disadvantages include the cost to set up. It is more difficult to set up; there is shared control via a board of directors and scrutiny by the public and incorporation as a nonprofit and setting up a federal 503c paperwork (Chen, 2013).

The main advantage of a for-profit business is income. The advantage of a for-profit business ownership is easier set up, and the net profit goes to the sole owner or owners. The benefit of a sole proprietorship is the owner is the boss and assumes all responsibility and liability. It is also the least complicated business type to set up.

Incorporation for solo practitioners or multiple partners can help limit the liability of the owners of the business. Each one has different tax burdens. We will go through each diverse type to help you decide what is best for you (Nash, 2018). For-profit businesses have less governmental regulation than nonprofits, though housecall practices have some restrictions through the State Veterinary board or veterinary regulatory board in the area. Liquidity of assets is another benefit of a for-profit business. If a company does not profit, it is easier to liquidate than for the nonprofit (Nash, 2018).

References: Find further information with Nolo books or other legal aid books.

Partnerships

Do you have a partner? If you have a partner, you will want to set up a partnership agreement. The partnership agreement should be treated like a prenupual agreement. You want to make sure everything is in writing about who gets what if you break up. It may not feel like that will happen when you are first beginning a business, but a partnership agreement can help define what your responsibilities are for the company and help you part ways if things don't go as planned between partners or for the business. There are many templates of partnership agreements online. The benefits of a partnership are that the income is only taxed once, and more than one person can handle the distribution of duties and funding to the business. The author strongly recommends discussing a partnership agreement with a lawyer and an accountant before entering a partnership (WSJ staff, 2018).

The partnership agreement should include:

1. Name of business.
2. The term of the partnership
3. The capital that each partner will provide to the business.
4. How the profits and losses will be split among the partners. The most common type between two people is 50/50.
5. How interest would be divided among the partners.
6. How the partners are going to take salaries.
7. How the partnership funds will be distributed.
8. The bookkeeping techniques of the partnership.
9. The different managerial duties of each partner.
10. What happens in the dissolution of the partnership?
11. What happens to the assets in the case of the death of one or more partners?
12. How the partners will notify one another of changes in the business.
13. Whether arbitration will be used in handling difficulties among the partners.
14. Integration of amendments to the partnership agreement. (NOLO, 2018a, 2018b).

And again with a partnership, you will need to decide whether you want to incorporate or not. You will want to check with your state to see what your liabilities are for each type.

Sole proprietor

Being a sole proprietor or a simple partnership is simple and straightforward, but it does leave you, the individual, open to financial liabilities. Setting up the sole proprietorship can vary from state to state. Check with your local veterinary regulatory board, and there is a NOLO book on setting up a sole propriertorship that provides information for all 50 states (NOLO, 2018a, 2018b). There are many steps to take to develop your legal status as a sole proprietor business.

1. You will need to pick a name, the name you will be doing business as, or a DBA.
2. You will need to visit your local city or county and obtain a business license and fill out a business name form. You will have to place an ad in a newspaper to signify that you are doing business as your business name and you will have to have a business name that the local government approves. Before filling out the paperwork, you must run a business name check to make sure there are no businesses with that name. You may want to trademark your business name.
3. Setting up a federal employer identification number or EIN through the IRS is simple. One can set it up online at https://www.irs.gov/businesses/small-businesses-self-employed/apply-for-an-employer-identification-number-ein-online
4. Taxes pass through the business and are the owner's tax burden. Discuss with a Certified Public Accountant (CPA) whether this is the best option for you.
5. Contact a business lawyer to ensure all the paperwork is done correctly. Utilizing the Small Business Administration in your area can also help the house call practice set up. (SBA, 2018) The Veterinary Information Network (VIN) also has extensive information on setting up a house call business.
6. Contact your state or local veterinary regulation board for a premise permit in addition to the veterinarian permit. They can help with the other regulatory boards that you may need to contact for other required permits. They may also have written instructions for boards to contact (NOLO, 2018a, 2018b).

Corporations

If you choose to have a corporation, you have different options available to you. Contact a CPA to discuss which one might be appopriate for you.

Limited Liability Corporations

Limited Liability Corporations or LLCs have some benefits over the sole proprietorship and the other corporate structures.

Advantages of an LLC:

1. Gives the owner limited liability protection.
2. There are fewer corporate rules to follow than an S or C- Corp.
3. It gives greater tax flexibility than other corporate types.
4. Gives managerial flexibility than other corporate types.
5. It is a Pass-thru entity.
6. It retains the flexibility of distributing assets to members.
7. It is an excellent corporate structure for holding appreciating assets. (Garrett Sutton, 2015)

Disadvantages are:

1. Some States charge additional fees for LLCs.
2. Some states do not allow professional businesses (veterinarians) to use an LLC.
3. There are restrictions on transferring the business to others.
4. Single-member LLCs face reduced asset protection in some states. (Garrett Sutton, 2015)

S-corp or C-corp

An S-Corporation or S-corp is a tax "pass-thru entity." Taxes are collected through personal taxes, not through the corporation. The C-corporation or C-Corp has taxes collected through the corporation.

Benefits of an S-Corp are:

1. Limited liability of the owners
2. The Pass-through taxation.
3. Investment opportunities.
4. Existence of the corporation past the leaving or death of the owner(s).
5. Once a year tax filing. (Incorporate Staff, 2018)

Disadvantages are:

1. US citizens and legal residents of the United States are the only owners of S-Corps.
2. Can have up to 100 owners.
3. Formation and ongoing expenses
4. Tax qualifications
5. Closer IRS scrutiny. (Incorporate Staff, 2018)

Benefits of a C-Corp are:

1. Best used for those who have a storefront and products (and less advantageous for housecall vets).
2. The most significant advantage is it has the broadest range of deductions and expenses (Corporate Direct, 2018).

Disadvantages are:

1. Double taxation of profit distributed to shareholders as dividends and again on personal taxes (Corporate Direct, 2018).

The key to deciding which tax and business structure work for you is doing further research and talking with a tax attorney about what would work best for your business.

Financing your business

Having your funding is the simplest way to start your business. If you have a nest egg, a savings account, minimize your start-up costs, which you should have developed in your business plan.

What other ways could you fund a business?

1. Finding investors. Friends and family or private investors can help sponsor your business.
2. Crowdfunding-there are many different crowdfunding sites. More frequently used with building nonprofits.
3. Requesting a small business grant. You can find out more at Grants.gov. or SBA.gov. There may be grants for women, people of color, LGBTQI.
4. Getting a bank loan. Many banks will send you information on loans as soon as you get a business license (McCreery, 2018).

What do you need to start working?

Once you have your business plan in place and decide what type of business liability you want to set up and finance, you can start implementing your business plan. Regulations are different from state to state, so you will want to check with your state board regarding the requirements for business licensing, premise permits.

Naming your business

You will need a name for your business, and it will need to clear trademark titles (at least in the United States). Pick a unique name.

A few things to think about when picking a name:

1. What will attract people? Does it sound good when spoken?
2. Whether you can get a domain that works with your name.
3. Branding. What does your logo look like, what colors might you use that compliment your business name.
4. Does it convey what you are doing?
5. Are you going only to be providing hospice, euthanasia, or other services? (Silver, 2012).

Licensing

Processing Business licenses can take a long time in some areas, so start filling out that paperwork as soon as you have a business name, and have it in the process as you are planning and implementing the rest. You may have to have more than one business license if you work in a major metropolitan area. Premise permits are another next step and are through the state board, and you may need a business license to start the process for your premise permit.

The Employer Identification Number or EIN is a number you will need if you are going to employ people, now or in the future. Call the IRS or go online and get an EIN.

If you carry anything taxable, you will have to contact your state for a resale license number. This is for sales tax purposes.

If you are going to start with employees, you will want to have:

1. Your federal EIN,
2. Check with your state and local governments for other licensing.
3. Mandatory Benefits include Social Security, Worker's compensation, Disability Insurance, Family leave benefits, and Unemployment insurance (all can be taken out of a paycheck, but these are companies that you will have to check with to provide insurance, some are federal, some are state, and some can be through private insurance companies).
4. Optional benefits for employees can include health care plans, retirement plans like 401K (SBA Staff, 2018/).

Your State Veterinary Medical Board will be where you can obtain a premise license. You may need a premise license even if you are home-based.

Some states may require a medical waste permit. Start with the state health department to find out which department in your state covers medical waste. Suppose you have a small amount of medical waste, such as sharps. In that case, you may have them disposed of through your crematorium or your local waste disposal, or another local private company.

Insurance

Insurance that you will need for your business as a sole proprietor or a sole business owner:

1. Malpractice insurance. You can find this through AVMA-PLIT, your state PLIT or personal insurance companies.
2. Business liability insurance is for things that may happen in the house you are visiting, bites, tripping over furniture, falling downstairs, for example.
3. Car insurance-You will need to let your insurance company know that you will be putting more miles on the car. And it may need to be under a commercial vehicle policy. Check with your insurance agent.
4. Homeowner's or renter's insurance if you are working out of your home with a rider for a home-based business.
5. A business owner's policy is to cover liabilities not covered with the other insurance.

Accounting software

Tracking your income and expenses in real-time assists the housecall practitioner to keep accurate books and make tax time easy.

Many different Accounting apps work with phones or tablets. Xero, FreshBooks, QuickBooks, Quicken, to name a few. A quick google search can provide you with a more comprehensive list of current accounting software. Utilize software you can use in your phone or tablet on the cloud and keep information available to you wherever you go. Back up the data regularly and have more than one backup plan. The author recommends software that will integrate with your other software, such as online scheduling.

Address

With a home-based business, using your home address for correspondence with clients can leave you open to having people show up at your house. To help set a boundary with clients, it is helpful to have a Post Office Box for most of your business information. The state board and the DEA will want your home address so check with your state licensing or other regulatory body.

Bank account

Setting up a bank account with your local bank. You will need your business name and EIN, your business license, and perhaps your premise permit. You may also need corporation information if you decide to set up a corporation. Check with your local bank to see if they need any other forms for you to set up a business account.

DEA license

You will have to contact the DEA in the United States or other controlled drug regulatory bodies in your municipality to set up an account number and licensing. Consider the drugs you need to carry and the types of scheduled numbers they are before you sign up. The author recommends getting approved for Schedule two to five drugs. Veterinarians are not allowed to be licensed for schedule one drugs (Marijuana and many products from marijuana are still schedule 1 as of this writing). The DEA website is: https://www.dea.gov/ There may also be additional state or local rules for controlled drug prescriptions. Check with your state or local regulatory bodies for more information.

Record-keeping

Doing end-of-life care, whether providing at-home euthanasia service or providing hospice and euthanasia or hospice or palliative only, extensive notes need to be made for your medical record. Keeping records can be time-consuming, and you may need to be called upon to have them available quickly. Remember, as you grow, you will want to have records readily available for others so that they can provide care from the doctor's notes and chart what was said and done at each visit. You can use paper records; however, they can be more difficult to carry as your team grows. Paper records do give you flexibility initially and minimize your risk of identity theft but carry cost and storage problems.

Online records may be easier to access for your team. Online records allow you to minimize your paperwork and be attached to your other software and scheduling.

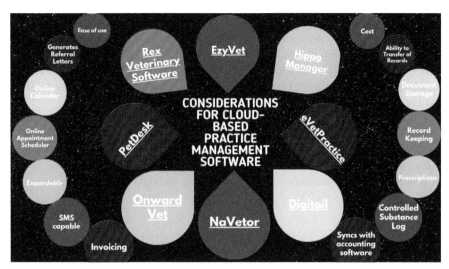

FIGURE 3.1

Considerations for Cloud-Based Practice Management Software and some examples.

Created in Canva by Lynn Hendrix ©2021.

The cost for online services may be more than paper records, depending on your needs and the company you choose. You are also able to send information to your referral hospitals and your clients easier.

Historically there have been several record-keeping apps and computer software. Computer programs change and update frequently and may not roll over to another software program if you decide to switch. Making a decision about which is best for you can be a complex choice. If you want to utilize online records, make sure you have the most critical security to prevent your clients' personal information from being stolen (Fig. 3.1).

Phone and phone number

Smartphones can include your accounting software, record-keeping, GPS, and mileage tracking, as well as your book, the ability to look up information on VIN and other platforms. And, it is your link to your clients.

Consider using your current personal phone and changing it to a business account. Or getting a second phone that is solely used for the business.

The phone expenses are part of the expense of your business, and keeping it separate can help with accounting and taxes.

In addition, you may consider having an online phone service as you grow. Online phone services can help separate your personal phone from your business, all while using the same phone. Online phone services may include Ring Central, Grasshopper, Vonage, Nextiva and more. A quick google search for a VoIP service will bring up a good list.

Computer-home, laptop, or tablet?

Next, you will have to decide whether to buy a home desktop computer, laptop, or tablet or use your existing equipment. The desktop is helpful to return emails and correspondence with clients and referral hospitals. Desktops tend to be faster and have larger storage capacity. Laptops are portable, and could be used in both office and in the field.

Utilizing a smartphone or tablet for in-field work is the most common practice. Smartphones or tablets can work with all the apps you may need.

Do you need a tablet if you have a smartphone? Ensure it will support all the apps you want to use and have local data (one with its own phone line). If you do not have wi-fi in the location, you may need the phone line to hook up to the internet.

Test or not to test

You may have clients who choose to continue with lab work and you would like to be able to provide lab work. Get an account with a lab that can run blood work. Or buy a machine to run your own. Purchasing a device can be a considerable cost, so if you want to keep costs down, setting up with a lab may be the way to go. If you want to have your own lab machine, consider finding a used one. Idexx or other labs may pick up at your home, or you may want to have a friendly clinic in town that would work with you to drop blood work off at to have picked up with theirs. If you are using a lab, setting up an online account allows you to get blood work back quickly and email the labwork and comments to clients.

If other diagnostic testing needs to occur, you could consider purchasing portable ultrasound machine or a portable X-ray unit or send the patient to their referral veterinarian. Referral back to their veterinarian establishes a relationship with your colleagues. Both of you can work together to make a better end-of-life experience for the pet and the family. Referral to specialists can also improve longer-term care for your patients. Palliative medicine can continue concurrently with curative treatment. Clients with hospice patients may forgo further testing and just want to provide palliative care.

Equipment to consider for the palliative house call veterinarian

You can find lists online for a start-up practice and ones that you can find for a house call practice, and even lists for a hospice house call practice.

But what do you NEED for a start-up hospice and palliative medicine housecall practice?

Vehicle

A small car or one with a trunk is probably not going to be your best vehicle. It may not appear right to clients to be placing their loved ones into a trunk. A small hatchback car would be better than one with a trunk, but you will have limited space. A better choice might be a hatchback SUV (these are large enough to carry big dogs) or a minivan. Some go even larger, like a truck or larger van or SUV. If you are going to buy one, consider getting a vehicle that has an automatic liftgate. You will want to consider the space for equipment, medications and if you will use it for family members when you are not working. Also consider how you are going to place a large animal in your car. Can you use a soft stretcher, a stretcher with wheels, a gurney in the car you want?

Equipment

Put a dog bed in the car. You could also use bathmats, blankets or other material that is appealing. Get a basket or cat bed for kitties and other small creatures. Use washable blankets to cover an animal and get a waterproof cover that will be underneath the other items for the area that you will have deceased animals. Consider using washable pee pads or crib sheets instead of disposable. You are going to need a safe or double-locked item to carry controlled substances. It needs to be attached to the car in some fashion, bolted, or locked to a bolted object in the vehicle. And you want to get a medical bag or suitcase, to bring medications, paperwork, or laptop, tablet, syringes, clippers, and muzzles. Carry disposable pee pads, additional clippers, clipper blades, blankets, or fleece, fluids, IV tubing, needles, and tape. Add in bandage material, sharps containers, controlled substance logs, sympathy cards, pens, clipboards, phones, or other point-of-sale equipment.

Medication

For palliative veterinarians, there are many ways to help clients obtain medications. Veterinarians can carry a pharmacy of medications in their home, or script out to local pharmacies. Veterinarians may opt for an online pharmacy for medication dispensing or local compounding pharmacies to make flavored medication, transdermal formulations, and treats to help get medicines into the patient with minimal stress.

The following pharmaceuticals are an essential list to get you started. You will add to it as you see a need or your practice grows and changes. This list was created to minimize your start up costs.

For a palliative/hospice practice—Pharmaceuticals that you will want for sure! (Order just a few bottles as you are not going to start with many patients).

1) Telazol®/Tiletamine/Zolazepam.
2) Acepromazine injectable and oral forms.
3) Butorphanol
4) Euthanasia solution of your choice.
5) Prednisone or Dexamethasone (or another steroid of your choice)
6) Furosemide

Pharmaceuticals you may want to carry some or all these instead or in addition to. You do not have to get all of these to start and many you can prescribe to keep your inventory costs low. Some may be used for a crisis kit which also may be prescribed out.

1) Ketamine
2) Midazolam
3) Medetomidine
4) Dexmedetomidine
5) Sileo® or Dormosedan® gel for sedation of difficult animals
6) Narcan or naloxone (not a must-have, but helpful if animals get too sedate from an opioid).
7) Methadone, Morphine, Hydromorphone, Buprenorphine, or another opioid of your choice.
8) Ondansetron
9) Cerenia®-maropitant
10) Reglan®-metoclopramide
11) NSAID of your choice
12) Antibiotic injectable and tablet of your choice.
13) Amantadine
14) Gabapentin
15) Amitriptyline
16) Vetmedin®—Pimobendan
17) Appetite stimulant—Mirtazapine, Entyce
18) Antidiarrheal of your choice
19) Vitamin B12 (cobalamin)
20) Oral viscous lidocaine gel or "magic mouthwash."
    a) Magic mouthwash may contain one or more of these items and can be made up at a compounding pharmacy according to what your patient needs:
    - An antibiotic
    - An antihistamine
    - Local anesthetic to reduce pain and discomfort
    - An antifungal to reduce fungal growth (not typical for animals)
    - A corticosteroid to treat inflammation (depending on what was going on inside the mouth)
    - An antacid (for humans to help coat the mouth, but maybe not necessary for animals, as they are not swishing it around) (Moynihan, 2018)
21) Eye, ear, skin ointments or creams

What do you need for a start-up euthanasia practice?

Pharmaceuticals that you will want for sure!

1) Telazol®/Tiletamine/Zolazepam.
2) Acepromazine injectable and oral forms.

3) Butorphanol or other opioids.
4) Euthanasia solution of your choice.

Pharmaceuticals you may want to carry instead or in addition to the above:

1) Ketamine
2) Midazolam
3) Medetomidine
4) Dexmedetomidine
5) Sileo® or Equine Dormosedan® gel for sedation of difficult animals

Veterinary telehealth

Veterinary Telehealth has gained popularity since the Covid-19 pandemic hit the United States in March of 2020. States moved to change the regulations on the veterinarian's ability to use telehealth to allow veterinarians and their team to stay safe as we learned more about the science of Covid-19. Many states chose to allow for telemedicine; other states have not.

Please be aware of the specific laws in your service area if you plan to use telehealth/telemedicine to provide veterinary services to patients. Many governmental bodies have utilized the AVMA guidelines on telehealth. Having a valid veterinarian—client—patient relationship (VCPR) is paramount when establishing care with a patient. The AVMA Model Veterinary Practice Act outlines the specific requirements that establish a VCPR and can be read in full detail online. The AVMA Model specifically details that "A Veterinarian—Client—Patient-Relationship cannot be established by telephonic or other electronic means." This means that the veterinarian must still provide an in-person examination and medically appropriate and timely visits while the patient is being managed. Without establishing a valid VCPR, the veterinarian may not use telehealth services alone to diagnose, prognose, or prescribe medication to patients. If you are interested in reading the guidelines in more detail, please read the AVMA guidelines for the use of telehealth in veterinary practice which may change post print (Staff of AVMA, 2021a,b,c).

Telehealth encompasses various virtual services, and a general overview of the different types of teleservices is available through the AVMA (Staff of AVMA, 2021a,b,c). The subcategories of telehealth are telemedicine, teleconsulting, telemonitoring, tele-triage, tele-advice, electronic prescribing, and mobile health.

Telemedicine provides veterinarians the option to set up virtual appointments with clients so that they can remotely monitor a patient's wellbeing. These appointments are typically set up through a mobile or web app and can utilize text, phone call, and video services and are particularly helpful in palliative and hospice cases. Telemedicine apps provide a way to regularly check in with patients and clients and allow for visual monitoring when using video-based services. In addition, families may be more interested in utilizing telemedicine services because they can be more cost-effective, for both client and veterinarian, than in-person visits. Telemedicine must be within the confines of a current VCPR in the United States at the time of this writing, though more states moved to change the rules for the pandemic needs.

Veterinarians, as well as, veterinary technicians or nurses can utilize tele-triage, tele-advice, and telemonitoring to help clients remotely care for their pets.

If you are looking to integrate telemedicine into your practice, there are a few things to consider when choosing the right app. Examples of what you should think about when investing in telemedicine include the following:

- Do you want to use a solely mobile app or one that can be used on a computer as well?
- What is the monthly cost of the app?
- Does the app allow you or your client to schedule appointments?
- Does it securely store records and the conversation you had with the client?
- How will clients pay for this service? Will they pay through the app or pay through a separate entity?
- How will you assess fees? Can you charge by the minute or charge per session?
- Can the app integrate with other services?

You can choose to use an all-purpose app or veterinary-specific app based on your answers to the earlier questions. Both can have pros and cons, and it depends on what best fits your needs.

Marketing for hospice, palliative medicine, and in-home euthanasia services

Setting up your website

Developing an excellent website is one of the essential marketing tools for the house call veterinarian. Setting up a website can be done by a web-savvy vet or finding a professional web admin to set one up and maintain it for you. You will need to know several things to set it up and maintain it, so this section is to help you do it on your own. In a way, it is like having an electronic puppy. You will need to routinely take care of it after you set it up.

If you want to set up your own website, there are several web developers you could utilize and different ways to help you set it up.

First, you will want a domain name. That is the name you will use for your website. The author has used their business name as an example. The business name is Beloved Pet Mobile Vet. The author could have chosen BPMV.com or Belovedpetmobilevet.com or.net or.org or any number of other endings. The author decided belovedpetmobilevet.com because it was one way to get the search engines to find my website. Keep that in mind when you are making your business name. There are also creative ways to get around a domain name that is already taken. For example, pethospice.com might be taken but you could create pethospice.net or pethospice.us, etc.

Second, your business name and your domain name are interlinked. Clients may look you up by your business name as you grow and if they cannot find you easily then you may lose business. If you choose a vague or common name, chances are, the domain name may have been taken. Search for your domain name before you get locked into a business name. Another issue that can occur outside of the United States is the limitations on the business name by the governing agencies involved in business formation. Check with your local government, small business association, or veterinary association for help in making a business name.

Pick a domain site to purchase or register your domain name. There are probably as many sites to buy or register your domain name as there are domain names. There are many website design sites to build your site, and you may be able to register a domain name directly with them as well.

Search engine optimization

Getting your website on the first page of a search, when people search for your business is particularly important. If you are difficult to find, you will lose business. Utilizing search engine optimization (SEO) is a significant way to increase the quantity and quality of visitors to your website. The goal is to have visitors that find your site organically, and appropriately managing your SEO can help you gain an audience. SEO is complex, and the author recommends doing your own research before starting to build your website. The essential SEO content that the search engines look for include the following:

1. Crawl accessibility allows search engines (like Google or Bing) to find and engage with your website. Make sure you have all the content about your services and information available on your website.
2. Keywords are words or phrases on your website that are going to be searched for frequently. For example, "housecall veterinarian" or "palliative vet" will become associated with your business.
3. User experience occurs when clients look at your website. Ensure that your site not only contains the information they are looking for and that it is easy for them to find the content. Having a website that loads quickly, is accessible, and is aesthetically pleasing are all things that contribute to the potential client's experience.
4. Links to your page on other sites (Fishkin, 2018). For example, you can share links to videos, businesses associated with you, and your social media accounts.

There is a great website dedicated to teaching you how SEO works, Moz.com, "The beginner's guide to SEO." (Fishkin, 2018) Websites like these will show you how to enhance your SEO from a basic to a more technical level.

Other marketing areas

Phone books are still significant to older adults, though more and more do not use them. The phone book companies will set an ad for the phonebook and add you to the directory online. Using the online phone book directory is one way to increase your SEO. This format may have a declining ROI.

Paid advertising

Yelp—Advertising directly on Yelp is another way to market. Yelp tends to market for the younger population. It will also increase your SEO.

Google AdWords—Google AdWords is a way to increase your visibility online and can put you on the first page as a paid account. The amount purchased is set by the business, and if you are in an area that does not have many who do what you do, you may not have to use Google AdWords. However, if you start in an area with more than one or a big corporate Hospice or Euthanasia practice, you will likely want to spend some of your advertising dollars on Google AdWords.

Bing Ads—Similar to Google AdWords, paying Bing to be at the top or near the top of the first page. It will depend on how many other veterinarians are also using this service and how high up on the page you may be.

Other online advertising ideas

Landing pages—Landing pages can be used as an ad, highlighting what product or service you would like to highlight. Landing pages can change monthly to highlight various aspects of service (Wordstream Staff, 2018).

Call tracking—Tracking where calls are coming from can be a way to focus your marketing. Your ROI can be streamlined with call tracking (Wordstream Staff, 2018).

Email marketing—Email marketing, or email blasts, can be a way to get your name out to a more significant population. You can purchase email lists to send to or you could accumulate your list with clients (Wordstream Staff, 2018).

Remarketing—This involves getting your ad on other sites and might require some more advanced training with computer technology (Wordstream Staff, 2018).

Social media

Social media can be a fantastic way to connect with clients and referring veterinarians. The top social media apps are free to create an account and use and connect you with an audience interested in your content. You can build long-term engagement and support for clients by providing online education, interesting stories and client-based posts. By utilizing various social media accounts, you can find different demographics of users interested in specific content. Many social media platforms link together seamlessly; however, you can use online services to connect your content using one link. Additionally, you can create more directed marketing campaigns on your business page and often start for free. Linking your social media to your website will also drive your SEO. You may also use paid ads on social media to reach an even larger audience. Social media is rapidly changing and the content here may not reflect the current trends.

Blogging

Some of the most successful social media veterinarians have utilized blogging to build a following. Examples of social media veterinarian influencers that have successfully integrated blogging for their audiences include Pawcurious.com, AndyRoark.com, Cody Creelman Cow Vet, and DrSueCancerVet.com. **Tumblr** is an example of a blog site connecting you with other people with the same interests.

Facebook

Facebook is social media used by veterinarians and clients alike. Building a practice page is significant to your SEO and is a way to inform and develop a practice. Practices can create fun medical challenges for owners to participate in or establish educational posts to promote aspects of their practice.

Facebook also has groups to join and communicate with other veterinarians in the community doing hospice, palliative medicine, or euthanasia. The Veterinarian Palliative Medicine group has grown exponentially. It is open to veterinarians from all over the world, with many small and large animal general practitioners, specialists, and university professors interested in learning more about palliative medicine. Specialists participate in conversations through Facebook Live events discussing different topics in veterinary palliative medicine. There are sister sites for students and technicians on Facebook as well.

Instagram

Instagram is an image-sharing platform with a range of ways to engage audiences. Add up to 10 pictures or videos per post with a caption to captivate your audience and an action button that may bring them more information or drive them to your website. Involve your followers in the post's comment section by asking for feedback on the pictures. For example, ask clients a funny story about a beloved pet or ask what topic they want to learn about in your next post. Videos on main posts can be up to 60 s. However, you can add longer videos (15−60 min) to IGTV (a section dedicated to long videos only) on your feed. In addition to your feed, post in the "Story" section of Instagram. Stories have three primary uses: short form (disappears after 24 h), long-form (as a story highlight that stays up on your page), and live (live video feed that gives you the option to save and repost or delete). Short-form stories are suitable for simple, brief posts. For example, you can show clients a "day in the life," and you can add-on questions to engage your audience via comments. Long-form story highlights can be used to provide posts that stay at the top of your page and make it easy for clients to access them instead of looking through average picture posts. For example, tell the story of your practice, or provide an "FAQ" highlight at the top of the page. Finally, like Facebook, Instagram allows veterinarians to post live videos with direct engagement to the audience. One can add people onto the feed in person or remotely. For example, add other veterinarians and specialists to live broadcasts if you discuss specific topics with a colleague. Finally, a critical addition to your Instagram posts is hashtags. Hashtags (# plus a word or phrase, ex. #veterinarian) can be utilized in the comment description and help reach a larger audience. Users can look up hashtags in the tags section on Instagram, so one needs to find hashtags that engage audiences looking for veterinary care.

LinkedIn

LinkedIn is a professional social media website. Building a professional following on LinkedIn can aid veterinarians in finding other veterinarians and professionals in a variety of fields. For example, you can find connections in advertising, marketing, computer programming, card stock, education, and others. To reach a larger audience, you can share your education, experience, licenses, and skills to find mutual connections with similar interests. You can also receive endorsements and recommendations from colleagues to boost your recognition on the site. Veterinarians can post blogs they have written, articles they find interesting, share that they are hiring, and more on LinkedIn.

Snapchat

Snapchat is remarkably like the Instagram stories feature. You can post short-form stories that last for 24 h or create a long-form episode that can remain indefinitely on your account. Snapchat stories can be recorded for significantly longer than 60 s. However, Snapchat automatically chunks the video into 10-s-long clips, making it difficult for a seamless transition in a long-form video. This app may be difficult to utilize to engage audiences with commentary. However, long-form episodes could be published on your page as educational tools. At the time of writing, Snapchat does not offer live broadcasts.

TikTok

TikTok is a relatively new social media platform at the time of this writing. However, it has seen incredible growth as a social media platform. Unlike other media platforms, TikTok is entirely video-based and provides users the ability to create short 60 s videos or go live for their audience. Veterinarians can use videos to provide educational content, show them what procedures look like, or answer questions about their practice. Users gain visibility by using trending sounds in their videos' backgrounds and using hashtags to find users with similar interests. Live videos are another great way to engage your audience, as they also have an open comment section that allows users to connect directly with the broadcaster and ask questions.

Twitter

Twitter has gained popularity and is another way to market and communicate directly with clients. You can use short phrases, up to 280 characters, in one Tweet. You can also attach pictures and videos to your posts that can entice clients to read and engage. Hashtags are beneficial on this platform, as they curate audiences interested in your content. Twitter has a "story" section where you can post pictures and videos that disappear in 24 h. Twitter is also a way to follow other veterinarians and educational websites.

YouTube

YouTube provides a platform that allows for primarily long-form videos (anything for a minute to several hours). Videos are a terrific way to improve your website and can be used to educate your clients. On YouTube, videos can include comments and direct feedback with a "like" and "dislike" button. You can consist of video playlists, a community page, and a related channels section within your channel. Video playlists make it simple for clients to watch related or story-based content that automatically plays one after the other. The community page is a way to post comments and pictures between video uploads and engage audiences with questions, links to articles, and more. The related channels page can connect you to channels with similar goals (education, client engagement) and can be used as a vast network to refer audiences to similar content. YouTube also has a live section to engage visually with audiences in between video posts.

Other sites you can utilize

Pinterest

Veterinarians can use Pinterest to post medical information and other pictures to help generate interest, provide education for your clients, and keep them interested in your practice.

Reddit

You can create a forum dedicated to your practice or area of interest. You can provide engagement by promoting topics like "AMAs" (Ask me anything) to educate your audience on what services you offer and where they can find support.

Navigating social media

There are many different companies that can help you navigate social media. An example is SnoutSchool.com, a social media guru who can help you design a social media plan for your business. They also have a Facebook page that offers free advice. There are many similar sources out there. Look for a social media planner who deals with veterinarian websites and social media.

Conclusion

There are many aspects of business to consider when setting up a hospice/palliative/euthanasia based housecall practice. This chapter has a brief overview of setting up a start up practice. If you would like more information there is a course online that goes into more depth, called The House Call Vet Academy. The focus now shifts to animal hospice and palliative medicine.

References

Chen, J. (February 1, 2013). *Should your business be non-profit or for-profit?* Retrieved from Harvard Business Review https://hbr.org/.

Corporate Direct. (2018). *C corporations: Learn the 11 advantages & disadvantages.* Retrieved from Corporate Direct https://www.corporatedirect.com/start-a-business/entity-types/c-corporation/.

Fishkin, R.a. (2018). *The beginners guide to SEO.* Retrieved from https://moz.com/beginners-guide-to-seo/how-search-engines-operate.

Garrett Sutton, E. (July 1, 2015). *Top 12 LLC advantages and disadvantages.* Retrieved from Corporate Direct https://www.corporatedirect.com/blog/top-12-llc-advantages-and-disadvantages/.

Incorporate Staff. (2018). *What is an S corporation (S corp)?* Retrieved from Incorporate https://www.incorporate.com/s_corporation.html.

McCreery, M. (2018). *The complete, 12-step guide to starting a business.* Retrieved from Entrepreneur.com https://www.entrepreneur.com/article/297899.

Moynihan, T. J. (February 2, 2018). *Magic mouthwash: Effective for chemotherapy mouth sores?* Retrieved from Mayo Clinic https://www.mayoclinic.org/tests-procedures/chemotherapy/expert-answers/magic-mouthwash/faq-20058071.

Nash, D. (2018). *Advantages and disadvantages of for-profit companies.* Retrieved from Chron http://smallbusiness.chron.com/advantages-disadvantages-forprofit-companies-24293.html.

NOLO. (2018a). *50-State guide to establishing a sole proprietorship.* Retrieved from Nolo.com https://www.nolo.com/legal-encyclopedia/50-state-guide-establishing-sole-proprietorship.html.

NOLO. (2018b). *Partnership agreements.* Retrieved from NOLO https://www.nolo.com/legal-encyclopedia/partnership.

SBA. (2018). *Small business administration.* Retrieved from Write your business plan https://www.sba.gov/business-guide/plan-your-business/write-your-business-plan.

SBA Staff. (2018). *Hire and manage employees.* Retrieved from US Small Business Association https://www.sba.gov/business-guide/manage-your-business/hire-manage-employees.

Schooley, S. (2021). *SWOT analysis: what it is and when to use it.* Business News Daily. https://www.businessnewsdaily.com/4245-swot-analysis.html. (Accessed 17 November 2021).

Silver, Y. (April 23, 2012). *7 tips for naming your business.* Retrieved from Entrepreneur https://www.entrepreneur.com/article/223401.

Staff of AVMA. (2021a). *Model veterinary practice Act.* Retrieved from AVMA.org https://www.avma.org/sites/default/files/2021-01/model-veterinary-practice-act.pdf.

Staff of AVMA. (2021b). *Tools of practice management.* Retrieved from AVMA.org https://www.avma.org/resources-tools/practice-management/telehealth-telemedicine-veterinary-practice/veterinary-telehealth-basics.

Staff of AVMA. (2021c). *Veterinary telehealth guidelines.* Retrieved from AVMA.org https://www.avma.org/sites/default/files/2021-01/AVMA-Veterinary-Telehealth-Guidelines.pdf.

The House Call Vet Academy, *An online course with Dr Eve Harrison.* Retrieved from https://www.thehousecallvetacademy.com.

Wordstream Staff. (2018). *Online advertising: How to create effective online advertising.* Retrieved from WordStream https://www.wordstream.com/online-advertising.

WSJ staff. (2018). *How to start a business with a partner.* Retrieved from WSJ How to Home Guides http://guides.wsj.com/small-business/starting-a-business/how-to-start-a-business-with-a-partner/.

Further reading

Amir Shanan, J. P. (2013, 2016). IAAHPC.org. Retrieved from Practice Guidelines https://www.iaahpc.org/resources-and-support/practice-guidelines.html.

DVM360.com staff. (November 1, 2014). *Veterinary practice software comparison chart.* Retrieved from DVM360 http://files.dvm360.com/alfresco_images/DVM360//2014/11/03/1baca57a-b9e7-4850-9251-7d0569a0c509/softwareguide_chart.pdf.

Your first appointment

Lynn Hendrix, AA, BA, DVM, CHPV [1,2,3,4]

[1]*Owner, Veterinarian, Beloved Pet Mobile Vet, Davis, CA, United States;* [2]*Former Board of Directors, IAAHPC, Chicago, IL, United States;* [3]*Consultant, Hospice, Palliative Medicine, End of Life, VIN, Davis, CA, United States;* [4]*President, Founder, World Veterinary Palliative Medicine Organization, Davis, CA, United States*

Prior to the visit

Your first contact with a client is going to be via a phone call, text message, or email. You choose how you want to be contacted. Make a message that is kind, and tells people the following information:

1. Who they are calling (which doctor, what practice).
2. Your hours available for phone contact, appointment contact—set up the expectation early.
3. A local emergency hospital to contact in case of crisis. Preferably one that is 24 h a day/7 days a week.
4. Ask to leave a message detailing what has been going on with their animal.
5. You may want to know who referred them (optional).
6. If you have an online scheduler, how to make an appointment through the online scheduler (this will save you time).
7. You may also want to define your service area (though you can do that on your website).

Once you have established contact with a client, finding out the details of the history, and current situation with the pet. The history may include what medications the animal is on, what tests have been run, diagnosis if any that have been made. It is helpful to establish previous veterinary care, and obtain records from their previous veterinarian to review prior to the appointment. You may get what their goals are in a phone call, though goals may change over time and can change with education on the specific disease, pain management, symptom management. Do not spend time on the call getting the goals, set up an appointment to go into goals and priorities. Supplemental information to collect may include who may be present at the appointment, whether there is parking readily available, if there are gate codes you might need, if there is limited access to their road. In addition, getting an address to calculate mileage, and to schedule based on the timing of the drive. Asking the client if the animal is fearful of strangers or vets, exhibits aggressive tendencies, and the extent of the disease, supports you in knowing what you may be walking into. Finally discussing the type of appointment they are looking for and when they are anticipating needing an appointment.

Setting up the appointment

Setting up the first appointment most commonly occurs with the initial contact, though occasionally several phone calls may take place before the client feels the animal is ready or the client is emotionally ready to set an appointment. If people are not making an appointment after the initial contact, they may not be emotionally ready or may go back to their regular veterinarian. They may not see the value yet, in what you do, and how you would be different from their current veterinarian.

People do not know or understand palliative care, or they may be concerned about hospice and do not feel like their animal is dying. They may think you are only a euthanasia veterinarian, and you may be calling for free advice before a euthanasia appointment. Offering a quality of life exam or a palliative consultation can support the client. Giving people options for end-of-life care and listening to their priorities and subsequently providing education takes time, and a consultation provides that time.

An online scheduler with a calendar can help you cut down on phone contact. It should be mobile and should work with your phone or tablet. An online scheduler can embed into your website, you can direct clients to make appointments there in your off hours. It can show a client when you are available (without having to call them to tell them) and when they will have to choose another vet or another way of helping their animal. Since society spends so much time on their phones, tablets and computers, online schedulers will save you and your clients time, in making appointments. Paper calendars or organizers are okay too if that is what you feel comfortable using.

> **Cancellations:** A word about cancellations. They will happen. They can happen frequently as you get busier. You may drive all the way to an appointment and have a no-show. Or make the effort and be half way there and have them cancel. They are frustrating. Reasons can vary. The animal may pass before you arrive, they may decide to take the animal to another vet, whatever the reason, make a cancellation policy to minimize cancellations. Make a cancellation policy from the beginning, whatever works for you and put it on your website. And any other literature you leave with people, including an online scheduler. Charge people for the appointments that canceled and you show up to or head towards. This will save you time and money.

First meeting in the home

The first consultation is your chance to meet people where they are, emotionally and physically in their home. Your first in-person meeting gives you the opportunity to educate and guide people in more depth with their pet's end-of-life experience.

Whether this is their first time with end-of-life care or death or they have been through other pet's deaths or euthanasias, this is your opportunity to improve the quality of life for both pet and beloved person. Finding out what their experience with death has been in the past is helpful to understanding their perception. Meeting people in their homes allows the veterinarian to be in a comfortable setting for both the animal and their people. The more you can do to help both parties relax, the better. Sitting on the ground with the animal is common, though I have sat on couches, at kitchen tables to do paperwork and for a palliative discussion, that will be much of your visit. Plan on at least 1−3 hrs to have an adequate time to discuss all that you need to discuss and allow for plenty of time for questions. Identifying where perceptions differ and meeting people where they are in life and listening to the complicated and sometimes complex emotional situation they live with, for example, the dynamics between the family members and the complicated relationship(s) with their pet in addition to assessing the often-multiple, and complex comorbidities, make this a challenging field of study.

> Helpful Hint—People will often offer food, water, or other beverages. Plan on whether you would like to take them up on the offer.

To be able to give the clients time to ask all the questions they need to and provide the information you need to convey, you need at least a 2-h appointment time; sometimes you will need additional time. It is crucial to provide enought time to cover the amount of information clients need and to plan for the future of the pet and to define the following things:

1. Introduction of team members if you have. This is a bonding time with people. Having them meet the team helps bond the relationship. Even if it is not everyone they might encounter, giving them contact points is a key component to establishing a relationship with your business.
2. Getting history from the caregivers and reviewing the previous medical history (this can also be done outside of the exam—the author takes time at the exam, to be paid for the time involved.)
3. Doing a physical exam on the animal.
4. Asking open-ended questions: What does the caregiver(s) understand about what is going on with their beloved pet?
5. What do they understand about the disease?
6. What are the client's concerned or, worried about, and fearful of with the future of the pet? This is a time to introduce disease trajectories.
7. What are the client's goals for care?
8. What are the client's priorities for care?
9. Are the caregivers all on the same page regarding care, priorities, and goals? If not, how are you going to help them? (This is an appropriate time to get a mental health person involved). This is a good time to review an advanced directive.

10. What outcomes are unacceptable to the client? What are you, the client, willing to have the animal go through and what are you and they not willing to let the animal go through?

11. Are they able to commit the time it takes to provide the care needed? Are they prepared for the potential cost of care? Take into account how many medications, non-medical interventions need to be provided. Will it work in their daily schedule? How can you adjust their plan to help both the client and pet?

12. Establishing goals of care together and providing a plan of action. Provide a written plan for the family to follow. It should include the following information:

    1. Establishing emergency/crisis plans.

    2. Having a comfort/crisis/emergency kit prepared (see Chapter 5).

    3. Establishing a medication regime. Let them know that it may be unlike curative medicine, this plan is going to change as the disease processes change and that this is your initial startup plan. Plan for the next follow-up appointment, whether it is by phone or in person. Inform owner of upcoming costs.

    4. Having written materials providing the caregivers information and backup of verbal information. Include cancellation policy, dealing with sharps, medications that may be left over, including what to do with controlled substances. Where to donate food and other items post death. What to do if the animal suddenly dies, crematoriums to contact.

13. Observation of the property to help establish ways to help the elderly animal get around better, looking at food dishes (do they have a stable surface to stand on to eat, are the bowls raised up so they do not have to put additional pressure on their joints?), what does the dog door look like, are there steps into, or out of the house, could they add a ramp?

14. Establish physical quality of life parameters and discuss the "Surprise Question?"

    a. Are they able to get themselves up?

    b. Are they pooping or peeing on themselves or in the house? Do the owners want to place them in diapers?

    c. Are they able to walk?

    d. Do the owners want to utilize harnesses, carts, wagons to get them around, are they physically able to help get them in one, or up and moving?

    e. Are they concerned about weight loss? Does it make the animal weak?

    f. Are they eating?

    g. Are they drinking?

    h. Are they stable in their disease or has it moved further along?

    i. What would a good day look like?

    j. (Surprise question) Would you (the clinician) be surprised if they were still alive in 2 weeks, 2 months, 6 months, or 1 year? This can help you and the client narrow down the approximate time you and the client believe this animal has left. Prognostication is not very accurate. The surprise question can help.

15. Establish emotional quality of life parameters
   a. Are they still happy, enjoying aspects of life? Identify aspects with the client.
   b. Are they still interacting with the family? Or have they gone into hiding? Are they super clingy? What is their mentation, is it declining?
   c. How long during a 24-h period are they interacting?
   d. What does the family think is important for their emotional quality of life?
16. What is their autonomy like?
   a. Are they able to feed themselves, drink on their own?
   b. Go out to go to the bathroom, or in a litter box?
   c. Can they clean, groom themselves?
   d. Are they able to move themselves from place to place or do they need assistance? Can they still jump up on things in the house?
17. Develop an advanced directive. This can help people establish parameters that matter to their family and can have end-of-life choices. Based on the legal document five wishes (Plummer, 2011) (the first wish is naming a power of attorney, which is not needed for animals), you could include;
   a. The kind of medical treatment or intervention the family wishes for their animal.
   b. Comfort or amount of distress that they are concerned about.
   c. Staying at home, do not resuscitate orders
   d. Aftercare plans

> Helpful Hint—This author has never spent less than 1 hour and believes that a minimum of 2+ hours is needed to provide time to answer questions and provide answers and a personalized plan.

Legal

The minimum number of legal forms that a house call vet will need include:

1. A client information sheet with a signature. This should include names of human family members, address, phone numbers, email address, pet's name, other pets (if you want), age, weight, color, breed, date of birth, reason for visit, how they heard about you (for tracking purposes).
2. A euthanasia form with a waiver for biting and rabies contact, and signature and date.
3. Body care information, (whether a euthanasia occurs, or they are dead on arrival or DOA), should have a signature, for what the client wants for body care. The author keeps their body care information on the same page so the client does not have to fill out multiple pages. The client should sign for body care (to minimize mistakes), and can include if they are donating a blanket or toy (so they do not

anticipate having them back and for any other extras they may want—a paw print, different urn other than the standard, and engraving done, as examples of extras).

4. Drug release forms. Drug release forms to obtain consent for—Use of medications off label. NSAIDs, Opioids or other controlled substances.

5. Hospice/palliative service agreement—include time needed to be seen (i.e., every 2 weeks, every 2 months ... etc.), costs (can be included on this one) Chapter 5.

6. Medical record.

7. Controlled drug record—the DEA requires drug logs to be maintained for all controlled substances separately. Schedule 2 drugs must be maintained separately from the Schedule 3,4,5 drugs and require Form 222 to obtain drugs. Controlled substance forms—Form 222, CURES forms (for California); inventory must be taken every 2 years. Drug logs must be kept for a minimum of 2 years (DEA Staff, 2018). Check with the DEA-in the United States, or other regulatory body for additional questions.

Informational white sheets

Informational forms are important to leave with the caregivers to have them refer to, as the first informational consultation is often fraught with emotion and an overwhelming amount of information. This gives them a framework of information to refer back to as they progress through the dying process with their animal. White sheets can also help the client refer to your information in times of crisis.

Information sheets to consider having are the following:

1. The plan you create together. It should include what to do in an emergency, what medications to give on a day-to-day basis, and what medications to give in an emergency. The parameters to contact you and an emergency clinic. End-of-life goals worksheet may be helpful to establish goals for the people involved.

2. Nutritional information. Food to try if they are not eating their normal diet, fluid parameters, and diverse ways to get medication into the animal if they are not eating. Animals who have tablet or capsules to take will need an alternative if they are not eating; transdermal formulations, liquid formulations, or injectables are all better ways to get medication into an animal that is not eating. Putting medication in a sticky substance, such as honey can be a McGyver way to get medications into an animal in a crisis.

3. Distress versus suffering. Define distress for clients. Suffering is a symptom, what one person can say to another and is based on emotion and personal history; distress is a clinical sign and as such is observable. More on this topic is discussed later in this chapter. Knowing observable signs empower clients as

to when to call the veterinarian. (the author will repeat this concept again in more detail) (Crisis kits—see Chapter 5).

4. Information on chronic pain and cancer pain. People do not always recognize chronic pain or cancer pain in their animals. Cancer does cause pain, though it may not always be apparent, like chronic pain, clients may not recognize the clinical signs of cancer pain. Helping clients recognize the signs of mild, moderate, and severe chronic pain, as well as acute pain signs, will help them know when to call the veterinarian.

5. Your availability. Having your availability in writing helps establish a boundary of when clients can contact you and when you will not be available. You do not have to be available 24/7 but the author recommends that you establish an emergency plan for the family or caregivers when you are not available. This can include a plan for emergency clinics, crisis kits, and other veterinarians in your area who can help them euthanize at home if there is a crisis. If you have a team, include them on the availablity whitesheet.

6. Mental health support. What mental health is available in your local area that can support people who need grief support and additional mental health support? Or if you have hired someone, have their contact information available. Utilize pet loss support hotlines around the country or your locale. In addition, a list of pet loss online sources, for example, The Association for Pet Loss and Bereavement (APLB) has an online chat room that is available for people for both anticipatory grief and postdeath grief. They also have educational tools for both the professional and the client (APLB Staff, 2018a,b).

7. Suicide information and complicated grief information. May want to obtain these from your local mental health professional (more in Chapter 11).

8. Disease trajectories. A graph of the expected course of disease until the end of life. Currently, we must use the human trajectories, because the veterinary trajectories mostly end in euthanasia. Veterinary trajectories are not helpful if someone chooses to have a palliated death; however, the human graphs can be informational.

9. Information on specific disease progression through the body (most helpful for cancer patients, though the bigger understanding of the disease to the end, will be helpful for making decisions on euthanasia or palliated death).

10. Assessment of approaching or/imminent death signs. This is one of the more useful white sheets as it contains the information that clients fear the most, what death may look like, and how will they know when it is time to call you, when is the animal in crisis. What is terminal delirium? This white sheet should include what terminal delirium might look like.

11. Cost information. A list of fees and services available, and a glossary of the services available. This may also be listed on your website.

12. List of medications available and common side effects, in California, there should be a complete list of side effects. Should be included in your plan.

13. Many veterinarians include a quality-of-life scale. More on quality-of-life scales is discussed later in this chapter.

14. Pain scales. More on pain scales is discussed later in this chapter and other chapters.
15. Wound care. Having various wound care descriptions can be helpful, from decubitus ulcers to craterous tumors, how to care for the individual wound, medications to use, bandaging material that would be helpful to buy, and a what to if checklist can be very helpful (not necessary to give to every client).
16. Household modifications that can assist their animal in getting around better in their house. May be included in the plan. Suggestions on items available, like rugs, yoga mats for grip, to lowering the dog door, to raising bowls, or placing a fan are all nonmedical strategies to make an animal feel better.
17. A calendar or journal, some type of daily logging system for the animal, to help both caregiver and medical staff assist and track the animal in changes to their needs. Pictures or videos can also be very useful to track progress of improvement or loss. Online apps may also be useful.
18. Crematoriums that you use or a list of crematoriums that you would send them to and what to do if the animal dies suddenly or unexpectedly.
19. Information on burial in your area, legalities, and fines possible.
20. What to do with the medications, sharps, bedding, and accessories after a death.
21. Ideas for memorializing. Scrapbooking, lighting a candle, ceremonies (especially if you have a nondenominational religious place you work with to provide rituals postdeath), writing about the animal, writing from the animals perspective about their life with the people, art, drawing, placing a picture a day on social media, and more.
22. How to talk with children about death and grief. Should include books that parents can use to help their child understand in an age-appropriate way.
23. Social media policies.
24. Zoonotic disease information for your local area (this part is optional unless … you have zoonotic disease present in the animal information if you have children or an immunosuppressed person in the household).

The exam
SOAP—how it might differ from the traditional exam
Subjective

The subjective aspect of the SOAP will encompass the history with the animal and with the family. Questions should include the previous history from other veterinarians, what is currently going on physically, socially, and psychologically for the animal. The palliative philosophy also includes the physical, psychological, social, and spiritual needs of the family or caregiver(s). The history of family's needs, their physical challenges (i.e., they work 12 h a day and the animal needs meds every 6 h), what their priorities are as the animal approaches death, and detailing what they are concerned about and fearful of can help guide the planning process. Adding to the comprehensive history, includes their previous experiences with death, what they understand of their animal's current condition, if they have been to a veterinarian, chronic pain signs they may have seen. Examining the house, the floors, the feeding area, the beds, the litter boxes, ways out of the house, things they might jump on or off, steps, and dog doors all need to be examined. This is an appropriate time to think about the surprise question. The surprise question asks, "Would you be surprised if the patient was going to die in the next few weeks, months, year" (The GSF Prognostic Indicator Guidance, 2011).

Objective

The initial objective exam is essentially the same as the physical exam for any other animal. It could include a complete physical exam, neurologic, orthopedic exam, and rectal exam that would be pertinent to the disease process you are seeing. Assessing how far along they are in the disease process, whether they have stable disease, have unstable disease, are in a deteriorating state, or are in their final days can be significant to discuss during the first visit. Assessing and documenting their current pain level, where they may have pain, whether it is mild, moderate, or severe, unrelenting or acute on chronic. Previous or current diagnostics can also be included in this section.

Assessment

The assessment will include a summary of the clinical signs and the rule-outs for each clinical sign as you see as with the traditional curative model.

Also included will be the assessment for the current state of pain, for psychosocial issues, mobility, incontinence issues, mentation, and disease state.

Plan

The plan is made together with the client or caregiver with the caregiver's priorities in mind. The plan will involve the previous assessments and comorbidities. Supportive care and medications that will target specific pain Chapter 5 and 6 and other clinical signs. Disease trajectory and progression and the state of the disease should be considered in making the plan.

Subsequent visits should be included and are to reassess where they are in their disease process again. Timing for future visits depends on the state of the disease and scheduling the next contact at the first consultation will keep the animal and the client in better support. Other aspects of the plan are in the subsequent pages.

Distress versus suffering

Every palliative veterinarian I have talked to gets this comment from families; "I don't want them to suffer." When I first began my journey, I often asked clients, "What does suffering mean to you?" It was difficult for the owner to put into words, exactly what they meant, most of the time they told me, it meant that they did not want their animal in pain, and they did not want to see them in distress. Suffering is really a symptom, it is subjective, and the definition varies from person to person and is based on their perspective and personal history (Cassell, 2014). Suffering can occur with animals, but defining it is difficult. Suffering can also happen with the people involved with the pet and can involve fear, anger, worry, emotional, and their own physical pain.

The author finds it more helpful for families to have clinical signs to watch for, the observable signs of distress. That is why the author prefers discussing the term distress. Distress is a more objective and a clinical sign, observable and can be defined by organ systems and we need to also define what causes possible emotional distress for animals. Clients are focused on the emotional aspect of quality of life whereas veterinarians tend to focus on the physical quality of life. Identifying the emotional aspects of distress can help a client empathize what their beloved animal may be going through. The author's list of distress signs are organized by organ system and emotional distress is in the last paragraph. This list is not comprehensive, and can be added to as the veterinarian sees fit or as more information becomes available.

Respiratory distress—dyspnea, respiratory rate-resting respiratory rates higher than 60 breaths in a minute or increasing over time (as monitored daily). Coughing frequently or in increasing frequency and intensity. Mucus membranes bluish, white, or pale pink can indicate respiratory problems. Wheezing or Stridor (teaching owners the sounds to watch for).

Body positioning—head and neck outstretched. Nostril flare can proceed open mouth breathing in cats (emergency). Abdominal breathing, paradoxical breathing (PetMD Staff, 2018).

Brain distress—seizures, that last longer than 3 min (emergency), have more than one seizure in a 24-h period or the seizures are getting closer together (increasing frequency), vestibular signs (head tilt, eyes bouncing back and forth, falling over, and circling), howling (especially in a kitty, although not always distress). Terminal delirum. Sudden blindness from hypertension.

Body positioning—head pressing, getting stuck in corners, seeming confused. Vocalizations. Sudden blindness.

GI distress—vomiting, diarrhea, especially with hematemesis, hematochezia. Constipation with straining to defecate. Regurgitation. Bloated abdomen with retching (emergency). Bloated abdomen with respiratory distress signs (also an emergency). Acutely painful abdomen (also an emergency).

Body positioning—praying posture. Licking or looking at abdomen, sleeping in a different position than typical, or unable to lie down. Can also be restless, lip licking (from nausea), retching with out production of vomitous.

Urinary stress—stranguria, hematuria, Pollakiuria, dysuria, lack of urine production (an emergency), crying when they urinate (can also potentially be an emergency, often pain).

Body positioning—squatting for extended periods of time in the litter box for cats or for dogs, going outside and standing or moving frequently in the urinating position with little to no production.

Cardiac distress—"saddle" thrombus, pulmonary thromboembolism, cardiac thromboembolism, cerebral thromboembolism, sudden death, and tachycardia >120 in dogs and >180 in cats Other abnormal rhythms, though the client may not be able to assess.

Body positioning—sudden loss of ability to move pelvic limbs, or one thoracic limb, knuckling, cold paw or paws. Sudden increased respiratory effort "racing" heart rate.

Musculoskeletal distress—musculoskeletal pain (acute pain, severe chronic pain) and difficulty getting up from a sleeping or sitting position, falling over when standing. Bone pain from osteosarcoma manifesting in, limping, not wanting to get up from a lying down position, or not laying down, not wanting to eat, can be a pain in teeth or jaw. Pain opening jaw.

Skin distress—decubitus ulcer(s), ulcerated or oozing tumors, acute moist dermatitis, urticaria, (can be pain related), and constant licking one spot (can be pain related). Maggots or other larva.

Emotional distress—(things that are emotionally distressing may also have a physically distressing component)—anything that can cause anxiety, strangers in the house, changes in routine, the animal cannot get up, is urinating or defecating on self, and is struggling to get up. Frustration, confusion, depression, avoidance behavior, withdrawing from family, and sleep disturbances may be a clinical sign of emotional distress, any change in behavior may be due to emotional distress (but can also be an indication of pain), obsessive behaviors (i.e., licking the same leg repeatedly), lacking energy can also be due to emotional distress, but should also look for a physical cause (Bouchez, 2018).

Quality-of-life scales

Quality-of-life scales are utilized in human medicine, and we have a few to use in veterinary medicine. The scales used in human medicine tend to be disease specific and are validated. QofL scales in veterinary medicine are not validated and are mostly based on physical quality of life. However, quality of life for people is broken down to physical and emotional quality of life. Veterinarians are trained to focus on the physical quality of life, while clients tend to focus on the emotional quality of life of their pet. The author believes the incongruity of decision making with end-of-life care pets comes from this disparity. Veterinarians tend to utilize QofL scales to assist the client on deciding on the right time for euthanasia. While they may have their place in end-of-life care, the author finds QoL scales limited. Clients invested in palliative care for their animals may utilize them, but the author has had clients overlook and cross things off, because they do not want the score to be low. For some clients, it may help them clarify the decline of the disease and can give an objective view of the situation. The author believes each of them to have limitations that do not take into account the whole scope of end-of-life care. In addition, they do not take the client's quality of life, nor the animal's will to live into account which is part of the euthanasia decision making.

The HHHHHMM scale

The HHHHHMM scale by Alice Villalobos was one of the first comprehensive scales in the United States for animals. HHHHHMM is the QofL scale developed by Dr. Alice Villalobos. The H's stand for Hurt, Hydration, Hunger, Happiness, Hygiene, and the M's stand for More good days than bad and Mobility (Villalobos, 2008).

Brambell's Five Freedoms

Brambell's Five Freedoms was another early look at the quality of life when talking about the end of life (Mellor, 2016).

Brambell's Five Freedoms are as follows:

1. Freedom from hunger and thirst
2. Freedom from discomfort
3. Freedom from pain, injury, and disease
4. Freedom to express (most) normal behavior
5. Freedom from fear and distress. (Mellor, 2016)

JOURNEY's quality-of-life scale

JOURNEY's scale was developed by Dr. Katie Hilst, owner of Journey's Home Pet Euthanasia LLC. She has a calculator on her website to help veterinarians or owners determine their patient's quality of life (Hilst, 2018). This quality-of-life scale does take into account some of the aspects of the human quality of life, which is affected by the animal's quality of life.

JOURNEYS quality of life scale for pets considers the following

J—jumping or mobility
O—ouch or pain
U—uncertainty and understanding (factors that affect YOU)
R—respiration or breathing
N—neatness or hygiene
E—eating and drinking
Y—you
S—social ability

Lap of Love quality-of-life scale

Lap of Love (a corporate business) has its own quality of life scale system.

It involves mobility, nutrition, hydration, interaction and attitude, elimination, and favorite things (McVety, 2017).

These are all adequate quality-of-life scales. However, the author believes veterinarians need an improved scale for palliative medicine to provide assessment not only for the quality of life, but will to live, ability to live, emotional quality of life, autonomy, quality of the dying process, human interaction, human quality of life, and nursing care involved (because the caregiver's quality of life and abilities to care for the animal also plays a role in decision-making) which needs to be validated to use adequately.

Animal advanced directives

Advanced directives for people are legal documents that help an individual make decisions regarding the end of their life, in the event that they are unable to make decisions for themselves. Currently, there are legal forms called advanced directives for pets that are legal papers people can draw up for the care of the animals after the death of the person.

However, another way of thinking of an advanced directive for animals would be to provide a document (not necessarily legal) allowing for the discussion of the wishes of the family for the animal, and/or the wishes of the animal, if those can be determined. Just like in human medicine, it is helpful to have an advanced directive to help make decisions for animals before a crisis occurs and subsequently a more emotional time, as the animal approaches death. It could also help facilitate a conversation among family members and help them define what is important. It can also be useful to help make a euthanasia decision if that is what the family chooses. Utilizing the animal advanced directive before a crisis can give caregivers backup to making decisions as they approach the more emotionally challenging time of the dying process. Making it a checklist can help owners identify needs and priorities.

The author's advanced directive is simple. What do you want to see your beloved able to do, and what you do not want to have to see them go through? They can be more complex, including what to do in emergencies, DNR (do not resuscitate) orders, and what you would like done with the body after death. Advanced directives can also include quality-of-life scales, emotional quality-of-life scales, and autonomy issues. Advanced directives can give people peace of mind, and in writing down their wishes, gives them their own path to follow. An advanced directive should also take into account the caregiver's quality of life, both what is working, and what is a struggle in caregiving. In the human literature, there are many caregiver scales that may be utilized.

Pain management plan (Chapter 6 goes into more detail)—building a pain management plan depends on several factors. What type of pain, is it visceral, neuropathic, inflammatory, cancer pain? Is there more than one location of pain? What is causing pain, are there multiple etiologies for pain? Is it acute pain, or is it chronic pain? Is the chronic pain, mild, moderate, or severe or unrelenting? Targeted pain therapy and multimodal pain therapies with pharmaceuticals and non-medical modalities are frequently used in palliative medicine.

Symptom management (Chapter 5 goes into more detail)—in addition to the pain management plan, the other clinical signs should also be taken into consideration. Clinical signs that are common are nausea, skin management, Upper respiratory infections, vomiting, diarrhea, oozing masses, bleeding from nose, gastrointestinal, lungs, spleen, liver, dyspnea, anorexia, and constipation. Less commonly and depending on the disease we see seizures (brain tumors, stroke, liver disease), pathologic fractures (occasionally with osteosarcoma, or bone metastasis), urinary tract infections, pneumonia, or more commonly with cancer, and heart failure, pulmonary edema or pleural effusion. An example for a specific disease, chronic renal failure, the client should watch for oral ulcers, urinary tract infections, weakness, and lack of appetite, in addition to anemia, weight loss and vomiting.

As different diseases have different comorbidities, personalizing the plan and changing it as different clinical signs arise is an important aspect of palliative medicine.

Prescribing medication in the home setting

Clincal veterinarians provide a pharmacy for their patients. Carrying pharmaceuticals are advantagous for the following reasons; 1. They can be a source of income for the veterinary clinic, 2. To have control over the medications prescribed. Making sure theclient gets what the doctor wants to prescribe and in the correct dose. The drawbacks for the house call veterinarian can be; 1. You have to carry inventory. 2. You need a variety of dose sizes and different medications, which for a startup business, can be a big outlay of money with possible waste from lack of use.

The house call vet is going to have to decide if they want to carry medications or just prescribe out to local pharmacies and if they are, what medications to carry. In this section, we will discuss the pros and cons of carrying medication inventory, versus other options to get medications to your patients.

- Carry with you—if you carry medications with you, you will have to stock an inventory and have a place to store medications. You will also need a place to store in your car.

Pros of carrying an inventory of medications—The veterinarian has medications readily available for clients. It helps the veterinarian the clients are getting the proper medications and at the dosing that you prescribe. Adds to your income (this may be nominal, compared to a brick and mortar).

Cons of carrying an inventory of medications—having to stock and keep inventory can take up space in your office/home. The veterinarian may have to carry with you in the car. Refills can be difficult and additional trips to client's house, which takes time out of the day (if you have a team, this could be one of their tasks, however, it would involve driving, and subsequently need insurance for their vehicle). Storage can be difficult (climate controlled and for controlled substances, need a safe bolted down). It opens you up to medication seekers (not common but do need to be aware).

- Local human pharmacy—can utilize local human pharmacies to provide many medications off-label. Some pharmacies do carry some veterinary preparations. Check with your local pharmacies.

> Pros of prescribing to a local pharmacy—often, it is cheaper for clients. Can be easy to call in or write or fax a prescription. You can utilize for some controlled substances.
>
> Cons of prescribing to a local pharmacy—problems can arise in the dispensation of medications. Pharmacies can be difficult to deal with and can have difficulty in understanding the human dosing versus animal dosing, and many do not carry veterinary-only products. Some pharmacies require an NPI number (it is a physicians database and veterinarians are not allowed to use it) or your DEA number (it is illegal for them to ask for this number for identification purposes. unless you are calling/faxing or sending in a controlled substance- and you can report them to the pharmacy board if they refuse to fill if you do not give them a DEA number). You can give them your office/business phone number and your state license number and that should be enough, check with your state pharmacy board for your state's legal regulations.

- Compounding pharmacies—compounding pharmacies are very useful to make up medications that you cannot find in human or animal preparations or that needs to be given in an unusual way that you are not able to find on the pharmaceutical shelf.

> Pros of compounding pharmacies—you can have many meds made up for cats and small dogs in high dose concentrations that can be given orally but in tiny volumes (0.1 mL) or into transdermal gels, to prevent giving oral medications, which can be difficult for some patients. They can also be flavored, which helps patient compliance and lessens their stress.
>
> Cons of compounding pharmacies—not all compounding pharmacies are the same. An accredited compounding pharmacy is preferred (There have been some compounding pharmacies in the news that have not followed adequate sterilization and have killed animals). Get to know the compounding pharmacy. If there is a current branded or generic preparation medication, compounding pharmacies cannot compound the same dose medication

- Online pharmacies—some house call veterinarians will utilize online pharmacies to help their patients and caregivers obtain medications. These can be pharmacies that directly ship to clients, which may or may not work with the veterinarian directly. A few examples:
- Vet's First Choice
- Vet Source
- MWI

> Pros—sometimes less expensive for owners, veterinarians can set up an online pharmacy to sell medications from their website. If set up through your website, can generate some income for the practice.
>
> Cons—Mistakes are more commonly made by online pharmacies. There are many disreputable online pharmacies, the AVMA has an up-to-date list.

Planning for death and body care

There is a chapter in the book dedicated to this subject. Discussion regarding the death is important to discuss in the first meeting. Do the caregivers want euthanasia? What are the factors owners are considering in considering euthanasia? Would they prefer a palliated death? What would they prefer for body care? Cremation, burial, and other rituals. Do they want the animal to lie in state for a while after the death? How could they accomplish that? Do they want you to come later and pick up or do they want to make their own arrangements?

Discussing grief—There is a whole chapter on grief later in the book. Grief is a very important aspect of end-of-life care, and some studies on the psychology of grief should be part of the education of a palliative or hospice-trained veterinarian or any member of their team. The veterinarian and team members will also need to know their limits of knowledge and be able to refer to trained mental health professionals. The team will deal with grief from the moment you walk in the door till after the death of the animal. Becoming better acquainted with grief will help you acknowledge boundaries and help you provide better care for your client(s). You can obtain certification in Pet Loss and grief through the Association for Pet Loss and Bereavement (aplb.org) (APLB Staff, 2018a,b).

What to do in a crisis

Part of the initial plan should include, what to do in a crisis. Comfort or crisis or emergency kits should be prepared based on the situation, the disease process, and what is expected to occur with the disease. There should also be a plan for what to do if the palliative veterinarian is not readily available. Instructions on what medications to give if certain clinical signs arise, and where to go or who to call if you do not have 24/7 capability. Give the owner their closest emergency clinic and provide that number so if and when they are in crisis it is easily accessible. If you are going to be out of town, give other house call veterinarians phone numbers that the client can contact to provide some continuum of care for the client and the patient. It is preferable if the animal does not have to leave the home a moment of crisis.

Wrapping up the consultation

Payment—obtaining payment can happen at the beginning or at the end of the consultation. If you have a flat fee, getting all the paperwork out of the way at the beginning can be useful, if you charge by the hour, then it will need to be at the end of the appointment. Have point of sale software for your phone or tablet and the ability to take credit cards. Online schedulers can be set up to do point of sale collection or integrate with your accounting and credit card software.

Financing options—house call veterinarians must decide whether they are going to take cash, check, or credit cards. Care Credit and Scratch Pay are two credit companies that can approve people for small short-term loans. They can be approved or declined over the phone or online.

Care Credit requires the vet to sign up, and it will take 5–7 business days and there is a fee for the veterinarian for signing up (check with Care Credit on service fees). There is an online sign-up available. They do run a credit check, and there is certification training. They do have promotional rates for people who pay off credit quickly and that can benefit someone who is not prepared for a large veterinary bill. The processing fees for each transaction, at the time of this writing (and subject to change) are 1.9%–14.9% (depending on various credit packages that Care Credit provides) (CareCredit, 2018).

Scratch Pay allows the vet to sign up for free, and there is no long-term contract.

There are no monthly fees for the veterinarian and no hardware involved (transactions are processed online), and there is a 5% processing fee for each transaction. Scratch Pay also donates 1% to animals in need (Scratch Financial, Inc., 2018).

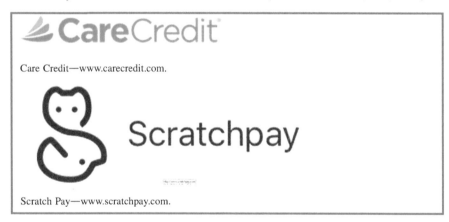

Care Credit—www.carecredit.com.

Scratch Pay—www.scratchpay.com.

There are also many different credit card companies available to process credit cards for a mobile/house call practice. Among them are Square, Cartwheel, QuickBooks mobile, Spark Pay, and PayPal Here. Many of them will sync with a mobile app for accounting that can decrease a paperwork step. Accounting apps may also have their own ability to take credit cards, saving the veterinarian time and step-in paperwork.

Accounting software—There are many different Accounting apps that work with phones or tablets. The top 10 cloud-based accounting tools are Intuit QuickBooks Online, FreshBooks, GoDaddy Bookkeeping, Zoho Books, Sage 50cloud, Kashoo, Xero, Wave, OneUp, and AccountEdge Pro (Yakal, 2018).

A quick google search can provide you with a more comprehensive list of accounting software. The ones that you can use on your phone or tablet are on the cloud and do keep information available to you wherever you go.

Making follow-up visits

Follow-up visits are at the discretion of the veterinarian. A suggested follow-up visit for stable palliative patients (those that are not close to death) is a monthly check-in, this may be done by phone, by email, or in-person, depending on the situation. For unstable palliative patients, at least weekly, and for degenerating patients, daily. If the patient is going to be supported to their death, the final days patient should be checked on at least once daily, if not more frequently. If you have a nurse or staff, they could check in on patients at these intervals.

Setting recheck appointments after the first consultation is helpful for many caregivers to feel they are being supported and gives you some feedback on how the treatments are working. The more often people check-in, the better it is for the caregiver and the animal.

One last thing …

Boundary setting—with the increase in suicides and burnout that happens in the field of veterinary medicine, boundary setting is so very important to veterinarians doing hospice and palliative care. It is very important to set up when you want to be available and be available for that time. This may be difficult when initially you do not want to give any new appointments away (and it is ok to take what you can when you start). However, once your business becomes more stable, it is very important to define those boundaries. The IAAHPC hospice guidelines recommend being available 24/7 (Amir Shanan, 2013). However, if you are a one doctor practice, this is not psychologically or physically healthy and can lead to burnout.

To start the boundary setting, I recommend setting times that you are available. If you have an interdisciplinary team then you may be able to do 24/7, if you do not, it is important to let people know when you are available and what you are willing or able to provide for care. Have it on your website and social media and your phone message. It is important to have a plan for after the first consultation, so caregivers know what to do when you are not available, and what you can do when you are available and to be upfront about costs of contacting you. When you meet with palliative clients for the first time, have that information in writing.

Set a plan for when you are not available—when you are working on the plan for people, they need to know what to do if an emergency should arise. If you have an emergency clinic that you can work with, or you are in a large metropolitan area, give them the closest emergency hospital to them. Give them the name and number in a readily available place on your plan. Have a crisis kit and specific instructions available.

Calendar your life

Another way to set boundaries is to schedule your life as important as your appointments. Make a calendar and place all your appointments on it. Schedule all that you have in life on the same calendar, kid's events, personal time, scheduled appointments, time with family, and even time to eat if you need to. This can help to set boundaries and can help compartmentalize your time for you. If you have put something personal on your schedule, think about it as being in an appointment. You cannot schedule two appointments at the same time. You cannot be in two places at once. Honor your time away as much as your time working. Personal time is just as important as clinical time (reminder: clients do not know what you have scheduled, just that you are unavailable at that time). This can take some time to shift your thinking about free time. For type A folks, we may feel like we have to work all the time in order to not feel lazy. Remember though, no one goes to the death bed wishing they worked more. Take time to be with family and friends and enjoy that time.

Work as much or as little as you would like to, but when you are off, step away from your phone, your computer, and any way that people can contact you.

Conclusion

You just made it through your first consultation. Congratulations. It will get easier every time you do one. And the rest of the book goes into more detail on how to care for each of the aspects of this chapter. Rest well, rejuvenate, and let's go onward.

References

Amir Shanan, J. P. (2013). *Guidelines for recommended practices in animal hospice and palliative care.* Retrieved from IAAHPC.org https://www.iaahpc.org/resources-and-support/practice-guidelines.html.

APLB Staff. (2018a). *APLB online seminars.* Retrieved from APLB.org https://aplb.org/training-courses/counselor-training/.

APLB Staff. (2018b). *Welcome to the APLB.* Retrieved from APLB.org https://aplb.org/.

Bouchez, C. (2018). *10 signs of an ailing mind.* Retrieved from WebMD.com https://www.webmd.com/mental-health/features/10-signs-ailing-mind#1.

CareCredit, C. F. (August 10, 2018). *Phone interview. (L. Hendrix, interviewer).*

Cassell, E. (2014). Suffering and human dignity. In R. P. Green (Ed.), *Suffering and bioethics.* Oxford.

DEA Staff. (2018). *Section IV – Recordkeeping requirements.* Retrieved from DEA.gov https://www.deadiversion.usdoj.gov/pubs/manuals/pract/section4.htm.

Hilst, K. (2018). *Quality of life scale for pets.* Retrieved from Journeys Home Pet Euthanasia LLC https://journeyspet.com/quality-of-life-scale-pets/.

McVety, D. (2017). *Quality of life scoring tools.* Retrieved from Lap of Love.com https://www.lapoflove.com/Quality-of-Life/Quality-of-Life-Scoring-Tools.

Mellor, D. J. (2016). Updating animal welfare thinking: Moving beyond. *Animals, 20.*

PetMD Staff. (2018). *Acute respiratory distress syndrome in dogs*. Retrieved from Pet MD.com https://www.petmd.com/dog/conditions/respiratory/c_dg_acute_respiratory_distress_syndrome.

Plummer, S. (2011). *Conversations/5 wishes: Relationship of living and dying well*. Retrieved from Alliance for living and dying well http://www.allianceforlivinganddyingwell.org/conversations5wishes.html.

Scratch Financial, Inc. (2018). *For clinics-the friendly alternative for client financing*. Retrieved from ScratchPay.com https://scratchpay.com/clinics.

The GSF Prognostic Indicator Guidance. (October 2011). Retrieved from The Gold Standards Framework https://www.goldstandardsframework.org.uk/cd-content/uploads/files/General%20Files/Prognostic%20Indicator%20Guidance%20October%202011.pdf.

Villalobos, A. (February 1, 2008). *Quality of life scale*. Retrieved from Pawspice https://pawspice.com/q-of-l-care/new-page.html.

Yakal, K. (July 31, 2018). *The best small business accounting software of 2018*. Retrieved from PC mag.com https://www.pcmag.com/article2/0,2817,2458748,00.asp.

Palliative symptom and disease management

5

Lynn Hendrix, AA, BA, DVM, CHPV [1,2,3,4]**, Mina Weakley, BSc** [5,6]

[1]*Owner, Veterinarian, Beloved Pet Mobile Vet, Davis, CA, United States;* [2]*Former Board of Directors, IAAHPC, Chicago, IL, United States;* [3]*Consultant, Hospice, Palliative Medicine, End of Life, VIN, Davis, CA, United States;* [4]*President, Founder, World Veterinary Palliative Medicine Organization, Davis, CA, United States;* [5]*Office Manager, Beloved Pet Mobile Vet, Davis, CA, United States;* [6]*Veterinary Student, College of Veterinary Medicine, Western University of Health Sciences, Pomona, CA, United States*

Veterinary palliative medicine's focus is to improve the patient's comfort, improve quality of life, and provide support and education for the families during the end-of-life stages of their beloved pet and for bereavement postdeath. Veterinary palliative medicine emphasizes symptom and pain management of advanced, progressive chronic, and late-stage terminal disease. Every veterinarian provides care at the end of the animal's life. However, formal training in palliative medicine is not provided in the current veterinary training. As a result, veterinarians do the best they can given the training they have received, or they may incorporate aspects of the palliative care paradigm that are available for human patients. Formal palliative medicine training for veterinarians could expand upon their current skills and knowledge base. Until then, expanding upon what veterinarians currently practice, with particular attention on symptom management, is the focus of this chapter.

Veterinary palliative medicine includes creating a medical plan for clients with continued medical follow through until the death of the animal. Veterinary palliative care also revolves around providing additional support for the caregiver experiencing grief following the loss of their their companion animal. Beginning with the first appointment, an initial medical plan is the primary goal. In this appointment, the focus is to establish client expectations that the treatment plan will be dynamic and ever-changing as the animal progresses through their disease. There are many factors that are also important to identify in terms of creating a comprehensive plan not only for the patient, but for their caregiver as well.

Animal Hospice and Palliative Medicine for the House Call Veterinarian
https://doi.org/10.1016/B978-0-323-56798-5.00003-5

Starting the conversation with client understanding of disease, their goals of care, client expectations, then moving into the psychosocial & possible spiritual needs of the family, the conversation may also include discussion of the physical abilities and greater support team for the family of the patient. Tools are needed to evaluate and reassess the patient as the disease progresses. Using validated pain scales or validated quality of life scales are preferred tools to help clients assess their pets progression. Simple tools, such as a video or pictures send via phone once a week, can also help the veterinarian assess how the patient is progressing. Telemedicine may also be another way to assess patients visually and give the veterinarian an opportunity to discuss the progress and changes to the plan with the client.

An advanced directive is another tool to begin the discussion of individual care with the client or family. In human medicine, advanced directives are used to determine the goals of care for the individual, if they are not able to verbalize their needs at the time of crisis. Advanced directives are also a legal form to establish goals of care. There has been no veterinary-based advanced directive system developed to date. The author has developed her own advanced directive system to help families determine in advance, what their goals of care are for their animal, in addition to their preferences for how the end of life experience will look. Examples of considerations for an advanced directive may include: what the family would like for their pet to be able to do and establish goals of care, what they do not want to see their animal develop or have to go through, medical interventions they do or do not want, as well as DNR status. The authors have found that developing an advanced directive can be more specific and inclusive to the needs of the individual family than a quality-of-life scale. Quality of life scales focus on the patient, and doesn't often address the family needs, concerns, expectations. A veterinary advanced directive may also take into account the client's quality of life, as a human being, including both positive and negative issues that arise from caregiving.

Palliative medical management of late-stage veterinary patients may deviate from the standard of care in curative medicine. For example, higher doses of an NSAID may be needed to achieve a palliated state, as compared to doses used more routinely. Clients should be made aware of the current standard of care, the deviation from the standard dosing, and the potential side effects. In addition, knowing when to add medications, when to change the plan is not covered in this edition, as it can be very individualized to the situation with the patient, and the client(s). Adding medications or other treatments should occur as the disease progresses and discussed with the client/caregivers.

Crisis kits otherwise known as emergency kits, or comfort kits may be recommended for animals receiving palliative care, as another aspect of advanced planning. Crisis kits need to have specific medications and instructions for use medications in an emergency. Crisis kits can help to relieve the fears that the caregiver may have and as a result, can also help veterinarians set a boundary. If clients are empowered with a backup plan and some steps they can take on their own to help their companion animals feel better in case of a crisis, then veterinarians will not have to be available at every moment. This is a mutually beneficial situation, ultimately, since being on call 24 hours a day, 7 days a week is not sustainable for any solo veterinarian.

Anxiety

Anxiety can be a key concern for elderly dogs and cats, particularly in the night hours. However, while, veterinary medicine studies have focused on anxiety behaviors for younger animals, there has been little work in senior dogs or cats on anxiety or the relationship of anxiety to pain as of this writing (Mills, D. D.-B., 2020).

Separation anxiety is the primary target of studies on anxiety in veterinary patients. Evaluating and reviewing human studies and understanding the neuropathic cause of anxiety from a neural-molecular basis may help us better understand anxiety-driven behavior in late-stage/end-stage animals and design research studies on late-stage anxiety in animal models and how it may relate to chronic pain.

Humans with anxiety may have early childhood stressors that affect their neurologic growth. There may be changes in the life of a young animal that also creates changes in the brain that may predispose animals to anxiety. There are also links between chronic pain and anxiety in people. It has also been shown that chronic pain in human and veterinary patients may induce a stress response. The stress response then causes anxiety which, in turn, increases pain levels, forming a positive feedback loop. The work done in human medicine may help us to understand why animals who have chronic pain may also have anxiety, and why anxiety may increase chronic pain levels.

Etiology/DDX

The normal response to stressful stimuli in humans, the processing of stress begins in the prefrontal cortex and then is further processed through the hippocampus and cingulate gyrus, which will up or down regulate the response. If the hippocampus stimulates the pituitary/adrenal axis, it causes a release of cortisol and epinephrine to prepare the body for a fear response (Herman, 2016). However, individuals with anxiety abnormally process perceived threats in the hippocampus and cingulate gyrus, which stimulates the amygdala, and in turn, leads to a maladaptive response to stress (Koga, 2015). The release of cortisol and epinephrine are due to a stressor real or perceived which can cause hippocampal cell death and in turn, suppresses normal responses to stressors (Koga, 2015). These abnormal neural pathways may begin early in life, with early stressful experiences affecting these pathways and continuation of the stress can further develop the abnormal response. Anxiety syndrome, recognized in teenagers, may extend into adulthood, may also involve changes in the neurotransmitters norepinephrine, serotonin, dopamine, and Gamma-aminobutyric acid or GABA. These changes may either be due to genetics or epigenetic changes with the early childhood stressors (Martin, 2009). More recently it has been recognized that the anterior cingulate cortex appears to be the targeted area in the brain that may induce anxiety syndrome in people. This synaptic plasticity creates pathways that prime the anterior cingulate cortex to be more reactive to stress. Chronic pain can create a stress response and may affect the perception of pain. It is hypothesized that chronic pain may potentiate the Adenylyl Cyclase subtype 1 (AC1), N-Methyl-D-aspartic acid or NMDA receptors, and Adenosine MonoPhosphate-α or AMPα postsynaptic receptors, as shown by the graphic (Fig. 5.1).

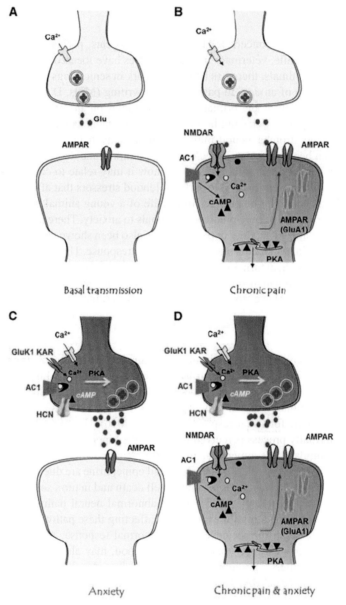

FIGURE 5.1

A hypothetical scheme for how synaptic plasticity may encode synergistic interactions between chronic pain and anxiety. (A) Basal transmission: the synaptic response, evoked by low-frequency stimulation, is due to glutamate activating α-amino-3-hydroxy-5-methyl-4-isoxazolepropionic acid receptor or AMPARs in the Anterior Cingulate Cortex or the ACC. (B) Chronic pain: peripheral nerve injury enhances excitatory synaptic

Researchers have found that acute pain did not produce the same effects with anxious patients as chronic pain did (Koga, 2015). Long-term potentiation and increased glutamate and NMDA receptors on the postsynaptic membrane and the increase of glutamate release from the presynaptic receptor may be significant for both anxiety and chronic pain (Koga, 2015). For animals that have had chronic pain for extended periods of time, may have developed an anxiety syndrome as can be seen in people with chronic pain, though more research is needed in veterinary medicine to evaluate this hypothesis.

Clinical signs

Human palliative medicine patients who have developed anxiety have developed it because of their physical symptom burden, including their difficulty in breathing, lack of mobility, nausea, or uncontrolled pain (Hofmann, 2017). Anxiety may also occur in humans because of grief-related stressors, for example, grief around the loss of abilities to do things they once did or losing their autonomy and because grief around the consideration of loss of their own life (Hofmann, 2017). In human palliative care, <10% of patients with anxiety-like behavior are clinically diagnosed with anxiety disorder (Bodtke, 2016).

For veterinary patients who don't have a history of anxiety, their new anxiety may also be associated with other clinical signs, such as pain and mobility issues, or cognitive dysfunction. It would be difficult to assess if veterinary patients are also grieving the loss of mobility or other clinical signs as a human would; however, chronic pain and the difficulty to breathe could certainly be stressors. The author hypothesizes based on the human research, that animals with chronic pain may develop anxiety, and that those who may already be predisposed to anxiety may behave more anxiously. Further research into how anxiety relates to changes in the brain of a dog or cat regarding genetics, epigenetics, structural neuroplasticity, and neurotransmitters may help veterinary patients with anxiety and chronic pain in the future.

◄───────────────────────────────────────

transmission through postsynaptic Long Term Potentiation or LTP. The activation of N-methyl-D-aspartate receptor or NMDARs leads to an increase in postsynaptic Ca^{2+} influx. The Ca^{2+} binds to calmodulin and leads to activation of Ca^{2+}-stimulated signaling pathways via Adenylyl Cyclase subtype 1 or AC1. The pathway leads to the enhancement of postsynaptic AMPARs containing the Glutamate A1 or GluA1 subunit and produces post-LTP. (C) Anxiety: normal anxiety enhances the release of glutamate, which feeds back onto presynaptic Glutamate K1 or GluK1 containing Kainate Receptor or KARs. The presynaptic Ca^{2+} influx via GluK1 KARs leads to activation of the Adenylyl Cyclase subtype 1-Protein Kinase A or AC1-PKA pathway, resulting in modulation of Hyperpolarization-activated cyclic nucleotide-gated or HCN channels, sometimes referred to as pacemaker channels, resulting in a long-lasting increase in glutamate release (pre-LTP). (D) Chronic pain and anxiety: nerve injuries and the associated anxiety activate both pre-LTP and postsynaptic LTP of excitatory transmission in the ACC. The synergistic interaction between pre-LTP and post-LTP underlies the heightened behavioral response.

Figure and legend from Koga et al., ©2015. Used with permission from Cell Press ©2021.

Behavior changes associated with anxiety/chronic pain

If new anxious behavior in a pet is noted by the client, a pain assessment may be appropriate. The author has observed the clinical signs in elderly pets that clients may describe as anxiety are often pain related. Anxiety behaviors may present as increased pacing or repetitive behaviors, especially at night. Panting heavily, barking abnormally, changes in body language, and avoidance behavior may all be signs of anxiety or dementia. However, those same signs can also be signs of chronic pain (Staff of Animal Surgical and Orthopedic Center, 2020).

Assessment of anxiety and chronic pain

Lincoln Canine Anxiety Scale (LCAS) is a validated separation anxiety assessment tool. It was developed for younger dogs with separation anxiety, and the researchers used fireworks anxiety as the basis of the scale. However, it is a tool to consider using as anxiety behaviors of other origins may behaviorly, manifest similarly to long term separation anxiety (Mills, D. M., 2020). Only one study has been published using the LCAS. There have been other studies that looked at pain and anxiety but not with the use of validated scales (Gruen, 2014; Nenadović, 2017). More research needs to be performed on chronic pain and how it relates to anxiety in companion animals. These tools, while not specific, may establish a baseline for developing more specific and validated tools that may contribute to our capabilities within palliative care for animals with chronic pain and/or anxiety.

Palliative management for anxiety

The current treatment for acute anxiety in both people and animals involves long-acting benzodiazepines. However, benzodiazepines may not address the primary issue which should be diagnosed and addressed and benzodiazepines should be used only in the short term, especially for cats (van Beusekom, 2015; Wright, 2020).

1. Alprazolam (Anxiety): Dogs—0.02—0.1 mg/kg PO prn for single dosing; q 4—6 h for repeated dosing. Cats—0.0125—0.25 mg/kg PO q 8 h; start at the lowest dose and titrate upward as needed.

To treat both anxiety and chronic neuropathic pain, adding onto the management protocol, an antidepressant, such as trazadone or amitriptyline, which may be beneficial to the animal. Additional therapies may be needed if antidepressants are not sufficient to manage clinical signs. Three antidepressents to consider include:

1. Trazadone for dogs—Give 2.5 mg/kg (max 150 mg) PO q 8—24 h for 3 d, then 5 mg/kg (max dose 300 mg) q 8—24 h as a maintenance dose (VIN Staff, 2017).
2. Amitriptyline: Dogs—1—4 mg/kg q 12—24 h, the higher doses treat chronic pain (3—4 mg/kg q 12 h) (VIN Staff, 2017).
3. Fluoxetine (Prozac): Dogs—1—2 mg/kg q 24 h, with behavior modification for anxiety and behavior changes. May be given with diazepam (VIN Staff, 2017). Cats—0.5—4 mg per **cat** q 24 h (VIN Staff, 2017).

Addjunctive therapy might include gabapentinoids. Gabapentin is also used in humans for anxiety, and it has been proposed for use in animals for both pain and anxiety (Bodtke, 2016).

1. Gabapentin—Dogs: 3—20 mg/kg PO 1—3 times per day. Cats: 3—10 mg/kg PO 1—3 times per day. (VIN Staff, 2017).
2. Pregabalin—Dogs (anticonvulsant dose): 2—4 mg/kg PO q 12 h. Cats: 1—2 mg/kg PO q 12 h (VIN Staff, 2017).

There is newer research into the NMDA antagonists being useful for anxiety/depression and chronic pain with humans (Gautam, 2020). It may be useful to consider NMDA antagonists for an animal with anxiety and chronic pain. More research is needed to assess the efficacy of NMDA antagonists and anxiety in animals.

1. Subanesthetic ketamine: (anecdotal dosing)—0.5—1 mg/kg Subcutaneous or SQ Pro Re Nata, which is Latin standing for "as the circumstance arises" or "as needed" or PRN can be given daily to monthly.
2. Amantadine: Dogs—3—5 mg/kg PO q 12—24 h. Cats—2—5 mg/kg PO q 24 h. Start with a low dose and increase as needed (VIN staff, 2017).
3. Memantine: 0.3—0.5 mg/kg PO q 12—24 h, start with a low dose and once daily, and go up as needed. Do not increase over 1 mg/kg (Scheidner, 2009).

Non-medical therapies to consider: For humans, changing the environment may also be helpful with anxiety. For example, utilizing music, decluttering, and exercise are ways to help ameliorate anxiety for people. For animals, we could consider utilizing music therapy, pheromone therapy, exercise, play, and environmental consistency (Bodtke, 2016).

Crisis kit for anxiety

The most common causes of crisis for newly diagnosed anxiety patient are pain and dyspnea (Mondino, 2021). For acute pain flare-ups, the crisis kit should include an opioid. Opioids may also help a dyspneic patient, so starting at a lower dose for pain might help both clinical signs. The crisis kit should also have a fast-acting benzodiazepine and gabapentin for genuine anxiety and an adjunct for pain. Acepromazine may be considered as an adjunct if the animal is becoming anxious at night and needs sleep, even though acepromazine does not help specifically with anxiety (Plumb, 2002).

Dosing information:

1. Acepromazine is not an anti-anxiety or pain management medication; however, it may help tranquilize an animal who is in crisis when used in conjunction with other anti-anxiety or pain management drugs. The author recommends utilizing a gabapentinoid or an opioid (or both) with acepromazine for this purpose. Dogs: 0.55—2.2 mg/kg PO, crushed-up tablets can help it work faster. Adding

the crushed tablets to a sticky sweet substance such as honey and rubbing on the gums can help apply medication, especially if the animal is anorexic. Another trick may be placing it in a gel cap because of the bitter taste. The injectable dose is 0.5–1 mg/kg SQ, IntraMuscular or IM. Although some clients may not want to give IM injections, Cats: 1.1–2.2 mg/kg PO, again crushed up tablets mixed with something sticky and applied on gums can help. The injectable dose is 0.05 mg/kg SQ, IM and it should not exceed 1 mg total per dose (written dosing in other texts). If considering euthanasia, higher doses may be used.

2. Gabapentin for crisis—Dogs: 20 mg/kg PO 1–3 times per day. Cats: 10 mg/kg PO 1–3 times per day (VIN Staff, 2017).
3. Alprazolam: Dogs—0.02–0.1 mg/kg PO prn for single dosing; q 4–6 h for repeated dosing. Cats—0.0125–0.25 mg/kg PO q 8 h; start at the lowest dose and titrate upward as needed (VIN Staff, 2017).
4. Opioids: For breathlessness and acute pain. Morphine, methadone, butorphanol—refer to the Pain Management chapter for more information.
5. Melatonin: Dogs—0.1 mg/kg PO q 8 h; Cats—0.01–1 mg/kg PO q 24 h (VIN Staff, 2017)

Ascites

Ascites is the pathologic accumulation of fluid in the peritoneal space. Ascites may be more common at end-of-life as a comorbidity with other late-stage diseases. If an animal develops ascites it is a poor prognostic indicator. Ascites may be difficult to manage at home as it progresses, however, there may be tools to help an animal with ascites live more comfortably. Ascites may also have comorbidities that may effect outcome.

Etiology/DDX of late-stage ascites

In dogs, the leading causes of ascites are right-sided heart failure, portal hypertension, hepatic neoplasia, splenic neoplasia, and carcinomatosis (Center, 2004). In cats, cancer, kidney and liver disease, pancreatitis, and right-sided heart failure, and Feline Infectious Peritonitis and trauma (not common at end of life), are causes of ascites (Cornell CVM Staff, 2020).

Dogs and cats may also develop ascites that is consistent with hemoperitoneum, bile peritonitis, or uroperitoneum.

Hemoperitoneum may be caused by hepatic neoplasia, splenic neoplasia, carcinomatosis, coagulopathies and hematomas of the spleen, liver.

Bile peritonitis and uroperitoneum may occur most commonly with trauma; however, bile peritonitis or uroperitoneum due to trauma is not commonly seen with terminally ill patients. Bile peritonitis for end-of-life veterinary patients may be due to cholangiohepatitis or extra-hepatic bile duct rupture. Uroperitoneum might occur in end-of-life patients due to a ruptured bladder from stones, or blockage of the urethra and/or ureters (Hunt, 2002). Transitional cell carcinoma may also lead to bladder rupture from erosive mural involvement (Hunt, 2002). These are more commonly seen at brick and mortar practices and are included here for completeness of the discussion with clients regarding differentials and disease trajectories for ascites.

Clinical signs

A distended abdomen may be the first clinical sign of ascites noticed by clients. Clients may believe the animal is just getting "fat" even though it is also often losing muscle mass, appearing thinner despite the larger abdomen. Differentials for a chronically distended abdomen may include Cushings disease, accumulation of fat, enlargement of organs, such as liver/spleen, neoplasia without ascites. Clients may also note a decreased appetite, difficulty breathing, or decreased exercise or lethargy. Ascites is often an end-stage clinical sign and a predictor of poor quality of life in people and animals (Goldstein, 2013).

Lab work will show ascites fluid to be a transudate or modified transudate. Transudate occurs when there are low proteins and increased hydrostatic pressure and reduced oncotic pressure (Rebar, 2009). Modified transudate is a fluid accumulation in the third space due to higher protein fluid and can indicate inflammation or lymph fluid or increased hydrostatic pressure. A quick lab check of ascites fluid looking for malignant cells might help you determine if a malignancy is present. Evaluating the fluid for an elevation in leukocytes, lactate, glucose level, and amylase can also help you determine malignancy (Glińska, 2007).

Malignant ascites also has an overproduction of vascular endothelial growth factor (VEGF) which increases vascular permeability (Hristov, 2019). VEGF also increases the number of small blood vessels going to the tumor. VEGF neutralizing antibodies or inhibitors may help decrease the amount of ascites produced with malignancy and have been used in women with ovarian cancer to decrease their ascites (Sangisetty, 2012). Matrix metalloproteinases may also contribute to increased vascular permeability and leakage of vessels and may be another target for treatment in the future (Ammouri, 2010).

Palliative management

The treatment of ascites may be challenging in the home setting. An abdominocentesis may be the most appropriate management of ascites for a number of other clinical signs; to help relieve pressure, decrease pain, and alleviate respiratory difficulties. However, it may be challenging to find a safe and aseptic place to perform an abdominocentesis in the home. A useful option may be a referral back to the animal's general practitioner for additional support. Pain management of comorbidites should be considered along with specific treatment for ascites.

Other medical options for ascites:

1. Furosemide (dogs and cats): 1–2 mg/kg PO, SC once to twice daily. Increasing the dose and frequency with the limiting factor of dehydration.
2. Spironolactone (dogs): 1–2 mg/kg PO (BID comes from the latin term "Bis In Die" or twice a day) BID; if no response in 4–5 days, double dose for an additional 4–5 days; if no response, may double again (4–8 mg/kg BID). The standard of care includes weighing your patients daily and not letting patients lose more than 0.25–0.5 kg/day nor allowing them to become dehydrated. Spironolactone (cats): if furosemide and ACE inhibitors do not control fluid accumulation: 1–2 mg/kg PO q12 h. If your cat patient has low serum potassium, you can supplement 1 mg/kg PO q12 h.
3. NSAIDs or steroids may also be helpful to decrease the inflammatory process for cats with FIP or neoplastia. Meloxicam can be given at 0.02–0.1 mg/kg q 24 h, and is to be used with caution in cats with chronic kidney disease (CKD). Carprofen 2–4 mg/kg PO BID for dogs or prednisone/prednisolone 0.5–1 mg/kg PO q12–24 h for cats or dogs are other alternatives to consider. Other steroids may be considered. When prescribing steroids, it is often helpful to start with higher doses and decrease to lower doses and frequency after 5–7 days for maintenance while minimizing side effects.
4. Sodium restriction is commonly used in human medicine for ascites from heart failure and may also help animals with heart failure. However, the author's clinical impression is that these animals may not be eating, especially in late-stage disease. Therefore, encouraging the animal to eat anything at all may be more beneficial than restricting sodium.
5. Indwelling peritoneal catheters to remove the ascites as it builds up may be a last resort palliative treatment for refractory ascites. However, these carry their own management challenges and potential side effects, such as infection and sepsis, should be discussed with the client and primary care veterinarian to determine the risk and benefit (Cooper, 2011).

There are newer treatments for people with malignant ascites. These newer therapies work on the blockade of Vascular Endothelial Growth Factor or VEGF, a monoclonal antibody that has decreased ascites in experimental animal models (Huang, 2000; Xu, 2000). Intraperitoneal immunotherapy interferon has helped women with ovarian cancer in stopping the development of ascites and should be further investigated in the animal model (Palaia, 2020). Matrix metalloproteinase inhibitors such as Batimastat may also be a consideration for some patients with refractive ascites (Sangisetty, 2012).

These may be useful for palliation of animals with malignant ascites; however, they may not be cost-effective for some clients at the time of this writing (Sangisetty, 2012). Treatment of ascites may be difficult and frustrating for both the client, pet and veterinarian, and a valid consideration for euthanasia in some situations.

Crisis kit

A crisis kit for ascites would focus on pain management and possible breathlessness. See those sections for further information. The best course of treatment for an abdomen with ascites causing pain or dyspnea would be to remove fluid via an abdominocentesis. This may be done as needed, timing defined by increasing respiratory rate and effort or chronic pain signs, as noted in other sections. However, treatment of the symptoms can certainly be initiated to help the animal feel better from a palliative perspective, until the fluid can be removed. Opioids would be the best medication to consider for the crisis kit, for both breathlessness and pain. Injectable lasix may be useful for heart failure patients.

The timing of a crisis may be a few days to several months in between each abdominocentesis. Given that ascites is a poor prognostic indicator, a discussion about euthanasia may be integrated into the discussion of the challenges of treating a patient with ascites.

Bleeding

Bleeding can develop in different areas of the body in a terminal patient, which may or may not be catastrophic. Bleeding can be a particular area of fear and concern for clients. For example, they may have been told, or read online, that their pet's spleen may rupture with hemangiosarcoma, and they will bleed to death. Or they may have witnessed a nosebleed or a bleeding dermal tumor. Planning can help alleviate fears and support clients in decision-making for their pets. A crisis kit is an essential part of the plan for an animal who may develop bleeding issues. This section is broken down to locations of bleed for easier look up.

Head and neck bleeding

Epistaxis

Etiology/DDX—Epistaxis most commonly occurs in an End Of Life or EOL patient due to the infiltration of blood vessels of the nasal passage by a tumor, infection, fungal or bacterial or trauma to the muzzle, or thrombocytopenia or coagulopathy (Bissett, 2007). Differentials include neoplasia with blood vessel invasion or a friable mass, bacterial or fungal infiltration, trauma, thrombocytopenia, nutritional deficiencies, medication, coagulation abnormality, and radiation therapy (Bissett, 2007).

Palliative management

Current treatment for epistaxis may include packing the nose (more commonly done in an emergency clinic), applying a drop or two of epinephrine topically, or providing other medications that cause vasoconstriction into the nose, such as Neo-synephrine®. Other treatments include raising the head above the heart with a pillow if possible, and using a cold compress on the muzzle, if practical. Packing materials to consider may include, gauze coated with petroleum jelly, a sponge made of hydroxylated polyvinyl acetate from Medtronic that swells with contact from fluid , or a packing agent with hydrocolloid coating from Arthrocare. For nasal drops, consider epinephrine or phenylephrine or diluted Cerenia to be included in crisis kits for animals that may be more likely to have acute episodes of external bleeding. Antifibrinolytics may also be used to achieve hemostasis. Fibrin-based intranasal drops or sprays may help provide hemostasis, and help with tissue healing. there are several available including, Tisseel (Baxter HealthCare Corp., Irvine, CA), Hemaseel (Haemacure, Sarasota, FL), Beriplast P (Aventis Behring, Marburg, Germany), Bolheal (Fujisawa, Pharmaceuticals Osaka, Japan) and Quixil (Omrix, Brussels, Belgium). (Both packing materials and fibrin based intranasal sprays are recommended by VIN consultant Dr Lester Mandelker with his permission).

Oral antifibrinolytics may be used to maintain stasis or prevent future bleeding. Commonly used antifibrinolytics in human medicine are tranexamic acid and aminocaproic acid. The Chinese herbal supplement. Yunnan Baiyao has been used widely in veterinary medicine as well.

Tranexamic acid inhibits the plasminogen on fibrin. It is a lysine-derived antifibrinolytic. An adverse reaction of tranexamic acid may be vomiting with IV administration (VIN staff, 2017). The dose in dogs is 10−25 mg/kg PO every 8−12 h (Osekavage, 2018). Nebulized tranexamic acid may also be beneficial to stop epistaxis. There is a human medicine case study that examined utilizing nebulized tranexamic acid and it showed benefits to it's use (Booth, D. Y., 2019). Additional studies are needed to assess the efficacy of nebulized tranexamic acid in companion animals.

Aminocaproic acid inhibits plasminogen and has antiinflammatory properties through interleukin inhibition. Like tranexamic acid, it is also a lysine-derived antifibrinolytic (VIN Staff, 2017). While generally well-tolerated in dogs, adverse reactions reported in humans are injection site reactions, malaise, seizures, renal failure, hypotension and bradycardia, and thrombosis (Kaseer, 2021). The dose is extrapolated from human medicine as there is no veterinary dose available and may not be accurate for animal patients. The human dosing is 100 mg/kg PO every 8 h for bleeding (VIN Staff, 2017). A study in dogs found that the dose of 100 mg/kg was more effective in clot formation than 20 mg/kg (Brown, J. C., 2016).

Yunnan Baiyao is a proprietary Chinese herbal blend formulated to stop bleeding with the proposed active ingredient of Notoginseng. Dosing—for dogs under 10 pounds, 1 capsule once daily, for dogs from 10 to 30 lbs. One capsule BID, dogs 30−60 lbs, 2two capsules BID, dogs over 60 lbs. Two capsules TID. Use the red pill in the center of the packet for an acute bleed (dosing is provided with the directions provided with Yunnan Baiyao) (Fig. 5.2).

This is a summary of studies looking at 40 years of research on the use of Yunnan Baiyao. Given that Yunnan can come in different blends depending on the manufacturer, and it is a secret proprietary blend of unknown herbs established by the Chinese government and there are adverse effects reported in people, it is difficult to ascertain the efficacy and the benefit of the use of Yunnan Baiyao (McKenzie, 2017). It has been reported that some blends have been found to have progesterone and other pharmaceuticals (McKenzie, 2017). Adverse drug reactions reported in people are urticaria, abdominal pain, vomiting, diarrhea, fever, nausea, rash, and anaphylaxis and should be monitored for with animals (Li, 2019; Whelan, 2021).

Study	N=	Rand	Blind	Control	Effect	Comments
Ogle, 1976[5]	54 (Rats) 10 (Rabbits)	N	N	Y	Y	YB reduced subjective bleeding time in cut rat livers and *in vitro* clotting time of rabbit blood more than saline or starch (applied topically or mixed w/blood)
Ogle, 1977[6]	? (Rats) ? (Rabbits)	N	N	Y	Y	YB reduced subjective bleeding time in cut rat livers and *in vitro* clotting time of rabbit blood more than starch solution (given by orogastric tube)
Graham, 2002[7]	6 (Ponies)	?	?	Y	Mixed	TBT-yes ACT-no 247 vs 318 seconds in TBT (oral use)
Epp, 2005[9]	5 (Horses)	Y	Y	Y	No	Many lab measures and clinical EIPH evaluated (oral use)
Fan, 2005[8]	17 (Rats)	Y	Y	Y	Y	Bleeding time cut tail tips 10.53-16.81 min wheat flour vs 7.1-14 13 min YB (topical use)
Murphy, 2017[27]	67 (Dogs)	N	N	Y	No	Retrospective, YB +/- aminocaproic acid with right atrial hemangiosarcoma, no difference in symptoms or survival (oral use)
Lee, 2017[10]	8 (Dogs)	Y	Y	Y	No	No change in lab measures of clotting (oral use)
Frederick, 2017[11]	8 (Dogs)	Y	Y	Y	No	No change in BMBT or lab measures of clotting (oral use)
MacRae, 2017[12]	6 (Dogs)	N	N	N	No	No effect on lab measures of clotting (oral use)
Adelman, 2017[13]	19 (Dogs)	Y	Y	Y	Mixed	Bleeding time after Bx (300+/- 12 sec YB: 367+/- 9 sec placebo) BMBT - no difference TEG (lab measure of clotting) - no difference Total blood loss - no difference
Ness, 2017[14]	12 (Horses)	Y	Y	Y	No	No effect on any *in vitro* measure of hemostasis

FIGURE 5.2

Chart review of Yunnan Baiyao Studies.

Created by Dr Brennan McKenzie© 2017. Used with permission from Dr. Brennan McKenzie ©2021.

Oral bleeding

Etiology/DDX—There may be many different etiologies of oral bleeding in the end-of-life patient. Differentials for late-stage patients can include oral neoplasia, tooth root abscess, gingivitis, coagulopathies, tooth loss or broken tooth, and stomatitis.

Palliative management—consider oral or topical tranexamic acid, "magic mouthwash,"—which can be made by compounding pharmacies into many different formulations based on your patient's need. "Magic Mouthwash"—for people with oral mucositis (similar to stomatitis) contains equal parts oral viscous 2% lidocaine, Benadryl, and Maalox. However, different formulations can be made containing some or none of the "common human formulation" can be made. Other substances such as, flavoring or sweeteners (ensure non-xylitol-containing flavoring or additives), or other medications such as sucralfate, antibiotics, an antifibrinolytic, steroids or other pain management, may also be added depending on the disease being treated. The authors recommend having a compounding pharmacy develop your "magic mouthwash recipe" based on the need of the animal and add flavoring, sweeteners in to make it more palatable for veterinary patients.

Bleeding dermal masses

Dermal masses may be challenging to treat, for both the client and house call veterinarian. Soft tissue sarcomas tend to grow slowly and may be locally invasive, and they may rupture and ooze or bleed. Mast cell tumors tend to grow more rapidly than soft tissue sarcomas, and may rupture, and bleed. Animals who have dermal masses may have had previous surgery or may have never seen a vet before with the current mass. The point when a dermal tumor bleeds or oozes, however, may be a point of consideration for euthanasia for a client. If the client elects to continue with treatment, there are treatments the veterinarian can employ to maintain the comfort of the animal.

Etiology/DDX

Mast cell tumor, mycosis fungoides (dermal lymphoma), dermal hemangiosarcoma, squamous cell sarcoma, soft tissue sarcomas, hygromas, pressure ulcers, and chronic open wounds/granulomas.

Palliative management

If there is active bleeding at the time of the appointment, consider using the following:

Tranexamic acid — Dogs: Current dosing in hospital: 10 mg/kg given by slow intravenous infusion (over 15−20 min). Subsequent doses: 10 mg/kg slow IV every 8 h for 24 h OR a continuous infusion of 10 mg/kg IV over 3−6 h; repeated every 8 h for up to 24 h (Staff of VetEducation, 2021). Recommended oral dosing at home: Dogs: 10−25 mg/kg PO q 8−12 h (Osekavage, 2018). Cats: In hospital dose: 10 mg/kg IV every 8 h (Girol, 2019).

Aminocaproic acid—Dogs: Although the dose is extrapolated from human medicine and may not be accurate for animal patients. 100 mg/kg PO every 8 h for bleeding may be considered (Brown J. C., 2016; VIN Staff, 2017).

Yunnan Baiyao—Dogs and Cats (anecdotal dosing): 12.5−25 mg/kg twice daily. Use the red pill in the center of the card for active acute bleed (Shmalberg, 2013).

Yunnan Baiyao is available in a topical aerosolized form. Apply a topical anesthetic to ease any local pain, and/or oral pain medication before applying topical antifibrinolytic. Opening the capsules and placing the herb directly on the tumor may also help, but it may be exacerbate pain. It may be useful to use oral viscous lidocaine mixed with an anticoagulant, though more research would be needed to evaluate the efficacy.

Consider using a topical dressing (if applicable, depending on location). Silver sulfadiazine, hydrogels, and hydrocolloidal preparations are topicals that may help moisten and heal the open area and a compression bandage if able to place (Campbell, 2006). Change dressings daily and monitor the wounds closely. Hygroma elbow covers may help decrease pressure on an elbow and help apply pressure on an open hygroma.

Palladia (Toceranib phosphate) can be used to treat mast cell tumors, melanoma, lymphoma, multiple myeloma, as well as many types of carcinomas and soft tissue sarcomas (VIN Staff, 2017). It has been shown to be effective in both dogs and cats (Berger, 2018; Yancey, 2010). Dose for Dogs: 2.5−2.75 mg/kg PO every 48 h. Cats: 2.7 mg/kg PO MWF. Use with caution and consult a oncologist when possible (VIN Staff, 2017).

With an active bleed or oozing mass, oral antibiotics should be considered to prevent secondary bacterial infections from developing.

Pain management should be taken into consideration with dermal bleeding masses. These are typically active ulcerations in the skin and should be treated as though the area is likely to be acutely or chronically painful. Additional considerations for pain management of dermal neoplasia or other dermal bleeding may include, size of mass, size of ulceration, inflammation, severity of pain, and progression of the disease associated with it. See the pain management chapter for options.

Palliative radiation may help shrink many types of dermal tumors and should be considered or discussed with clients as a first line palliative option (Bodtke, 2016). Palliative radiation has potential side effects and drawbacks such as time in the hospital, anesthesia, so that some clients may not wish to put their animal through this treatment. See the pain management section for further information on palliative radiation.

Bleeding internal organs
Etiology/DDX

Cardiac-—Hemangiosarcoma, chemodectoma, paraganglioma, and lymphoma (Treggiari, 2017).

Hepatic—Hemangiosarcoma, hemangioma, lymphoma, mast cell tumor, adenocarcinoma, cholangiocellular neoplasia, fibrosarcoma, metastasis from ovarian, uterine, mammary, renal carcinoma, and soft tissue sarcomas (Vilkovyskiy, 2020).

Renal—hemangiosarcoma, lymphoma, renal cell carcinoma, transitional cell carcinoma, anaplastic sarcoma, or carcinoma, nephroblastoma, and polycystic kidney disease (VSSO Staff, 2021a,b).

Splenic—Hemangiosarcoma, hemangioma, hematoma, nodular hyperplasia, lymphoma, and mast cell tumors (VSSO Staff, 2021a,b).

Gastrointestinal—Lymphoma, adenocarcinoma, leiomyosarcoma, gastrointestinal stromal tumors, plasmacytomas, adenomas, adenomatous polyps, carcinoids, GI ulceration due to bacteria, medication, hepatic failure, and hypoadrenocorticism (Willard, 2011).

Urinary bladder—Transitional cell carcinoma, kidney, bladder stones, crystals, FLUTD (though not as common an issue with EOL patients). (VSSO Staff, 2021a,b).

Palliative management

A general pain management plan should be considered for any internal bleeding tumor. Bleeding into a third space can create inflammation, which, in turn, may lead to pain. We may consider an antiinflammatory pain medication, such as an NSAID or steroid. But it is also important to consider that either of these medications may cause bleeding to worsen due to their inhibition of platelet aggregation and promotion of vascular fragility, respectively. Medications like gabapentin or opioids might be a more common choice to use when treating discomfort that is due to internal bleeding. Discussing options with the client regarding the possible side effects and the benefits of use is significant to any pain management plan. Neoplasia needs multimodal pain management. Consider using the WHO cancer pain ladder and evaluate mild, moderate, or severe pain to create a plan for multimodal pain management as indicated.

Targeted plans

Cardiac-based tumor—Drain pericardial sac as needed. The client needs to be prepared to drain frequently and it may be a point to consider euthanasia. Though surgical intervention is not necessarily considered a palliative treatment, it may allow both pet and caregiver some better-quality time together. Consider surgery for a surgical window placed into the pericardium and then place the animal on a antifibrinolytic medication. Treat for any existing heart failure. Treat for inflammation and neuropathic pain as well.

Hepatic bleeding—If early in the disease process or there is disease/neoplasia in a single lobe, consider palliative surgical removal of a liver lobe. If there is late-stage or multifocal disease, place the patient on pain management, and antifibrinolytics. Consider clotting issues that may occur with liver dysfunction. Patients may require vitamin K1, vasopressin, platelet, or plasma transfusions. Nutraceuticals that may be therapeutic to the liver may be considered. Doses for nutraceuticals: Dogs and cats can be placed on Silybin (a component of silymarin, which is found in Milk Thistle) 1.2—4 mg/kg/day in combination with SAM-e at 15—38 mg/kg/day PO. The dosing of silymarin is 20—50 mg/kg/day PO (VIN Staff, 2017). Denamarin is a combination of SAM-e and Silybin/silymarin. Monitor for coagulopathies and liver failure.

Renal bleeding—Treat kidney failure with appropriate fluid therapy. Additional medication may be needed for uremia, hyperphosphatemia, as well as electrolyte changes. Use antifibrinolytic therapy for bleeding. Pain management should include an antiinflammatory, and consider acetaminophen or paracetamol in dogs for early pain management. See pain management section for additional information.

Splenic bleeding—Remove spleen surgically if there is no obvious macroscopic metastasis. Surgery could still be considered palliative therapy as removal of the spleen will help with pain, even with metastasis if bleeding has occurred. This may also give the animal additional time before another bleeding episode. However, the client needs to be made aware of the possibility of any metastasic tumors bleeding subsequently. Monitor for hemorrhage and give antifibrinolytics daily. Pain management should be given as indicated. Animals with bleeding into the abdomen have pain and should be treated for pain.

Gastrointestinal bleeding—Upper GI—consider giving sucralfate, H2 blockers such as famotidine, or proton pump inhibitors such as omeprazole. Enrofloxacin may be considered in cases of potential gastric infection, postbleed for 7—10 days (Bodtke, 2016). In human medicine, the drug octreotide, a somatostatin analog, is used for the palliation of gastrointestinal bleeding. We may consider using this medication in the future if more research becomes available on it's use in dogs and cats). Lower GI- Used in humans with palliative care, adding in sucralfate paste or enema rectally along with other upper GI and coagulopathy treatements (Liao, Johnstone, & Rich, 2021).

Urinary bladder bleeding—If possible, surgery, chemotherapy, or radiation may be appropriate therapeutically. Treat for urinary tract infections as needed. Use an oral antifibrinolytic to help control bleeding. Pain management should be provided.

Hemoptysis

Patients with hemoptysis may have a history of a cough and may be tachypneic or dyspneic upon presentation (Bodtke, 2016).

Etiology/DDX

Hemoptysis is the expectoration of blood and may occur with lung cancer, bronchopneumonia, pulmonary thromboembolism, left-sided heart failure, pulmonary hypertension, coagulopathy, lung torsion, and heartworm disease in veterinary patients (Bailiff, 2002).

Palliative management

Nebulized tranexamic acid (human dosing—500 mg diluted in 5 mL saline solution 0.9% TID for 5 days) may help the bleeding from head and neck neoplasia, as well as pulmonary masses that may bleed (de Oliveira, 2020).

Oral tranexamic acid, aminocaproic acid, or Yunnan Baiyao may also be considered to minimize bleeding. See earlier section for dosing.

If bleeding is from one side of the lung field, placing the patient into a position where the bleeding lung is gravity-dependent may help with coughing or may slow bleeding. Veterinarians could also consider more invasive procedures (such as bronchial lavage with saline, epinephrine, or bronchial embolization, as used in human medicine); however, this is not practical for most of our house call patients (de Oliveira, 2020).

Disseminated intravascular coagulopathy and other coagulopathies

Disseminated intravascular coagulopathy (DIC) is an end-stage complication that may be an indicator that death is approaching. Disease processes in which DIC may more commonly occur include liver failure, pancreatic cancer, and hemangiosarcoma. Other neoplasia may also predispose animals to DIC. DIC may also be seen with sepsis, severe pancreatitis, and hepatic lipidosis as well (Couto, 2002; Venugopal, 2014).

Treatment for DIC can be complex. For treatment, patients require blood products, as well as case management in a critical care facility. DIC may be a point at which the client needs to be prepared for euthanasia and education of the client on options is recommended.

Crisis kit for bleeding

A crisis kit for bleeding should include one or more antifibrinolytics, and possibly Yunnan Baiyao, as well as supplemental oxygen. Epinephrine or phenylephrine may ameliorate epistaxi or bleeding from the mouth (ie: tooth loss or oral ulcer). Sucralfate may be helpful for oral, esophageal, and gastrointestinal bleeding. For gastrointestinal bleeding, famotidine may help reduce discomfort in a crisis. Rescue oxygen may be beneficial in the short term as well. Pawprint oxygen canisters (short term), oxygen concentrators, or compressed oxygen (for longer term) for a modified oxygen cage at home may be established in case of a nasal or pulmonary bleed. IV or SQ fluids or a blood transfusion may help stabilize a patient if the client is not prepared for euthanasia, though this would need to be done at a hospital, as blood transfusions are not typically offered in the home (aside from SQ fluids). Sedation and pain management should be utilized to minimize the distress of the patient (and subsequently mitigate the stress of the client/caregiver).

Dosing information:

Tranexamic acid—(for bleeding, epistaxis) inhibits the plasminogen on fibrin. It is a lysine-derived antifibrinolytic. The dose is 10—25 mg/kg PO every 8—12 h (Osekavage, 2018). It may cause vomiting if given IV (VIN Staff, 2017).

(For bleeding dermal masses) Dogs: Current dosing in hospital:10 mg/kg given by slow intravenous infusion (over 15—20 min). Subsequent doses: 10 mg/kg slow IV every 8 h for 24 h OR a continuous infusion of 10 mg/kg IV over 3—6 h; repeated every 8 h for up to 24 h (Staff of VetEducation, 2021). Recommended oral dosing at home 10—25 mg/kg PO q 8—12 h (Osekavage, 2018). Cats: In hospital dose: 10 mg/kg IV every 8 h.

Epinephrine—1—2 drops in the affected nostril to treat epistaxis (anecdotal).

Neosynephrine—1—2 drops in the affected nostril for epistaxis (anecdotal).

Sucralfate—Dogs: 0.5—1-g P.O. 2—4 times per day; for patients with severe gastrointestinal blood loss, give an initial loading dose of 3—6 g and then resume lower dose. If also using an H2 blocker, administer sucralfate 2 h before or 1 h after other medications.

Cats: 0.25—0.5 g PO q8-12 h (VIN Staff, 2017).

Omeprazole—Dogs: 0.5—1 mg/kg PO once daily, for dogs >20 kg do not exceed 20 mg/dog, for dogs <20 kg do not exceed 10 mg/dog PO once daily. For severe ulceration unresponsive to H_2 blockers and severe esophagitis unresponsive to metoclopramide.

Cats: 0.7 mg/kg PO q 24 h.

Famotidine 0.5—1 mg/kg PO q 12—24 h.

Yunnan Baiyao—Dogs and cats (anecdotal dosing): 12.5—25 mg/kg twice daily. Administer the red pill in the center of the card for active acute bleeding (Shmalberg, 2013).

Oxygen supplementation— It is possible to utilize an oxygen concentrator and cage or mask in the home. Pawprint Oxygen may be used as well. These are small canisters of oxygen that may be utilized for a brief time (5—20 min is reported depending on the flow used.)

Breathlessness

Breathlessness for people is defined as the feeling that one cannot breathe, catch a breath. It is a perception of having a hard time breathing, regardless of cause. Dyspnea, or having difficulty breathing can contribute to the feeling of breathlessness, as can anemia, tachypnea, weakness. Breathlessness can be a primary cause of anxiety for people with end-stage disease. Breathlessness may contribute to anxiety-like behavior in animals when they lie down to sleep. Soft tissues begin to relax, which may contribute to difficulty breathing, which in turn, may cause restless nights. Breathlessness may also be seen with anemia or with exercise intolerance due to heart or pulmonary disease. Breathlessness may be classified in terms of the cause such as dyspnea, hyperpnea, tachypnea, or increased effort in breathing due to weakness and anemia.

Etiology/DDX: The pathway for breathing is initiated in the brainstem via central and peripheral chemoreceptors and mechanoreceptors in the lung and chest wall. Chemoreceptors sense changes in pH, pCO_2, and pO_2. The mechanoreceptors sense changes in blood pressure in the carotid and aortic bodies. There are additional receptors in the trigeminal nerve in the nasopharynx that sense cold and airflow. The airways and the lung parenchyma have *c* nerve fibers that sense changes in the wall tension, irritants, chemicals, embolisms, and infections. There are feedback loops seen in the algorithm (Fig. 5.3) (Booth, S. J., 2019).

Breathlessness may occur when the brain processes both afferent and efferent nerve signals, or there is a V/Q mismatch. The perception of breathlessness occurs in several areas in the brain including the association cortex, limbic system, insular cortex, anterior cingulate, amygdala, and cerebellum. Some common diseases that can cause breathlessness at the end of life include lung tumors, congestive heart failure, pleural and pericardial effusion, pleural carcinomatosis, and pneumonia. Additional causes may be anemia, pulmonary thromboembolism, cachexia (causing weakness of the diaphragm and intercostal muscles), asthma and ascites or other space occupying abdominal mass.

Assessment of breathlessness

The initial assessment for the palliation of breathlessness may include the primary diagnosis from the referring veterinarian, current medications, and the effects breathlessness has on daily living for both pet and caregiver. When obtaining the history, evaluate additional potential triggering factors, such as cigarette or marijuana smoke, or other particulate matter or allergens in the home.

Tools for the client to help with assessment

Tools that may help assess breathlessness in the home, such as pulse oximeter, can help a client monitor O_2 saturation. Phone apps may also be useful in monitoring resting respiratory rate and effort. Cardalis is one phone app that is easy to use and is available on both Apple and Android and other operating systems. Cardalis

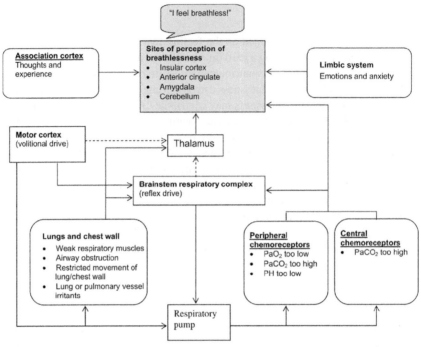

FIGURE 5.3

Central control of breathlessness.

From the European Journal of Oncology Nursing. Used with Permission from Elsevier Thomas, S. B. (2011). Breathlessness in cancer patients — implications, management and challenges. European Journal of Oncology Nursing, 459–469.

can graph the respiratory rate measured by the client and can be sent to the veterinarian to monitor the respiratory rate over time. A pulse oximeter could be rented to a client and the respiratory monitoring app can help both the client and the veterinarian monitor the pet. A technician or veterinarian can teach the client how to use both appropriately. The figure below shows an algorithm for the care of breathlessness (Fig. 5.4).

General symptoms that may occur with breathlessness
Etiology/DDX

Bronchorrhea is an excessive pulmonary fluid with mucus that can occur with primary lung cancer or metastasis, chronic bronchitis, COPD, and heart failure. Typically, associated with a cough that brings up the excess fluid, and fluid may be blood-tinged or clear. Bronchorrhea differential list can also include asthma,

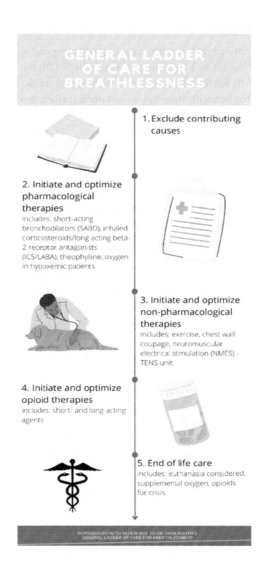

GENERAL LADDER OF CARE FOR BREATHLESSNESS

1. Exclude contributing causes

2. Initiate and optimize pharmacological therapies
includes: short-acting bronchodilators (SABD), inhaled corticosteroids/long-acting beta-2 receptor antagonists (ICS/LABA), theophylline, oxygen in hypoxemic patients

3. Initiate and optimize non-pharmacological therapies
includes: exercise, chest wall coupage, neuromuscular electrical stimulation (NMES) - TENS unit

4. Initiate and optimize opioid therapies
includes: short- and long-acting agents

5. End of life care
includes: euthanasia considered, supplemental oxygen, opioids for crisis

REPRODUCED WITH REFERENCE TO DR. SARA BOOTH'S GENERAL LADDER OF CARE FOR BREATHLESSNESS

FIGURE 5.4

General ladder of care for breathlessness.

Created on Canva by Mina Weakley © 2021. Booth, S. J. (2019). Improving the quality of life of people with advanced respiratory disease and severe breathlessness. Breathe, *198–215.*

organophosphate poisoning, and scorpion stings though these are less likely to be seen by a palliative or hospice veterinarian.

The workup for a bronchorrhea diagnosis may include thoracic radiographs, bloodwork, bronchoalveolar lavage, or transtracheal wash.

Palliative management

Palliative management of bronchorrhea may include atropine, nebulized corticosteroids, or nebulized NSAID and antibiotics if needed (de Oliveira, 2020). Octreotide and Epidermal Growth Factor Receptor (EGFR) targeted medications are also used in human medicine for bronchorrhea but would need further investigation regarding the efficacy in animals (Marks, 2017).

Cough

A chronic cough may significantly impact the animal's quality of life. The coughing dog or cat may also pointedly impact the client's quality of life, which may provoke a premature euthanasia decision. Treating coughing in animals can help both the client and the pet and strengthen their bond.

Etiology/DDX

Differentials for animals with a cough toward the end of life include pulmonary edema (cardiogenic or noncardiogenic), canine chronic bronchitis, allergic bronchitis, bacterial bronchitis or pneumonia, aspiration pneumonia, and severe fungal pneumonia (Hawkins, 2021). Collapsing trachea or laryngeal paralysis may also elicit a cough in patients with later-stage disease. For patients with tracheal collapse, surgery and intraluminal stenting may be a possible treatment. Surgery is also an option for laryngeal paralysis. For clients who may not want surgery, palliative medical treatments may help.

Palliative management

Pulmonary edema may be treated with diuretics, furosemide, spironolactone, or hydrochlorothiazide (Rozanski, 2009). Diuretics should not be used if pneumonia is suspected.

1. Furosemide, dogs: dosage ranges from 1.1 mg/kg PO every other day to 4.4 mg/kg PO q8h when animal in severe heart failure. In cats: dosage ranges from 1.1 mg/kg PO every 2–3 days to 2.2 mg/kg q8-12 h. Cats that are difficult to treat orally can be given doses up to 6.6 mg/kg q12 h or 15.4 mg/kg PO once daily (Grobman, 2016a,b).
2. Spironolactone, dogs, and cats: use when furosemide and ACE inhibitors do not control fluid accumulation: 1–2 mg/kg q12 h PO. Specifically for cats: can provide 1 mg/kg q12 h PO when serum potassium is low (VIN staff, 2017).
3. Hydrochlorothiazide: use in both dogs and cats in combination with furosemide, utilize when patients become refractory to furosemide alone. Dogs: 2–4 mg/kg PO q12 h. Cats: 1–2 mg/kg PO q12 h (VIN staff, 2017).

Palliating a cough with low doses of opioids can help with the feeling of breathlessness. However, if there is significant fluid production, indicating pulmonary edema, or bronchorrhea, opioids may make the animal dyspneic, so use with caution.

Opioids that may be used for a coughing dog are butorphanol, codeine, and hydrocodone; for cats, buprenorphine may also be beneficial.

1. Butorphanol: 0.05—1 mg/g PO q6-12 h with the goal to suppress coughing without causing excess sedation, up to 0.5—1.2 mg/kg PO twice to 4 times per day.
2. Codeine: 1—2 mg/kg PO q6-12 h
3. Hydrocodone: 0.22 mg/kg PO q6-12 h with the goal to suppress coughing without causing excess sedation.
4. Buprenorphine: for cats, start lower, for dogs double the cat dose 0.01—0.05 mg/kg IM, IV, transmucosal administration.

If there is additional pain involved and you need to add to your multimodal pain plan, acetaminophen (or paracetamol) with codeine or hydrocodone could be utilized for both pain and to ameliorate coughing in a dogs. The acetaminophen dose for dogs is 10—15 mg/kg q 8—12 h PO, and the dosing should be based on the acetaminophen. Acetaminophen or paracetamol should never be used in cats due to low LD50 in cats.

Gabapentin has also been used in human medicine to treat chronic cough (de Oliveira, 2020; Ryan, 2012). Although it has not been studied specifically for cough suppression in animals, it may be useful for refractory coughing. It is hypothesized that there may be a central sensitization component to chronic coughing (Ryan, 2012).

Cerenia (Maropitant) It has been hypothesized cerenia could be considered as a treatment for cough due to amount of substance P receptors in the lung. There is one study that looked at the use of Cerenia in dogs with chronic bronchitis and found that it did not decrease the inflammation in the lungs. The authors of that study concluded that further review was the necessary regarding the antitussive properties of Cerenia (Grobman, 2016a,b). Dosing: Dogs 2 mg/kg PO q 24 h, Cats 1 mg/kg PO q 24 h.

For tracheal collapse, crisis medication may include opioids, or tranquilizers for patients if they are coughing or panicking. Tessalon Perles (benzonatate) can be given to help with a refractive cough. Tessalon Perles dosing is 100 mg PO per dog q 24 h and must be swallowed without chewing. Overdoses can lead to seizures, cardiac arrhythmias, and death (VIN Staff, 2017). There have been anecdotal reports of the use of Doxepin for laryngeal paralysis, however a small, double blinded study in Labrador retrievers was published in 2021, that showed no difference for cough or clinical signs due to laryngeal paralysis with the use of Doxepin (Rishniw, Sammarco, Glass, & Cerroni, 2021).

Dyspnea

Etiology: Dyspnea or difficulty breathing can have multiple etiologies. The common differentials for late and end stage patients include congestive heart failure, pneumonia, primary lung cancer, or metastasis, or secondarily by cachexia, intercostal muscle loss and weakness, distention of the abdomen with ascites, or anemia. Animals with tracheal collapse and laryngeal paralysis can also become dyspneic.

Palliative management: Opioids—It has been proposed that opioids change central perception, decrease anxiety around dyspnea, and may also affect the opioid receptors in the lung (Mahler, 2013). A meta-analysis of literature in human medicine found that opioids did not improve dyspnea in cancer patients. However, the feeling of breathlessness was improved, and the conclusion was that they still benefit some patients (Feliciano, 2021). Benzodiazapines have been used around anxiety and dyspnea however the evidence for use in dyspnea is weak in humans and may increase mortality with higher dosing (Finney, 2019).

Cold air or a fan may also help with dyspnea. It is preferable to have the fan directed on the dog or cat; however, they may get up and move away and so being in the same room as the fan may be helpful. It is the authors experience that if the fan is started on low first, and moved up as needed, it is better tolerated by the animal. It is hypothesized that the passive airflow helps to stimulate the sensory afferents of the trigeminal nerve (Baker Rogers, 2020). Cooling the house, especially at night may also be useful for breathless patients.

Pain: Many patients who experience breathlessness also have pain related to their illness. More than 50% of humans who have breathlessness also report pain (de Oliveira, 2020). Veterinary patients who are experiencing breathlessness may also be experiencing pain even though it may not be noticed by their caregiver as they may be focused on the breathless behavior. A plan for a breathless animal may include a multimodal pain plan.

Specific diseases that may cause breathlessness in end-of-life patients

Congestive heart failure (CHF): There are several different etiologies to heart disease in dogs and cats. End-stage heart disease will have similar concerns regardless of the pathophysiology, and therefore the author will not discuss the specifics prior to late-stage disease.

End-stage heart failure in humans is defined end-stage when it becomes refractory to standard treatments. Patients with heart failure may be referred to palliative care early, when they begin to have clinical signs, before they become fatigued, dyspneic, or develop peripheral edema. Early palliative care may improve overall outcome, and can help support the family as well as the patient (Sood, Dobbie, & Wilson Tang, 2018).

End-stage heart failure human patients report generalized pain (Johnson, 2007). People may be referred to the emergency room, hospital or a hospice when they are considered end-stage. They may also be referred for hospitalization or to hospice with the history of supraventricular or ventricular arrhythmias, unexplained syncope, and stroke (Al-Khatib, 2018). Chronic Kidney disease or CKD can be present with Congestive Heart Failure or CHF and monitoring for clinical signs of CKD with CHF is appropriate. CKD can make palliation of heart failure more complex.

The psychological effects of heart failure for people may include fear and uncertainty because of the disease's waxing and waning nature. This may be the case for animals, further studies are warranted. These patients often visit the hospital unless they have clear instructions or a palliative or hospice plan in place and an advanced directive for discontinuing any further intervention.

For congestive heart failure patients sudden death may occur because of a fatal arrhythmia or thrombus. If sudden death does not occur, death may occur due to hypoperfusion of organs leading to multiorgan failure or pulmonary edema leading to dyspnea and hypoxia, which may also include pleural effusion that decreases the capacity of the lung and leads to further hypoxia which leads to death.

For veterinary patients, like human patients, curative medicine treatments, such as pacemakers and inotropes, diuretics, ACE Inhibitors, and β-blockers, are appropriate care. Starting palliative care early may also be helpful (Sood, Dobbie, & Wilson Tang, 2018). Nonmedical treatments for CHF that may be useful in veterinary palliative medicine may include fans, salt-restricted food, fluid restriction (sometimes), raising head or limbs above the heart with pillows or tilted beds, and supplemental oxygen. Oxygen concentrators can be afairly inexpensive way to get increased oxygen levels to an animal. Home providers could consider renting to clients, or they may find other means of rental online. Oxygen chambers or nasal cannulas for larger patients can be implemented to help accomodate the increased day-to-day oxygen needs of the late stage patient. NSAIDs are not utilized for pain in humans due to interactions with ACE inhibitors; however, discussing the benefits and costs with clients can help them decide whether to utilize NSAIDs for comorbidities with an end-of-life veterinary patient.

Depression is a significant sequalae in humans with CHF, and the use of antidepressants, SSRIs, are used to help with pain and depression. Progressive mental withdrawal is common in humans with end-stage heart disease, and with time, recumbency, and then the need for recumbent care becomes significant. In one study, people in congestive heart failure reported severe pain and dyspnea near death (Levenson, 2000). For veterinary patients, it is more difficult to assess depression; however, withdrawal from the family, and sleeping more may occur and be earlier signs clients can watch for before breathlessness may take over the lives of the pet and their family. Withdrawal from the family and life may be a clinical sign caregivers want to watch for to make a euthanasia decision.

Clinical signs

People describe the feeling of breathlessness with congestive heart failure as working at breathing, and tightness of their chest. Clinical signs noted in animals that caregivers can monitor for in dogs and cats may include nostril flair, increased thoracic effort, abdominal effort, a resting respiratory rate that is increasing over time or is greater than 50–60 breaths per minute, or development of a cough. Nostril flare precedes open mouth breathing in cats. Open mouth breathing is an end-stage clinical sign with a cat in congestive heart failure.

Palliative management

Technology can help improve monitoring the patient's resting respiratory rate. A phone app called Cardalis is an easy tool to use and can help the client and veterinarian to keep track of the daily resting respiratory rate. There are also other apps that may be used for monitoring. Teaching the client to use the app is easy with a demonstration by a technician or veterinarian. The client can also use Cardalis to schedule medication times and send the veterinarian a graph of the resting respiratory rate they have measured. The client could also obtain a video of their pet's respiration effort to help the veterinarian evaluate any changes. Keeping a video diary can also help the client see changes as they occur and may help with the treatment plan.

Nebulized medications have been used with people in end-stage heart failure. Nebulized furosemide was compared to IV furosemide in people with congestive heart failure. The conclusion was that IV furosemide was more effective than nebulized furosemide; however, nebulized furosemide had less hemodynamic changes (Barzegari, 2021). Veterinarians could consider nebulizing furosemide to assist in anxiolysis from dyspnea in addition to doing injectable or oral treatments (Diehl, 2021). Late-stage congestive heart failure will likely need supplemental oxygen and opioids to help relieve the feeling of breathing harder by relaxing the airways and affecting the perception of breathlessness in the CNS. Smaller animals may be accommodated with an oxygen cage and an oxygen concentrator, or for larger animals, nasal cannulas can be placed, and extension tubing allows them a limited area to be able to move. Pawprint oxygen makes short-term canisters of oxygen that may be used in crisis. They also rent oxygen concentrators. The need for oxygen may also be a point in which the client may want to consider euthanasia.

Anxiety is also associated with breathlessness. Benzodiazepines may reduce anxiety in people with dyspnea but do not decrease dyspnea and may make it harder for the animal to breathe (Baker Rogers, 2020). Opioids may be a better choice for anxiety and breathlessness. Gabapentin is also used for anxiety, though it may make the animal weaker and make dyspnea worse.

Crisis kit

Concerns that may arise with heart failure patients in crisis are pain, breathlessness, night waking, restlessness, and nausea. The crisis kit should include medications for these concerns. If the animal is not on oxygen regularly, the crisis kit should also contain short-term oxygen, or an oxygen concentrator. Morphine/hydromorphone/butorphanol/methadone—see pain management for dosing. Consider using for breathlessness, increases in pain, night waking and restlessness.

Furosamide is a rescue drug, and a higher dose than what they may currently be on might help get the animal through the night, though it may cause dehydration. A check in appointment would be recommended the following day if the client had not opted for an emergency visit.

Cerenia might be a good option in a multimodal plan to help with cough and nausea for CHF patients.

End-stage pulmonary disease
Etiology/DDX

pulmonary diseases seen in late-stage breathless patients include lung cancer, pneumonia, COPD, restrictive diseases such as asthma, and other interstitial lung diseases (Sharp, 2011) (asthma is less commonly seen with end-stage patients as a primary disease; however, it may be a secondary issue or they may have developed pulmonary fibrosis or chronic bronchitis).

Human patients with late-stage breathlessness tend to be referred to palliative care for dyspnea, when they become unresponsive to bronchodilators, and have multiple infections or hospitalizations, hypoxia on room air, right-sided heart failure, progressive weight loss, and resting tachycardia (Zhou, 2015). Veterinary patients may come home from the hospital and be referred to a house call veterinarian for palliative care or euthanasia. Animals with pleural effusion or pulmonary edema may be refractive to treatment. If the client does not elect euthanasia at the time of the first home appointment, then making the animal comfortable is the goal of care for end-stage pulmonary disease. If the animal is not in distress at the time of the appointment, directing the conversation about specific signs to watch for can support the caregiver of a potential breathless patient. End stage pulmonary disease may be a point at which the client considers euthanasia.

Pulmonary neoplasia

Etiology/DDX: For veterinary patients the etiology of pulmonary neoplasia include: adenocarcinoma, squamous-cell carcinoma, bronchial gland carcinoma, and alveolar-cell carcinoma and metastasis from other neoplasia (Moulton, von Tscharner, & Schneider, 1981). For human lung cancer patients, the final clinical signs observed may include pleural effusion, pulmonary edema, bronchiolar obstruction, hemorrhage in the bronchioles and hemoptysis, fatigue, and pain (Farbicka, 2013). The final stages in companion animals is consistant with what is observed in people. Clinical signs that indicate lung cancer is progressing may encompass increasing breathlessness, decreasing appetite, increasing pain, dysphagia, change in voice, peripheral edema, or pulmonary edema, which are late-stage signs. Most frequent metastasis sites for lung cancer is to brain, bone, or liver (Keuhn, 2018). Death occurs because of respiratory failure from tumor burden, hemorrhage or pulmonary edema or infections, or organ failure from metastatic disease. Average life span for dogs with primary lung tumors is 2 months with metastatic disease, and 12 months with no obvious metastatic disease (Keuhn, 2018).

Palliative management

In addition to the general recommendations for breathlessness, steroids may help palliate animals with late-stage lung who are breathless. However, a recent study showed human patients with late-stage lung cancer had a shortened life span when steroids were used (Skribek, 2021). The client should be made aware of the benefits and the costs of utilizing steroids. Late-stage lung cancer patients may also need oxygen supplementation. Pain management may be started early, at the time of diagnosis. Late-stage pain and cough/breathlessness management should include adding in opioids and multimodal pain management for metastasis.

Crisis kit concerns that arise with pulmonary disease are the patient's sudden increase in pain, breathlessness, air hunger, dyspnea, restlessness, and night waking.

Opioids-late-stage disease, see pain management chapter for further dosing information.

Should have rescue oxygen for crisis and need longer term oxygen source if considering doing a palliated death with this disease.

If having an active bleed, place the bleeding lung-dependent side down (Bodtke, 2016).

COPD

COPD is a common ailment in end-stage pulmonary disease for humans. Risk factors for dogs may include chronic bronchitis and dogs who have been exposed to cigarette smoke (Rozanski, 2020). Progression in COPD is a worsening cough, increased wheezing, increased respiratory rate, increase in mucus production, fever, lethargy, and peripheral edema.

Long-term palliative management: A β-adrenergic agonist and muscarinic antagonists may reduce COPD symptoms in humans and could be considered for use in veterinary patients (Baker Rogers, 2020; Chapman, 2008). Steroids may also help decrease inflammation, as well as nebulized furosemide for COPD (Baker Rogers, 2020). Long-term oxygen can help palliate hypoxemic patients with breathlessness (Baker Rogers, 2020). Use of an oxygen concentrator at home with an oxygen cage or long lines of tubing can allow an animal to stay with their caregivers while maintaining their quality of life.

Bronchodilators may also be helpful in the treatment of COPD for dogs and cats and lower airway disease (Hoshino, 2009).

Treatment of a COPD related cough can include an opioid. Some common opioids used for cough include, oral hydrocodone, codeine (±acetaminophen), butorphanol, or buprenorphine TransMucosal (TM).

Monitoring their oxygen levels can be maintained with a rented or purchased by client, pulse oximeter.

Crisis kit for COPD: Concern for COPD patients may be sudden dyspnea, pain and distress from ruptured bulla and the development of a pneumothorax. Should include short-term oxygen source (if they are not already on oxygen), an opioid to be given by injection or transmucosally. See the pain chapter for opioid dosing. Inhaled/nebulized steroids and albuterol are rescue drugs that may lessen clinical distress signs.

Late-stage pneumonia

Late-stage pneumonia is not likely to be seen in the home setting except for euthanasia. Most late-stage pneumonia is going to be diagnosed in the emergency room or at a general practitioner's office. However, pneumonia may be a sequalae or comorbidity to the disease the veterinarian may be treating and if that occurs, these are some tips for care. Pneumonia may be a point the client considers for a euthanasia decision.

Having specific criteria for decision-making can help support clients who may be struggling with making decisions for their animal's disease. For example, respiratory distress may include a resting respiratory rate greater than 60 breaths per minute, or open mouth breathing for cats. Utilizing a validated QoL scale developed for people with respiratory issues may be considered until a scale is developed for animals and validated. The human respiratory quality of life scale can be found at https://www.semanticscholar.org/paper/Chronic-Respiratory-Disease-Questionnaire-Analysis-V alero-Moreno-Castillo-Corull%C3%B3n/c39d499369247c26a9ed3de28321446a93 bbff45.

Aggressive intervention may need to occur for pneumonia, such as being on a ventilator in a hospital. This may be a point where the client might consider euthanasia.

Clinical signs for the client to monitor—cough, fever, dyspnea, pain, tachypnea, and crackles. An increasing respiratory rate, effort, abdominal effort to breathe, nostril flare and open mouth breathing are all points that should be defined for the client for decision making.

Palliative management—mild pneumonia—antibiotics that would be appropriate for the disease, oxygen for a crisis, pain management to include opioids, NSAID.

Moderate-to-severe pneumonia patients—in addition to the mild treatment, the family needs to be prepared for more aggressive treatment such as a possible ventilator, needing an oxygen cage, and future hospitalization or consider euthanasia before respiratory distress becomes fulminant.

Crisis kits for pneumonia—should include a short-term or long-term oxygen source, opioids, and +/− acepromazine. The client needs to be prepared with clinical signs to monitor for and prepared for euthanasia if they are in the late stages of pneumonia. The clients should be educated on imminent death signs that may include gasping, agonal breathing, and that it may be extended. These may be considerations for euthanasia and euthanasia earlier in the disease would be appropriate for a pneumonia case that is progressing.

Cachexia and other muscle loss in the end-of-life patient

"They are just getting old, doc" is a common phrase clients might utter about weight or muscle loss in their pet. Clients often believe muscle and weight loss is a normal part of the aging process. However, muscle loss can be a significant sign of disease and may contribute to a declined or poor quality of life in aging animals. Muscle loss can cause weakness, changes in ability to maintain body temperature, increasing immobility and concern about falls and injury. Sarcopenia is defined as muscle atrophy and can occur in the elderly person or animal due to disuse, hormone, and cytokine changes, decreased protein intake and synthesis, and neurogenic disease (Freeman, 2012;Larsson, 2019). While veterinarians traditionally focus on an overall body condition score, adding a muscle condition score to the medical record for elderly patients may help identify muscle loss earlier that may occur. The figure below is the World Small Animal Veterinary Association Chart proposed in 2017 regarding muscle condition (Fig. 5.5).

Cachexia is defined as the unintended loss of body mass, both fat and muscle, due to complex changes associated with disease (Freeman, 2012). Sarcopenia occurs with cachexia. Late-stage cancer, heart disease, and renal failure are the most common later stage diseases in animals. Cachexia has also been observed with chronic respiratory diseases in animals (Freeman, 2012). In human medicine, cachexia has been shown to decrease the quality and quantity of life of a patient (Kasvis, 2019). The concern is that cachexia will also decrease the quality and quantity of life in the veterinary patient, and there is cause for concern. Cachexia may contribute to fatigue in cancer, heart failure and renal failure patients (Powers, 2016). Cachexia may also contribute to increased morbidity and mortality in the animal patient (Freeman, 2012).

Cachexia may also be a prognostication tool. Cachexia may indicate a poor prognosis for long-term survival, especially when it is late stage, or severe muscle wasting. However, clients may not notice the muscle loss in their pet until the later stages of disease and therefore it may be difficult to slow or reverse and contribute to a poor prognosis. A caregiver may believe a distended abdomen is their animal is gaining weight despite the increase in muscle wasting (Freeman, 2012). Cachexia may contribute to a euthanasia decision as the animal gets weak, so identifying it and slowing the progression early can improve quality of life. Palliating patients with later-stage cachexia may help the animal feel better and contribute to ability to move, though the goal is to slow the progression prior to later stages.

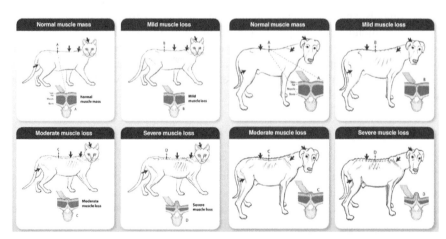

FIGURE 5.5

Cat and dog muscle condition.

Identifying factors involved in cachexia

Cachexia when studied in humans and mouse models shows a shift in mitochondrial function, increased collagen content, and changes in the muscle fiber from type I to type IIb using glycolic metabolism (Wang, 2013). When these changes occur these fibers are more likely to atrophy. Muscle atrophy may not become apparent until later-stage disease (Wang, 2013). In dogs and cats, the muscle groups that veterinarians should focus on are the epaxial, gluteal, scapular, or temporal muscles (Freeman, 2012). Depending on the disease, there may be an increase the energy requirements while decreasing appetite, change in the cellular metabolism, and decrease in the absorption of nutrients. The loss of lean body mass can also change the immune function and ability to heal, and the animal becomes weaker as they lose muscle (Freeman, 2012). For this text, we will focus on the differences of cachexia between cancer, congestive heart failure, and renal failure. The graphic is a proposed definition of Pre-Cachexia in people, which we will utilize for the purpose of this discussion (Fig. 5.6).

The proposed signs in humans for precachexia may assist veterinarians in determining early cachexia in veterinary patients. Instituting therapy in the precachexia stage may help slow the progression. The second figure is the proposed definition of cachexia for humans which may also be useful for veterinarians to adapt (Fig. 5.7).

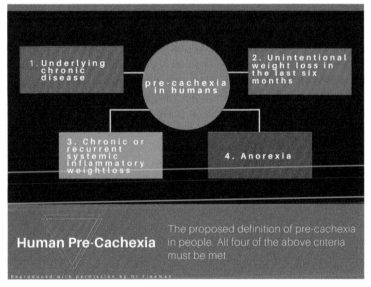

FIGURE 5.6

Used with permission and with attribution from Journal of Veterinary Internal Medicine, Dr. Lisa Freeman ©2012. Created on Canva by Lynn Hendrix and Mina Weakley ©2021. Cachexia and sarcopenia: Emerging syndromes of importance in dogs and cats. Journal of Veterinary Internal Medicine, *3–17.*

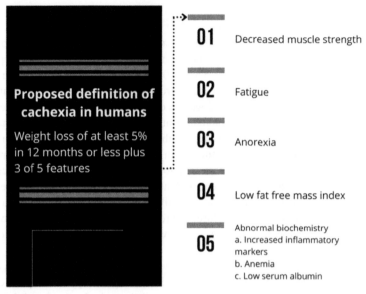

FIGURE 5.7

Proposed definition of cachexia in humans.

Reproduced from article by Dr. Lisa Freeman. ©2012 Created on Canva by Mina Weakley ©2021, Used with permission and with attribution by Freeman, L. M. (2012). Cachexia and sarcopenia: Emerging syndromes of importance in dogs and cats. Journal of Veterinary Internal Medicine, *3–17.*

If the animal meets the criteria for precachexia, then having the clients observe them for the clinical signs of cachexia may be crucial to monitoring the progression. The proposed definition of cachexia in humans may also be similar in animals (Freeman, 2012).

Cancer cachexia produces many cytokines however TNF-α, IL-6, IL-1β, and ILF-δ have been identified that contribute to anorexia or decreased food intake and further inflammation (Powers, 2016). These cytokines activate the ubiquitin-proteosome pathway that contributes to protein breakdown (Dev, 2017). The inflammatory processes also generated by these cytokines increase energy consumption that drives increases in cellular protein metabolism and decreased protein synthesis (Powers, 2016). Cancer cachexia subsequently has muscle and fat breakdown due to these changes (Dev, 2017).

Cardiac cachexia has different proposed mechanisms. There may be dysfunction of the autonomic nervous system, a systemic inflammatory response, deviations of the renin-angiotensin axis, and variations in the immune response (Lena, 2019). These changes can affect the skeletal and cardiac muscle and may also cause fibrosis of the heart (as seen in humans) whereas cachexia in cancer patients tends to decrease the muscle mass of cardiac muscle (Lena, 2019). There is an obesity paradox noted in people, while obesity is a risk factor for developing cardiac disease, it also "protects" patients with heart failure from cachexia. A similar obesity paradox phenomenon has been observed in dogs and cats (Freeman, 2012).

Kidney failure associated cachexia may occur with protein loss (Koppe, 2019). The four changes they all may have in common are an elevated metabolism, malabsorption of nutrients, hyporexia or anorexia, and biochemical changes in metabolism.

Elevated metabolism

While people living with congestive heart failure may have an elevated metabolism due to changes in respiration, sympathetic activation, and tachycardia, they also tend to have exercise intolerance so their elevated metabolism may be minimal in contributing to their cachexia (Lena, 2019). It is unclear as to the significance of this in dogs and cats, as some literature finds no difference in metabolism between healthy and unhealthy animals with cardiac disease.

With cancer patients, cytokines may increase metabolic needs in about 50% of human patients (Dev, 2017).

Malabsorption of nutrients

Cancer patients can have decreased bowel function from medications, autonomic changes, or paraneoplastic syndrome that may affect their ability to absorb nutrients. It has been documented that there are alterations in the metabolism of nutrients in dogs with cancer (Ogilvie, 1998). People with congestive heart failure may have decreased circulation to the bowel that may decrease the absorption (Lena, 2019). However, the etiology is unknown. This has not yet been established in animals.

Hyporexia or anorexia

Patients with neoplasia, congestive heart failure (CHF), and chronic kidney disease (CKD) may modify their food intake. Decreased food intake with CKD may be due to medications, increases in Blood Urea Nitrogen (BUN), fatigue, dyspnea, and pain (Freeman, 2012; Koppe, 2019). Cancer, CHF and CKD may also have alterations in both orexigenic and anorexigenic factors (Freeman, 2012).

Cancer patients may have hyporexia or anorexia due to medications affecting the gastrointestinal tract, functional change to the bowel from cancer, paraneoplastic syndrome or other proinflammatory cytokines, and changes in neuropeptide Y/agouti-related peptide and the regulatory hormones. The decrease in the regulatory hormones was hypothesized to contribute to cachexia so that ghrelin agonists might be helpful in improving cancer cachexia (Johannes, 2021). In a cochrane review, ghrelin agonists had no statistical difference in increasing appetite or improving cachexia for cancer patients (Al-Khatib, 2018).

For human cardiac patients, ghrelin has been shown to be increased; however, the satiety factors are also increased suggesting that there is a dysregulation in hunger hormones (Freeman, 2012; Lena, 2019). Research in human patients with congestive heart failure has shown improvement in cachexia using ghrelin agonists (Lena, 2019). Treating with ghrelin agonist (Entyce® or capromorelin) may help stimulate appetite but also help may help slow the progression of cachexia by stimulating growth hormone and IGF-1 (Rhodes, 2017).

There is a rat model of long-term critical illness that shows that while ghrelin helps increase body mass and food intake, it did not increase muscle mass nor improve muscle function (Hill, 2017). Omega 3 fatty acids may also help maintain weight (Freeman, 2012). Ace inhibitors may also slow the progression of cachexia in cardiac patients (Freeman, 2012). More research needs to be done to see if this will be a valuable tool for end-of-life veterinary patients.

Biochemical changes in metabolism

Cancer, heart, and kidney failure all influence the development of cachexia due to changes related to each of their varied inflammatory processes. Patients with cancer have increases in proinflammatory cytokines, catecholamines, cortisol, insulin, and glucagon that contribute to inflammation and subsequently, cachexia. The tumor-induced proinflammatory cytokines identified in humans are TNF-α, IL-1β, IFN-γ, TGF-β, and IL-6 (Biswas, 2020). For patients with cardiac disease, the chief cytokines that are involved in cachexia are TNF, IL-1β, and IL-6 (Freeman, 2012). With cardiac cachexia, there are also changes in hematocrit, hemoglobin, and CD4+ and CD8+ lymphocytes (Freeman, 2012). Another significant pathway that may result in cachexia, identified in people, is the Ubiquitin-Proteasome pathway. Other biochemical contributors may include the renin—angiotensin—aldosterone system, epinephrine, and cortisol (Azhar, 2013). Additional studies with cats and dogs may help elicit how these pathways could be altered to improve patient care and slow the progression of cachexia.

Palliative management

Identifying and preparing for cachexia in the early stages of cancer, cardiac, and renal failure may help slow the progression of muscle loss (Penet, 2015). Evaluation of muscle scores, instead of an overall body condition score, and monitoring the muscle loss throughout the course of the disease can help evaluate the progression of cachexia. Having tools for the client to measure and monitor muscle loss and begin to adjust their needs accordingly. Nutritional supplementation may slow the progression; however, it will not reverse the course. Omega-3 fatty acids may help decrease the production of IL-1 and TNF. A nutrition evaluation by a board-certified veterinary nutritionist to create a better-balanced diet for the pet based on the disease and what may be palatable to increase the likelihood of continued proper intake. Increased protein and increased caloric density may be needed to slow the progression (Ali, 2014). Smaller portions given more frequently may help with decrease intake.

Adding a ghrelin agonist may help slow the progression with cardiac cachexia (Lena, 2019). More studies are needed to evaluate the efficacy of adding ghrelin agonists in companion animals to slow the muscle loss.

With humans, weight training, exercise, and physical therapy contribute to minimizing loss over time (Biswas, 2020). Exercise and rehabilitation may also help maintain muscle mass, and physical therapy techniques can help assist the animal in continuing to move along with pain management (Freeman, 2012).

Emerging treatments in human medicine for appetite loss with end-stage patients include IV vitamin C, infliximab, and other -mab(TNF antagonist) drugs. Cannabidiol or CBD has been found to be helpful with people in combination with THC to help with cachexia however like the other emerging treatments, the use of CBD with cachexia in companion animals would need further evaluation to asses the efficacy (Wrede-Seaman, 2019).

Crisis kit

A crisis kit for cachexia is not needed as this is a chronic, not a crisis disease. See sections on cancer, congestive heart failure, chronic kidney disease, pulmonary disease and mobility issues for additional information.

Carcinomatosis

Carcinomatosis may occur in the thoracic or peritoneal cavity. This finding has been associated with a poor prognosis in both cats and dogs.

Etiology/DDX

Carcinomatosis of the peritoneum in people has been shown to arise from various abdominal cancers, mammary, and lung cancer, malignant melanoma (Desai, 2021). Thoracic cavity carcinomatosis arises from lymphatic infiltration and are associated with cancers of the chest and may also be seen in colon and blood borne cancers (Ajith Kumar & Mantri, 2021).

Clinical signs

Peritoneal carcinomatosis may cause an inflammatory response that may cause distention of the abdomen from ascites, and can include nausea, and pain. Pleural effusion and dyspnea are the most common clinical sign of thoracic carcinomatosis (Lambert, 2018).

Carcinomatosis may also cause generalized or referred pain in humans. There is a mouse model that shows increased substance-P receptors in the dorsal root ganglion being expressed and a decrease in μ-opioid receptors being down-regulated in the same neurons (Suzuki, 2012). Pain may also occur from the pressure of ascites or pleural effusion (Suzuki, 2012). Other concerns with carcinomatosis may be dyspnea from the distended, fluid filled abdomen or plural effusion, bowel obstruction and constipation or diarrhea, nausea, lethargy, and cachexia (Suzuki, 2012).

Palliative management

Carcinomatosis is inflammatory, and an antiinflammatory should be included in a treatment plan.

1. Carprofen is 2–4 mg/kg PO q 12 h, and meloxicam is 0.1 mg/kg PO q 24 h. Other NSAIDs can be used as well.
2. Prednisone dose should start on the higher end and work down to the lowest possible dose for maintaining clinical signs with minimizing side effects. Recommended dosing is 0.5–1 mg/kg PO q 12–24 h.

Neuropathic pain (gabapentin or pregabalin) should also be a consideration on a treatment plan.

1. Gabapentin should be started at a low dose and increased over time and with need. Gabapentin dose for dogs or cats is 3–5 mg/kg PO q 12–24 h to start and can move up to 10–20 mg/kg PO q 8–12 h or higher PRN.
2. Pregabalin: Dogs—2–4 mg/kg PO q 12 h, Cats 1–2 mg/kg PO q 12 h.

Substance P receptors are increased and the author recommends considering Cerenia (Maropitant), for visceral pain in addition to other pain adjuncts; though it should not be the sole treatment.

1. Cerenia dose is 2 mg/kg PO in dogs, 1 mg/kg PO in cats. Cerenia, ondansetron, or both should also be on a treatment plan for nausea.
2. Ondansetron dosing can be 0.5–1 mg/kg PO q 12–24 h PRN for nausea or vomiting.

In addition to pain management, treating constipation with a stool softener like lactulose or Miralax (Polyethylene glycol 3350) can help relieve discomfort.

Diarrhea may also occur secondarily to ascites in late-stage disease. See the ascites or diarrhea sections for additional management information.

Chronic kidney disease, end-stage
Etiology/DDX

Renal disease is one of the most common metabolic diseases that veterinarians treat, and CKD patients are cared for by veterinarians all around the world. Since veterinarians tend to be well versed in CKD, this chapter will focus on late, and end-stage CKD. Late-stage chronic kidney disease (LSCKD) may be of particular interest to the end-of-life house call veterinarian. The International Renal Interest Society or IRIS has developed a staging system to help veterinarians stage this insidious disease. Each of the stages evaluates a fasting serum Creatinine with at least two measurements, fasting symmetric dimethylarginine (SDMA), then substages based on proteinuria and blood pressure. Per the IRIS website, treatments are meant to slow the progression of the disease and improve quality of life but not reverse the course of the disease (Staff of IRIS, 2021).

Animals may be euthanized before LSCKD; however, if you have a patient who has moved into Stage 4 disease, evaluating additional palliative management for those patients may help improve their quality of life. People with LSCKD may have multiple symptoms that need additional treatment and monitoring.

There is a myth in medicine that CKD is an easy way to die. It is a myth because people have significant symptom load and palliative management to make the death "easier." According to one text, it is of utmost importance to begin palliation for CKD patients as early as possible to manage syptoms (Germain, 2011). The early clinical signs have been established by IRIS and will not be reviewed in this text. Late-stage disease for this book will be based in the additional therapies available for human patients with late-stage kidney disease.

Renal disease, late-stage clinical signs, and comorbidities

Chronic kidney disease will likely be treated by the general practitioner until the later stages of the disease. As the animal starts to progress to stages 3 and 4, clients may elect home support. As the clinical symptoms progress, the need for care progresses. Clinical signs that may be seen with later stage CKD:

1. Oral changes—halitosis, oral ulcers, stomatitis
2. Gastrointestinal signs—vomiting, nausea, anorexia, hyporexia
3. Systemic hypertension—monitoring the blood pressure in the home may help get a more accurate reading than in the clinic. Sequelae of hypertension can be retinopathy/choroidopathy, hemorrhage, hyphemia, secondary glaucoma, and blindness. Systemic hypertension may also cause a stroke or encephalopathy. Changes in behavior like disorientation, vestibular signs, or seizures may also occur. It may damage the heart, contributing to left ventricular hypertrophy, heart failure, and a rare aortic aneurysm/dissection (Acierno, 2018). People do report headaches with hypertension.
4. Proteinuria may be present and should be monitored.
5. Pain—nearly 60% of people with renal failure report pain, 50% of those reporting it to be moderate to severe pain (Yennurajalingam, 2016). The types of pain people report is classified as musculoskeletal, some cellulitis, neuropathic or a mixture of somatic and neuropathic (Yennurajalingam, 2016).
6. Fatigue, weakness—in addition to all the other clinical signs, people report fatigue and weakness. CKD dogs and cats can also develop lethargy and weakness due to sarcopenia, anorexia, and renal cachexia (Brown, C. E., 2016).
7. Neurological changes—seizures, sleep disturbances, altered taste, smell reported in people (but may contribute to lack of appetite in CKD patients?), and peripheral neuropathy have been reported in cats (Brown, C. E., 2016).
8. Musculoskeletal changes—bone pain from renal osteodystrophy is reported in people, muscle twitching, cramps reported in people, cachexia. Changes in potassium levels can cause a hypokalemic polymyopathy (Bartges, 2012).
9. Dermatological changes—while not well understood in people, dermatological changes and pruritus are hypothesized to be due to chronic inflammation and abnormalities in calcium and phosphate depositing or mast cells affected. Other hypotheses are alterations of nerves due to uremia (Yennurajalingam, 2016).
10. Hematological changes—later stage changes in bloodwork of note include hypercalcemia, anemia, hyperphosphatemia, hypokalemia, in addition to increases of BUN, creatinine, and SDMA (Brown, C. E., 2016).

Comorbidities of CKD may include diabetes mellitus, cardiac changes (in cats, hypertrophic cardiomyopathy), hypertension, pancreatitis, inflammatory bowel disease, hyperthyroidism, and osteoarthritis (Brown, C. E., 2016).

Palliative management

Slow the progression and improve quality of life

Fluid therapy, whether provided orally, SQ, or IV, is significant to the treatment of LSCKD. Fluid intake is a daily living requirement, and any fluid supplementation needs to be given daily unless the patient is imminently dying. Common clinical signs of overhydration are weight gain, peripheral edema, pulmonary edema, pleural effusion, and ascites. Supplemental oral fluids may be utilized if the client wants to be diligent in measuring and tracking both fluid intake and weight and the animal is willing to drink. If they don't, doing SQ fluids daily to supplement or replace fluids may be useful. IV fluids, while the most effective means of supporting kidney health, are not as easy to provide in the home. Additional types of fluids may also be useful, such as no salt broth, or broth that has potassium added, ice water, or warm water depending on the preference of the animal. Occasionally, it may help to warm any drinking water (lukewarm), especially for cats with oral ulcers and dental disease.

The IRIS stage four recommendations are to discontinue any nephrotoxic medications. However, if the animal has late-stage disease and has other comorbidities, such as arthritis, and the medicines will palliate them, then having an open discussion with the client about the pros and cons of any medication use is warranted. Clients can then make an informed decision and sign a waiver, acknowledging they are aware of the side effects, the costs, and benefits of continuing treatment with that medication.

IRIS also recommends measuring and monitoring blood pressure, weight, and urine protein. Discussing the costs and benefits with the client regarding measuring or monitoring blood pressure, weight, and urine protein is warranted.

Oral changes—oral ulcers, stomatitis:

1. For oral changes, a "magic mouthwash" that may be helpful; 1 part sucralfate and 1-part oral 2% viscous lidocaine, +/− an antibiotic, other pain medication and flavoring made up at a compounding pharmacy may be beneficial to heal and ease the pain of oral ulceration or stomatitis.

Gastrointestinal changes that may be seen with a late-stage CKD are vomiting, nausea, and anorexia. For LSCKD, adding ondansetron and Cerenia for both cats and dogs may help ease nausea and vomiting. Starting with one and add the other in if there is continued nausea or vomiting. Ondansetron may be better at managing nausea, Cerenia better as an anti-emetic (VIN staff, 2017). The dose of Cerenia is: Dogs 2 mg/kg PO q 24 h or 1mg/kg SQ q 24 h, Cats 1 mg/kg PO q 24 h or 0.5 mg/kg SQ q 24 h (VIN staff, 2017). Ondansetron : Dogs 0.1−1 mg/kg PO, SQ q 12−24 h, Cats 0.5−1 mg/kg PO, SQ q 12 h (VIN staff, 2017).

Anorexia or hyporexia may be late-stage signs of CKD. Adding mirtazapine, either as an ear gel or orally, may not work, and the client should be made aware that the animal may not eat. It may be a clinical sign that clients consider for deciding on euthanasia.

1. The dose of Mirtazapine is 0.5–1.5 mg/kg PO q 24 h, not to exceed 30 mg/dog/d
   3.75 mg per dog PO q 24 h for dogs <5 kg body weight.
   7.5 mg per dog PO q 24 h for dogs 5–10 kg body weight.
   11.25 mg per dog PO q 24 h for dogs 10–15 kg body weight.
   15 mg per dog PO q 24 h for dogs 15–30 kg body weight.
   22.75 mg per dog PO q 24 h for dogs 30–50 kg body weight.
   30 mg per dog PO q 24 h for dogs >50 kg body weight (Casamian-Sorrosal, 2010; VIN Staff, 2017). For cats, 1.88 mg/cat q 24–48 hrs for renal insufficient cats. Mirtaz® is 2 mg/cat or 1/2 inch ribbon transdermally. Most commonly placed inside the ear pinna on the non-haired area (VIN staff, 2017).
2. Gastroprotectants such as sucralfate dogs 0.5-g–1-g PO every 8–12 h for 5–7 days, cats 25 mg PO in a slurry every 8–12 h for 5–7 days may help with GI ulceration (VIN staff, 2017).
3. Famotidine 0.5 mg/kg PO, SQ q 12–24 h (VIN staff, 2017).

Hypertension: Monitoring animals monthly to adjust medications as needed, sooner if they are symptomatic.

1. For cats, amlodipine 0.0625–1.25 mg/cat PO q 24 h or Telmisartan 0.5–1 mg/kg q 24 h, Can increase by 0.25–0.5 mg/kg to maximum daily dosage of 5 mg/kg (VIN staff, 2017).
2. For dogs—benazepril 0.5 mg/kg PO q 24 h or other ACE inhibitor may be helpful, add in amlodipine 0.1–0.6 mg/kg PO q 24 h if needed for dogs whose blood pressure is not well controlled. Or Telmisartan 0.5–1.0 mg/kg PO q 24 h. Can increase by 0.25–0.5 mg/kg to maximum daily dosage of 5 mg/kg (VIN staff, 2017).

From the American College of Veterinary Internal Medicine Consensus Statement:

Protocol for Accurate Blood Pressure (BP) Measurement:

Calibration of the BP device should be tested semiannually either by the user, when self-test modes are included in the device, or by the manufacturer.

The procedure must be standardized.

The environment should be isolated, quiet, and away from other animals. Generally, the owner should be present. The patient should not be sedated and should be allowed to acclimate to the measurement room for 5–10 min before BP measurement is attempted.

The animal should be gently restrained in a comfortable position, ideally in ventral or lateral recumbency to limit the vertical distance from the heart base to the cuff (if more than 10 cm, a correction factor of +0.8 mm Hg/cm below or above the heart base can be applied).

The cuff width should be approximately 30%−40% of circumference of the cuff site.

The cuff may be placed on a limb or the tail, taking into account animal conformation and tolerance, and user preference.

The same individual should perform all BP measurements following a standard protocol. Training of this individual is essential.

The measurements should be taken only when the patient is calm and motionless.

The first measurement should be discarded. A total of 5−7 consecutive consistent values should be recorded. In some patients, measured BP trends downward as the process continues. In these animals, measurements should continue until the decrease plateaus and then 5−7 consecutive consistent values should be recorded.

Repeat as necessary, changing cuff placement as needed to obtain consistent values.

Average all remaining values to obtain the BP measurement.

If in doubt, repeat the measurement subsequently.

Written records should be kept on a standardized form and include person making measurements, cuff size and site, values obtained, rationale for excluding any values, the final (mean) result, and interpretation of the results by a veterinarian.

Acierno (2018)

Pain managment: Because the pain is nociceptive, neuropathic, or both with CKD, gabapentin and pregabalin may be first-line pain medication. Antidepressants would be a reasonable second choice for neuropathic pain. There is much debate about treating CKD patients with NSAIDs for comorbidities, such as arthritis. The client should be informed of the cost and benefit of using an NSAID, and it should be confirmed that the animal is hydrated and not proteinuric. A lower dose, 0.02 mg/kg, can be given daily of meloxicam. The changes in survival times are not significant between animals getting NSAIDs and animals who are not (Monteiro et al., 2019). More studies are needed to evaluate whether the efficacy seen at higher doses may be achieved with these lower doses(Monteiro et al., 2019).

Additional pain medications may also be used with animals with CKD. Steroids may be used sparingly in healthier cats with CKD. With late-stage disease, steroids may be needed for other inflammatory comorbidities, such as arthritis or to help to stimulate appetite. Gabapentin and pregabalin may also be considered for neuropathic pain. Consider lowering the dose for late-stage renal patients, especially if they are gabapentin naïve (Raouf, 2017). As of this writing, anti-nerve growth factor antibodies have been reported to help both cats and dogs with O.A., lasts 4—6 weeks, and may be used with CKD patients. However, it is not yet on the market in the US as of this writing (Lascelles, 2019). It is available for cats in Europe under the name Librela® (bedinvetmab) and for dogs in Europe, Solencia® (frunevetmab).

Pain management: Oral or transmucosal pain medications should also be part of a plan for CKD.

1. Buprenorphine 0.01—0.05 mg/kg PO every 8—12 h for both dogs and cats for as long as they have active ulcers or mouth pain. Transmucosal will help acute pain with active ulcers and stomatitis (VIN staff, 2017).
2. Oral gabapentin (made up by a compounding pharmacy) may also help, start at a low dose to prevent drowsiness, 3—5 mg/kg and go up to 10—20 mg/kg PO q 8—24 h for dogs and up to 10 mg/kg for cats PO q 8—12 h (VIN staff, 2017).
3. If there are comorbidities, such as arthritis, consider NSAID. Meloxicam Dogs: 0.2 mg/kg initial dose PO, SC, or IV, then 0.1 mg/kg q 24 h PO. Cats: 0.1 mg/kg initially, then 0.05 mg/kg/d, then reduce dose to every other day, or 0.02 mg/kg PO q 24 h (VIN staff, 2017).

Fatigue: weakness is reported in human CKD patients (Davey, 2020).

Neurological changes: seizures, sleep disturbances, altered taste, smell reported in people (and may contribute to lack of appetite in veterinary patients?), and peripheral neuropathy can be treated with gabapentin or pregabalin.

Musculoskeletal changes: bone pain from renal osteodystrophy—reported in people—treat for pain, muscle twitching, cramps reported in people, cachexia. If noted, consider hypokalemia, and treat with potassium.

1. Potassium supplementation can happen with SQ fluids or IV fluids, or orally. The oral dose for dogs is 0.44 mEq/kg PO q 12 h. For cats, 0.21—1.6 mEq/kg q 24 h of potassium gluconate.

Dermatological changes: Pruritus in humans is treated with topical immunomodulators, gabapentin, UVb phototherapy, and naltrexone, among other methods (Weisshaar, 2012). There is little in the veterinary literature regarding pruritus in CKD patients.

Anemia: while late and end stage disease may receive some benefit from erythropoietin, it is more likely going to be given in earlier disease.

1. Darbepoetin: 0.45—1.8 mcg/kg (for cats) 0.45—1.5 mcg/kg (for dogs) sq once weekly then taper to q 2—3 weeks.

Proteinuria: Telmisartan a Angiotensin II (typeAT1) can help with the reduction of proteinuria in CKD cats. May help control systemic hypertension.

1. Telmisartian—Dose in dogs and cats 0.5—1 mg/kg PO q 24 h. Can increase the dose 0.25—0.5 mg/kg over time to a maximum of 5 mg/kg (VIN Staff, 2017). Reduction of proteinuria and systemic hypertension is 1 mg/kg PO q 24 h for both dogs and cats (VIN Staff, 2017).

Crisis kit

Pain—An opioid is going to help with any acute pain crisis. Morphine, hydromorphone, and methadone may be helpful in the short term to get them more comfortable. If you do not carry schedule 2 drugs, you can utilize Buprenorphine at 0.05 mg/kg for cats transmucosal or 0.05—0.1 mg/kg TM in crisis every 6—12 h for dogs, as this is for crisis, prescribing at least 24 h of dosing to allow the animal comfort until they can get them to an emergency hospital or have a house call veterinarian to their house. In preparation for euthanasia, use it with another pain medication, such as gabapentin—crisis dose 100 mg/lb (for sedation) given every 8—12 h as needed for sedation.

Dehydration—If they are not already giving sq fluids, they may want to keep a bag of lactated ringers or Normosol R to give to their pet if they become moderately or severely dehydrated or constipated with instructions on when to provide and how to give it. The client should also be shown how to give SQ fluids prior to a crisis so that they feel comfortable giving if the house call veterinarian is not readily available.

Nausea/vomiting—Cerenia injectable Dog 1 mg/kg SQ, Cat 0.5 mg/kg SQ, or ondansetron meltaway tablet- 1 mg/kg on gums in crisis for dogs and cats (VIN Staff, 2017).

Diarrhea—see Diarrhea section.

Constipation—see Constipation section.

Oral ulcers—consider a sucralfate/oral 2% viscous lidocaine mouthwash in the crisis kit even if the animal does not have oral ulcers at the first visit. Recommend having a compounding pharmacy make the formulation with flavoring.

Constipation
Etiology/DDX

Patients toward the end-of-life may develop constipation. Constipation is defined as infrequent bowel movements that may be difficult to pass. Obstipation is severe constipation and needs medical intervention. Constipation most frequently occurs and is a clinical sign of dehydration (Scherk, 2018). Constipation may occur with increased water loss, such as in vomiting, polyuria with CKD, Diabetes mellitius, diuretic medication, or obstruction such as happens with neoplasia, metastasis (to lymph nodes), carcinomatosis, adhesions from prior surgery, postradiation, bowel damage, inflammatory bowel disease, decreased motility of bowel due to inflammation, neoplasia, diabetic neuropathy, or other neurologic disorder, such as megacolon and low fiber diets may also play a role (Yennurajalingam, 2016, Scherk, 2018). Recumbency and pain may also play a role in the development of constipation (Dzierżanowski, 2018). A partial or total bowel obstruction may occur with cancer patients, causing an accumulation of stomach fluid, biliary and pancreatic enzyme secretions and regurgitation or vomiting in addition to constipation. There may be a decrease in the absorption of water and sodium in the intestinal lumen. With opioid use, decreased motility is a factor and minimizing or discontinuing the opioid and substituting an alternative analgesic may help constipation. Slowed bowel movements may not necessarily indicate constipation or obstipation, though clients often are concerned about lack of bowel movements. Decreased appetite, anorexic, and postoperative patients may have a decrease in the amount and volume of bowel movements.

Clinical signs

Signs for clients to watch for are straining to defecate, leaking diarrhea, especially if straining, lethargy, abdominal distention, nausea, vomiting, agitation, or anxiety-like behavior.

Palliative management

Medical management of constipation may help before enemas and digital removal. Modification of the diet such as adding fiber to the diet can be helpful if there is a history of constipation or constipation is anticipated due to the disease.

1. Fluid therapy is a significant first step, SQ, IV Fluids are recommended or moderate or severe constipation, increased oral fluids are recommended if mild constipation or concerned that constipation may occur.
2. Osmotic laxatives such as Lactulose 0.22 mL/kg PO PRN for dogs and cats or Miralax® ¼- ½ tsp PO mixed in water or broth every 12—24 h for cats, ½ tsp2 tsp for dogs (VIN Staff, 2017) (use to effect—go down in dose if it develops diarrhea, go up if still confirmed to be constipated).
3. A prokinetic can be added to the treatment plan as well for neurologic constipation (metoclopramide, cisapride, erythromycin).
4. Enema if needed. Special caution is needed for patients with cancer and neurological conditions. Lubricants may help pass the stool.
5. If needed, digital removal of the stool if obstipated and none of the other treatments worked. It may also be a consideration for euthanasia depending on the cause for constipation (e.g., neoplasia) (Scherk, 2018).

Delirium

Delirium is defined in humans as a state of incoherent behavior, that may be associated with fever, drugs, or other etiologies that can include restlessness, vocalizations, and hallucinations. Animals who may exhibit delirium-like signs, may stand in a corner and bark, vocalize at apparently nothing, and seem incoherent or restless. These may be signs of other disease or pain; however, keeping delirium on the list of rule outs to help treat this frustrating symptom. Delirium may be a

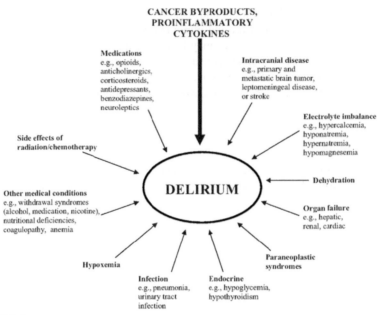

FIGURE 5.8

Causes of delirium in human beings.

Used with permission by Bush, S. H. (2009). The assessment and management of delirium in cancer patients.
The Oncologist, 1039–1049.

late-stage clinical sign that is distressing to clients. If an animal develops delirium, it may be a point of euthanasia decision-making for clients. There can be many different etiologies. However, not every case that may be on the list is going to develop delirium. The following is a list of etiologies for people with delirium (Fig. 5.8). Etiology/DDX: Medication, such as opioids, neoplasia cytokines/paraneoplastic syndrome, primary or secondary intracranial disease, organ failure, such as liver, renal or heart failure, endocrine changes, such as hypoglycemia, hypoxia (Bush, 2009).

Palliative management

The treatment for humans is a neuroleptic medication, haloperidol (Bush, 2009; Yennurajalingam, 2016). Haloperidol is not commonly used in veterinary medicine, however, the mechanism of action is dopamine receptor antagonism. A veterinary medication that has a similar mechanism of action is acepromazine or chlorpromazine, which are also dopamine receptor antagonists (VIN staff, 2017).

Options for management of delirium in dogs and cats may be acepromazine and chlorpromazine. Acepromazine dosing for both cats and dogs is 0.5—2 mg/kg PO q 8—12 h (may cause profound sedation. Start with low dose, but give your clients permission to increase dosing if needed) (VIN staff, 2017).

Chlorpromazine dose is 0.55—2 mg/kg PO PRN for delirium (may cause profound sedation. Start on low end of dosing) (VIN staff, 2017).

If it is related to medication use, change to alternatives for pain management to opioids or decrease dose and use adjuvants for pain management. Consider changing pain management plan.

Treat the primary disease. Ensure that the animal is hydrated and electrolytes are normal and adjust medications that may cause delirium, check oxygen levels, and blood glucose levels.

Crisis kit

Consider a neuroleptic medication such as acepromazine or chlorpromazine if all other causes have been ruled out.

Discontinue opioids to rule out dysphoria.

Dementia

Veterinarians may find dementia one of the most challenging diseases to manage in end-of-life medicine. Clients may find it onerous to choose a time for euthanasia as no single day is dramatically worse than another, and the disease process tends to be slow and progressive. Dementia is heavily studied in human medicine and has been drawn on for this section for comparison and therapies as well as veterinary literature.

There are different types of dementia seen with both people and animals. There are different clinical presentations for dementia in humans which we will review. Alzheimer's disease is a dementia most commonly evaluated in people, between 60−80% of cases. Alzheimer's dementia has clinical signs that are slowly progressive and have short term memory loss in the early stages, with eventual long term memory loss. Alzheimer's has beta amyloid plaques and neurofibrillary tangles that initially affect the entorhinal cortex, the area of the brain that connects the hippocampus and neocortex. Veterinarians hypothesize based on brain lesions, most dementia in both cats and dogs are similar to Alzeimer's disease (Duong, Patel, & Chang, 2017).

The second most common type of dementia seen is vascular dementia. Vascular dementia tends to have a more sudden onset, and can have a cardiovascular event associated with the onset, such as stroke and in people , tend to have arthrosclerotic comorbidites, such as heart disease, diabetes, hypertention. Vascular dementia can be due to a significant stroke, or occur more gradually with smaller or transient strokes. Patients with vascular dementia tend to have significant changes in their executive function (Duong, Patel, & Chang, 2017). Lewy-body dementia (LBD) is signified by alpha-synuclein proteins (also known as Lewy-bodies) developing in neurons. Lewy-Body dementia is associated with Parkinson-like movements and significant behavior changes, associated with executive function and visual hallucination. People with LBD have more sleep wake disturbance, disengagement with their environment, body rigidity and changes in rapid eye movement sleep. And then there is frontotemporal dementia, as the name suggests, affecting the frontal and temporal cortex associated with significant personality and behavior changes (Duong, Patel, & Chang, 2017). While the majority of dogs and cats have changes similar to either alzeimer's disease or vascular dementia, it remains unclear if they are affected by Lewy bodies.

Veterinary patients with dementia may be palliated differently depending on the stage. Early treatment may slow the progression, while there may be little change as the animal approaches later stages. End stage dementia may be challenging to palliate to the end of the disease for animals due to the need for significant nursing care. Palliative sedation may be warranted in the late stages of disease. Palliative sedation may need to be provided in the hospital setting to have 24/7 care. Setting up expectations for the caregivers early in the process and reviewing the progress and trajectory of the disease frequently as it progresses can support the caregiver in decision-making. More on palliative sedation in the pain management section.

Etiology/DDX
Changes seen in the brain

Canine cognitive dysfunction (CCD): Elderly dogs may have normal aging variations due to a reduction in neurons, decreased neurogenesis, changes in vasculature, decreases in myelin, cholinergic function, and altered gene expression (May, 2019). With canine cognitive dysfunction (CCD), there is an accumulation of β-amyloid(Aβ) plaques in the cerebral cortex, and there are different configurations of Aβ (For example: Aβ42, Aβ40, Aβ21). Tau phosphorylation may also play a role in Alzheimer's disease and frontotemporal dementia in people. Fibrillar deposits of phosphorylated tau have been identified in dogs (Prpar Mihevc, 2019). In one study, they looked at the difference between Senile Plaques(SP) and Cerebral Amyloid Angiopathy (CAA) and found that there was no correlation between SP and Canine Cognitive Dysfunction (CCD). They also found CAA did corelate with CCD and that CAA increases with age. They concluded in that study the role of Aβ is unclear in CCD (Ozawa, Chambers, Uchida, & Nakayama, 2016). Dogs also have a lack of the neuro fiber tangles that have been found in human pathology (Dewey, 2019). NMDA receptors are upregulated and excessive NMDA receptor activity may also accelerate neuron death (Wang, 2017). Alterations in mitochondrial function may diminish metabolism in the brain and contribute to the amplified production of free radicals (May, 2019). The changes seen in the CCD dog brain are most similar to the changes seen with human Alzheimer's disease (Prpar Mihevc, 2019).

Feline cognitive dysfunction (FCD): In FCD, researchers have noted chronic inflammation in the brain, oxidative changes, microglial stimulation and neuronal loss similar to Alzheimer's disease. Neuronal loss has been noted in the cerebellum and caudate nucleus with progressive atrophy of the cerebral cortex and basal ganglia in cats. There is an increase in ventricular size and there can also be vascular changes that occur. There is also lipofuscin accumulation, amyloid-β (Aβ) deposition, and τ hyperphosphorylation seen in cats (Sordo, 2021). Cats tend to have an accumulation of Aβ42 plaques, differing from humans that have pathology with both Aβ42 and Aβ40. The lack of Aβ40 plaques may be due to higher solubility and metabolic turnover in the cat brain, however cats with CAA have an accumulation of Aβ40 plaques. These differences need further evaluation as to the effects on cats and whether it affects the development of FCD. Cats have a reduction in cholinergic neurons and a loss in the locus coeruleus, similar to the changes seen in humans with dementia (Sordo, 2021).

Behavioral changes seen with dementia

There may be many behavioral changes seen with CCD or FCD. There are stages of dementia in humans. No studies found as of this writing have categorized CCD or FCD into stages but it may be useful for veterinarians to become familiarized with the human stages. The stages in human medicine (and proposed veterinary patient behaviors that may be consistent with and translated for the veterinary patient in this text—similar behaviors in people with dementia) (Staff of Alzheimers Association, 2021) are as follows:

1. Mild dementia
   a. There are mild changes in behavior in humans. (Clients may not notice changes or believe they are part of the aging process).
   b. Changes noted in people may include, forgetting commands, more difficulty performing normal tasks. (These changes in dogs and cats may be subtle initially and may not be noted by the client or considered part of a normal aging process).
   c. The person may be more anxious, or painful, but changes are subtle. (This may also be the case for animals in the early stages of dementia and changes may not be noted or considered part of the normal aging process).
2. Moderate dementia
   a. People start noticing they are seemingly more forgetful, disoriented, and confused. (Clients may start noticing changes in behavior of an animal, that may include disorientation, confusion, and seeming forgetful).
   b. People may start having urinary or fecal incontinence (Clients may notice urinating and defecating inappropriately or incontinence).
   c. People have changes in sleep patterns with moderate dementia. Sundowner's syndrome may be noticed more with moderate dementia. (Sundowner's syndrome or changes in sleep patterns may be noticed in cats and dogs with dementia).
   d. Moderate changes in behavior are noted in people. (Other changes in behavior may be noted in veterinary patients).
   e. Wondering and pacing become more frequent in human patients. (Wondering and pacing become more frequent in veterinary patients).

3. Severe dementia
  a. People need more help with daily care, may go to the bathroom where they lay and not realize it. They may need diapers to stay clean. People may also need assistance eating, or drinking. (Dogs and cats with dementia may be more fecal and urinary incontinent, need to be hand fed, or encouraged to eat or drink).
  b. People with severe dementia signs may have delirium. (This may also be true for dogs with dementia with delirium-type signs, barking at walls, getting stuck under furniture).
  c. People develop dysphagia. (Dogs and cats with dementia may also develop dysphagia).
  d. People have more difficulties with mobility, more sleep/wake disturbances. (Sundowner's syndrome may get worse, mobility declines).
  e. People may stop vocalizing. (Dogs and cats who were previously vocalizing, may stop as they get closer to death).
  f. People are more frequently forgetful, disoriented, confused. (Dogs and cats progress with disorientation, confusion).

More studies are needed to examine possible staging of CCD or FCD to evaluate the similarities to the stages identified in people. In humans with dementia, both seizures and transient vestibular events (may also occur with CCD or FCD) have been reported (Dewey, 2019). The common acronym DISHAA, which stands for; Disorientation, social Interactions, Sleep/wake cycle, Housesoiling/memory loss, Activity and Anxiety is commonly used to identfy changes in behaviors associated with cognitive dysfunction.

Dogs with dementia signs that may include behaviors such as confusion, changes in the sleep-wake cycle, anxiety, or aggressive behavior, getting stuck in corners or under furniture, pacing (especially at night), inappropriate elimination, vocalization (especially at night), decreased interactions with the family, difficulty eating, or drinking. Pain may be present in dogs with dementia signs however it may go underreported and unrecognized by the client (Prpar Mihevc, 2019).

Cats with dementia signs may include behaviors such as: increased vocalizations (especially at night, and may also be due to other causes including pain, hypertension, hearing loss), inappropriate elimination (may also be because of pain), attention seeking, disorientation, staring into space, getting stuck in corners, changes in learning and memory, and changes in sleep—wake cycle (Sordo, 2021). Pain may be also present in cats with dementia signs however it may go underreported and unrecognized by the client (Sordo, 2021).

DDX/etiology: Other possible causes of changes in behavior should be ruled out first. Differentials for changes in behavior associated with dementia like signs—hypertension, brain neoplasia, stroke, pain, chronic kidney, liver failure, endocrine disorders such as diabetes, hyperthyroidism, infectious disease such as FIV, FELV, distemper, and inflammatory disease (Sordo, 2021). Diagnosis: While dementia may be difficult to diagnose in the early stages, we can rule out other differentials with bloodwork, X-ray, ultrasound, and MRI.

Testing for CCD and FCD

Obtaining a comprehensive history from clients and signalment is the first step to diagnosing CCD or FCD. Food-searching tests or problem-solving tests may assist the clinician in assessing an animal for CCD or FCD. Using the DISHAA scale may help clients identify behavior changes. There are also a few validated scales that may also be useful for the clinician to further identfy cognitive dysfunction.

There is a validated scale for CCD called Canine Cognitive Dysfunction Rating Scale. It was developed by researchers at the University of Sydney (Barnette, 2020) and validated in 2011 (Salvin, 2011).

Another validated screening tool is Canine Dementia Scale, validated in 2015 (Madari, 2015).

An MRI is used to evaluate changes in the brain consistent with CCD or FCD (Dewey, 2019). Visual Evoked Potential (VEP) tests are used in humans with Alzheimer's and may be of use in dogs and cats. A 2015 study done on pomeranians found changes in 8/28 dogs that confirmed CCD on MRI, 2 had confirmed brain tumors and that there was a difference between CCD and brain tumor with VEP test (Hamnilrat, Lekcharoensuk, Choochalermporn, & Thayananuphat, 2015).

Medical Management of CCD or FCD

Selegiline, an MAO b inhibitor, may help improve behavior changes in the early to midstages of CCD (Dewey, 2019).

NMDA antagonist: NMDA antagonists may also help slow the progression of clinical signs in Alzheimer's like dementia and vascular dementia. Memantine is used in human dementia patients. Consider SQ subanesthetic dose ketamine, or memantine for palliative patients—more research needs to be done in veterinary medicine to evaluate the efficacy in veterinary patients (Wang, 2017). Gabapentin may be helpful for anxiety and agitation (Megna, 2002). It may also help the animal sleep, decrease neuropathic pain, which may not be recognized because of the changes in behavior with dementia. The author has noted that gabapentin can have a paradoxical effect with some dementia patients and may worsen mobility of dogs with CCD.

1. Amantadine 2—5 mg/kg PO q 12—24 h. Start on the lower end and increase as needed.
2. Subanesthetic ketamine SQ 0.5—1 mg/kg SQ PRN (anecdotal. May need to be given monthly or more frequently. Studies need to be done to assess the efficacy)
3. Subanesthetic ketamine in CRI 0.5 mg/kg bolus then CRI of 10 mcg/kg/minute for about 2 h.
4. Memantine 0.3—0.5 mg/kg q 12—24 h (Wright, 2017)
5. Consider an antidepressant such as trazodone or amitriptyline (Dewey, 2019).
6. Avoid Benzodiazepines with cognitive dysfunction patients as they may worsen cognitive function (Rochon, 2017).

7. Dietary changes: In human dementia patients, it has been found that the brain has a decreased capacity to use glucose sources for energy. The brain is still able to utilize ketones and medium-chain triglycerides as energy sources (Taylor, Swerdlow, & Sullivan, 2019). In addition, free radicals are hypothesized to contribute to dementia in humans (Taylor, Swerdlow, & Sullivan, 2019). Adding anti-oxidants to the human diet have been shown to help slow the progression of dementia. Veterinary diets have been developed to include antioxidants and ketones and medium-chain triglycerides. Examples include BrightMinds, Hill's B/d, Purina Neurocare (May, 2019; Pan, 2018). Other nutrients found to help are omega-3 fatty acids, arginine, branched-chain amino acids, and L-carnitine. The combination of nutrients and anti-oxidants may make a difference in the quality of life of the CCD or FCD patient (May, 2019).

8. In addition to dietary changes, some nutritional supplements have also been used in people and pets and may help slow progression, including Senilife (a blend of several different neuroprotective nutraceuticals), phosphatidylserine, SAM-e, Ginkgo Biloba (free radical scavenger, used in humans), vitamin B6 (cofactor in neurotransmitter synthesis), Resveratrol (may decrease Aβ production), and vitamin E (may help enhance Ginkgo's effects). Apoaequorin may be another neutrceutical that may be effective and a double-blinded study showed improvement in patients with cognitive dysfunction with cognitive tasks more than selegiline affected CCD patients. However apoaequarin is not currently available as of this writing. The use of nutritional supplements may have little to no impact and are primarily based on human trials (Dewey, 2019). Further studies in veterinary patients are needed to examine the benefits of these nutritional supplements.

9. There may be an neuroinflammatory component to CCD, and NSAIDs may be considered (Dewey, 2019).

10. A hormonal supplement that has been studied for use with patients with Alzheimers is melatonin. Melatonin may help with the sleep—wake cycle of dogs or cats with dementia, though further studies need to be done to further evaluate the efficacy (Cardinali, 2010).

11. CBD may also be useful for sleep—wake disturbance; however, additional research needs to look at the efficacy with CCD.

Nonmedical therapies

There is evidence that obtaining novel skills or knowledge may slow the progression of human dementia. Behavioral therapies may include adding to the enrichment of the animal's environment, regular exercise and varying the routine of walks or play, puzzle feeders, and novel toys may help lessen symptoms and slow the progression of dementia. In addition, continuing some routines, including sleep—wake habits, can also help improve the quality of life for both pets and their people (Yennurajalingam, 2016).

Acupuncture and physical therapy/rehabilitation may help improve clinical signs for people with dementia and may help with both dogs and cats. Additional double-blinded studies need to be done to further evaluate the efficacy with cognitive dysfunction veterinary patients (Kowalska, 2019; Yu, 2020).

Crisis kit

1. Gabapentin: Dogs: 3—20 mg/kg PO 1—3 times per day. Cats: 3—10 mg/kg PO q 8—24 h (can go higher if needed, the higher doses are more likelyto be sedative) (VIN staff, 2017).

2. Trazadone: (anxiety/chronic neuropathic pain/delirium): Dogs: in dogs, there is a range of doses. They include 2.5 mg per pound per day to 15 mg per pound every 24 h. The average dose is approximately 3.5 mg per pound per day. Lower doses are used when combined with other behavioral modification medications. Most veterinarians prescribe trazodone at the lower dosage range to minimize side effects and may gradually taper the dose up after 3—5 days. Cats: trazodone has been infrequently used. The documented dose used in cats is 50—100 mg total dose for short-term use(VIN staff, 2017).

3. If acute pain occurs, opioids should be included. See pain management for opioid dosing.

4. Consider acepromazine for delirium: 0.025—0.2 mg/kg IV; maximum of 3 mg or 0.1—0.25 mg/kg IM. If considering euthanasia can go higher(VIN staff, 2017). If seizures are a concern, intranasal or rectal midazolam could be utilized. However, dementia signs may worsen.

5. CBD: Hemp-based CBD dosing 1—2 mg/kg q 12 h. Seems to be more bioavailable in dogs than cats (Deabold, 2019). CBD is not regulated and may not contain the content that the label has listed; monitor FDA warning letters to identify products that have been found to be labelled differently than the measured dose. More research is needed to look at the efficacy of CBD and seizures. At the time of this writing, it is not legal for veterinarians to prescribe or recommend cannabinoids to be given to our patients. Check with your local regulatory board for more information.

Diarrhea

Diarrhea can be one of the most frustrating and difficult symptoms/sequelae to treat for the end-of-life patient. Patients with inflammatory bowel disease or lymphoma may have chronic diarrhea. The end of life patient may develop acute diarrhea with a dietary indiscretion or change in medication. This section will explore therapies to help patients with diarrhea, whether chronic or acute.

Etiology/DDX

Osmotic diarrhea: Exocrine pancreatic insufficiency, small intestinal bacterial overgrowth, dietary indiscretion, some fruit, vegetable ingestion (Marks, 2013).

Secretory diarrhea: Clostridium, cryptosporidium, giardia, IBD, diabetes mellitus, carcinoid syndrome, non-beta pancreatic islet cell tumor, gastrinoma, pancreatitis, parvovirus (though not typically seen in older veterinary patients). Increased mucosal permeability—ulcers (Marks, 2013).

Changes in motility causing diarrhea: Radiation-induced diarrhea, surgical resection, chemotherapy, constipation, bowel obstruction, diabetic neuropathy, bowel neoplasia.

Medications such as antibiotics, laxatives (Marks, 2013). Stress-induced colitis may be possible in some circumstances, though less likely to be seen in late-stage veterinary patients.

Clinical signs: soft to fluid stool, with or without blood or mucus. Secondary symptoms may be abdominal pain, serosal pain, distention of abdomen or bowel, borborygmi, flatulence, PU/PD, tenesmus, weight loss, dehydration. There may also be changes in appetite and vomiting may occur (Marks, 2013).

Management of diarrhea

If diarrhea occurs and the patient is currently on laxatives or antibiotics, lower dosing, if applicable, or discontinue medication.

End-stage veterinary patients may need fluid therapy if the animal has lost significant amounts of fluid with diarrhea and is dehydrated, has decreased fluid intake, or is moribund. For patients who are not vomiting and have secretory diarrhea, oral fluids that are supplemented with glucose, amino acids and electrolytes may be useful (Candellone, Cerquetella, Girolami, Badino, & Odore, 2020).

Antibiotics such as metronidazole and tylosin may be helpful for some secretory or osmotic types of diarrhea (Marks, 2013).

Opioids may modify motility and help with pain management. Transmucosal buprenorphine or codeine or hydrocodone with acetaminophen (for dogs only) may help improve both diarrhea and pain management of comorbidities. Lomotil may also be a consideration for chronic diarrhea patients (VIN staff, 2017).

Consider starting patients on Cerenia for secondary serosal pain management. 2 mg/kg PO q 24 h for dogs, 1 mg/kg PO q 24 h for cats. Cerenia should be used with other pain management medications (VIN staff, 2017).

Prebiotics, foods that contain fermentable fiber, are recommended for diarrhea due to changes in motility and inflammatory bowel disease (Alves, Santos, Jorge, & Pitães, 2021). Fiber may create more gas, fluid/diarrhea as the bacteria develop an affinity. Soluble or mixed fiber sources may be useful for acute diarrhea. One source recommends 7–15% dry matter of diet as a fiber source (Candellone, Cerquetella, Girolami, Badino, & Odore, 2020).

Probiotics, adding bacteria to the diet, have been used for diarrhea. However, the evidence may not support the continued use of probiotics for chronic diarrhea (Jensen AP, 2019).

Hydrated calcium aluminosilicate, a clay product, may help with some diarrheas, (ie: chemotherapy-induced diarrhea) (Fournier, 2021). More research may need to be done for other types of diarrheas.

Octreotide is used in human medicine for secretory diarrhea. There is some information in the older literature about its use in veterinary patients with gastrinomas. However, it seems to have lost favor in the veterinary patient over time.

"Octreotide is an octapeptide that mimics natural somatostatin pharmacologically, though it is a more potent inhibitor of growth hormone, glucagon, and insulin than the natural hormone" (Vetbook Staff, 2012). Other physiological effects include reducing splanchnic blood flow, inhibition of release of serotonin, gastrin, vasoactive intestinal polypeptide, secretin, motilin, and pancreatic polypeptide.

Octreotide is primarily used in canine medicine to treat gastrinoma, insulinoma, osteosarcoma, and acromegaly. The recommended dose for dogs is 10–40 mg/kg IV every 8–12 h (Vetbook Staff, 2012). There is no published oral dose for dogs. It has been used in cats for chylothorax, gastrinoma, and acromegaly and may decrease growth hormone. There is a case report on a cat with hepatic masses that was stabilized with IV fluids, maropitant, pantoprazole, and octreotide for the gastrinoma (Lane, 2016). There are no published oral doses for cats either. This would be a novel, and off label use of Octreotide.

For a patient receiving palliatve care, Octreotide may be a helpful treatment for diarrhea as a last resort. Although the use in humans with secretory diarrhea has an evidence basis for use, there is not yet evidence of its use in veterinary patients for secretory diarrhea.

Fecal transplants may also be considered (via rectal administration or with orally administered capsules). If rectal administration of a fecal transplantation is elected, the general practitioner or a specialist in a brick and mortar practice may be able to facilitate (Chaitman, 2021).

Consider SQ Vitamin B 12(cobalamine), for palliative treatment for patients with diarrhea. The dose for cobalamine for dogs less than 15 kg is 500 mcg SQ q 7 days, greater than 15 kg 1000 mcg SQ q 7 days, for cats, 250 mcg SQ q 7 days. For animals with chronic diarrhea, continue Vitamin B12 weekly (VIN staff, 2017).

Another recent novel approach that may need further investigation, is the use of antioxidants and polyphenyls (Candellone, Cerquetella, Girolami, Badino, & Odore, 2020).

Dysphagia

Patients that a house call veterinarian may help may have dysphagia or difficulty prehending and painful swallowing. Dysphagia may have a primary cause or be a secondary sequelae. Managing these patients may be a challenge for both the client and veterinarian.

Etiology/DDX

Dysphagia is the obstruction or dysfunction of the oral cavity, pharynx, or esophagus (Chilukuri, 2018). Oropharyngeal dysphagia may be structural, with a deficit in the teeth, hard or soft palate, tongue, or the cricopharynx or upper esophageal sphincter. Oropharyngeal dysphagia may be due to a neuromuscular or vascular, or trauma-based etiology (although trauma is less likely with late-stage and end-of-life patients). Oral dysphagia differentials include stomatitis, severe periodontitis, caries, tooth root or retrobulbar abscess, head and neck neoplasia, geriatric onset laryngeal paralysis and polyneuropathy (GOLPP)/degenerative myelopathy, stroke, CCD, FCD, uremic oral ulcers, and temporal-masseter myositis. Calicivirus, viral rhinotracheitis, lingual, or glossal foreign objects may be secondary sequelae (Chilukuri, 2018).

Pharyngeal dysphagia may be caused by head and neck neoplasia, myasthenia gravis, brain stem lesions, cranial nerve X, XII dysfunction, esophagitis, and fractured bones in cricothyroid (Chilukuri, 2018).

With esophageal dysphagia, the deficit may be structural or neurologic. Differentials for esophageal dysphagia may include megaesophagus, lung neoplasia, dilated cardiomyopathy, myasthenia gravis, or gastroesophageal reflux disease or GERD (Chilukuri, 2018).

Clinical signs

Patients who have developed oral dysphagia, may drop food or have difficulty chewing food and become subsequently hyporexic or anorexic. Patients who develop neurologic deficits may get food impactions of the pharynx, reflux into nasal passages because they are not swallowing properly. Prehension problems may also occur with stroke patients, animals with head/neck tumors, and severe periodontal disease (Chilukuri, 2018).

Patients who have esophageal and pharyngeal dysphagia may include simlar clinical sings as oral dysphagia and be more at risk for aspiration pneumonia (Chilukuri, 2018).

Palliative management

Palliative management concerns for patients with dysphagia include pain management, motility of the esophagus, infection. Patients with oral dysphagia from painful teeth, oral ulcers, stomatitis or neoplasia may be helped with "magic mouthwash" and transmucosal pain medications. Palliating pets with moderate to severe dental disease may include encouraging clients to do a dental cleaning for their pet despite their advanced age. Pets who have severe dental disease and the client elects to not move forward with a dental prophylaxis, adding oral antibiotics may help decrease the infection in the mouth and alleviate pain. Veterinarians must consider antibiotic stewardship guidelines in the use of oral antibiotics.

Patients with oral dysphagia may need a feeding tube placed. A feeding tube can bypass the need for oral feedings and help with the comfort of the patient. Nasoesophageal tubes could be used in the short term with a liquid diet. If the feeding tube needed to be longer term, esophageal feeding tubes may be the feeding tube to consider and discuss with the client.

If there is pharyngeal or esophageal dysphagia, feeding meatballs and the use of prokinetics may help these patients pass food. Consider using Percutaneous endoscopic gastrotomy tube or PEG tubes. Treat suspected gastroesophageal reflux disorder (GERD) with prokinetics, famotidine in the short term, omeprazole for longer-term use, and sucralfate if ulceration is suspected.

If the client does not want to pursue feeding tubes, it may be a point for decision-making time with clients for euthanasia.

Crisis kit

If there is a crisis with dysphagia, it would likely be pain related, and the crisis kit should include pain management.

Dysrexia

Dysrexia is defined as a disruption in food intake, anorexia is defined as absent appetite, and hyporexia is defined as decreased or waning appetite with an unbalanced diet (Cook, 2020). Dysrexia occurs frequently with end-of-life patients A brief review the normal pathways for hunger and satiety can help further define the possible changes that may happen with dysrexia. The neurons in the hypothalamus which are involved in the drive of eating or satiety, include the orexigenic neurons, drive hunger and food seeking behavior, and the anorexigenic neurons which will depress appetite. Ghrelin, primarily produced by the stomach, affects the orexigenic neurons, stimulating hunger. Thyroid hormones and cortisol can also play a role in food seeking. The neuroendocrine system also is involved in the regulation of hunger/satiety. The inflammatory process can changes the regulation of the anorexigenic neruons. Inflammation and the dysregulation of satiety hormones may occur with animals who are approaching death. This may also explain why animals who are dying also develop symptoms like cachexia, dysrexia (Cook, 2020). Animals can live on average 8–21 days, without eating if they are getting adequate fluid intake (possibly up to 8 weeks) (Kottusch, 2009).

Physiologic changes that may occur with extended periods of dysrexia include: changes in motility, such as delayed gastric emptying, and ileus, changes in the intestinal bacterial populations. These shifts may then create changes in mucosal integrity and death of enterocytes, adding to concerns about dysrexia, nausea, diarrhea, sepsis. We have to consider the etiology of the individual disease, and the physiologic drives of hunger to treat dysrexia (Cook, 2020).

Etiology/DDX

Animals with dysrexia can have a multi-factoral basis for dysregulation of hunger. Factors may have a physiologic, environmental, medication, pain, or psychological cause. The common differentials for dysrexia in patients in end-of-life stages may include orapharyngeal or esophageal dysphagia differentials, CKD, pancreatitis, neoplasia, heart failure, liver disease, diabetes (and possible sequalae) pain, dehydration, stress and anxiety and side effects from medications—either the medication themselves or the route they are given may contribute (Cook, 2020).

Palliating the dysrexic patient

Consider the possible etiology. Are they likely to have nausea, pain from their disease? Are they in the hospital or at home, what are new changes to their environment? Changes to the environment by adding pheromones, giving the animal space, such as a cardboard box or stairs to their favorite chare or bed, may be helpful. *Nausea*: For the dysrexic patient, treat for nausea first, even if they are not exhibiting apparent signs of nausea. The symptomatic changes of nausea for end of life patients may be subtle. Cerenia can given for nausea and vomiting: Dogs: 2 mg/kg PO q 24 h for dogs or 1 mg/kg SQ q 24 h, Cats: 1 mg/kg PO q 24 h, 0.5 mg/kg SQ q 24 h. Ondansetron (meltaway tablets are available) 0.1–1 mg/kg PO q 12–24 h for dogs or 0.5–1 mg/kg PO q 12 h for cats or Dolasetron 0.6–1 mg/kg PO or SQ q 24 h for dogs and cats (VIN Staff, 2017). Cerenia can be used in conjunction with ondansetron or dolasetron.

Using appetite stimulants: A nauseous or painful animal will not eat with appetite stimulants alone. Treat for nausea for 24–48 h before treating with an appetite stimulant. Appetite stimulants may include a ghrelin agonist (Entyce®) for dogs and Elura for cats FDA approved Oct 2020, an SSRI (mirtazapine) dose 0.5–1.5 mg/kg PO q 24 h for dogs (not to exceed30 mg/dog/day), for cats 1.88 mg per cat q 12–24 h or 2 mg per cat administered topically on the inner pinna of cat (VIN Staff, 2017; Quimby, 2018), or an antihistamine (cyproheptadine) 0.1–0.2 mg/kg PO q 12–24 h in dogs, 1–4 mg per cat PO q 12–24 h (VIN Staff, 2017). Other ways to stimulate the appetite may include, steroids (prednisone, prednisolone) 0.5–1 mg/kg PO q 12–24 h for dogs and cats, benzodiazepine (diazepam) 0.05 mg/kg IV for cats and put food in front of the cat (Cook, 2020; VIN Staff, 2017).

Prokinetics: Include a prokinetic if emptying of the stomach or gastrointestinal tract may be an issue (Cook, 2020). Reglan or metoclopromide can be given to dogs or cats at 0.2–0.5 mg/kg PO, SQ, IV, or a CRI- 0.01–0.02 mg/kg/hr IV constant rate infusion (VIN staff, 2017). Or Erythomycin for dogs to increase gastric motility 0.5–1 mg/kg PO q 8 h, cats 0.5–1 mg/kg PO q 8 h (VIN staff, 2017).

Proton pump inhibitors: Proton pump inhibitors may be used in the short term. Dogs and cats: pantoprazole (1 mg/kg IV q24h) or omeprazole (0.7 mg/kg PO q12h) (Cook, 2020).

Feeding Tubes: Although it is unusual for end-of-life patients to get them, a feeding tube may help a pet with a head and neck tumor or animals who cannot or are not taking appropriate amounts of nutrition if they are otherwise stable. Tube feeding an animal who may be within days to a few weeks from death may cause ethical/moral issues to arise for clients or veterinarians. Discussion about the pros and cons of the use of a feeding tube should be part of the future planning. Note: Humans who are toward the end of life become hyporexic then anorexic, so be aware for animals who are having a palliated death, the animal may not need additional food as they are approaching death (Thomas, 2019).

Changing the food: Warming foods, adding fluid, water, or no-salt bro th, and making a "gravy" or buying store bought gravied food can help stimulate the appetite. Giving novel foods to hyporexic or anorexic patients may stimulate the appetite, offering one novel food at a time.

Comfort food: Toward the end of life, animals may only eat small amounts of of novel food. Foods the author has tried include cooked fish, both white fish and salmon, cheesecake filling, vanilla pudding, ice cream (beneficial for cats with mouth pain), baby food, cooked and raw hamburger. (Please make sure to avoid products with xylitol sweetener). These foods are only tried when nutritionally balanced foods are no longer working, and animals are in their end stages and dysrexic.

Fever

Human palliative patients may experience a fever and it is a common problem in human medicine. However, when reviewing the veterinary publications, the literature regarding fevers focuses on younger patients, with infections and inflammation as typical. Studies do recognize that paraneoplastic syndrome is a cause of fever in elder patients. Typically, late-stage fevers may go unrecognized by clients or the symptoms they note may include the animal behaving unusually, with decreased or absent appetite, or lethargy.

Etiology/DDX

Patients with neoplasia may have a fever due to paraneoplastic syndrome. Patients with neoplasia develop a fever due to the pyrogenic cytokines, primarily IL-1, IL-6, and TNF-α (Harkin, 2016). These cytokines induce the Cox 2 conversion of arachidonic acid creating Prostaglandin E2 (PGE2) which raises cAMP, which acts on the hypothalamus to change the set point (Harkin, 2016). The most common types of neoplasia that the palliative veterinarian may encounter that may cause a fluctuating fever include canine and feline lymphoma, lymphoid leukemia, acute and chronic plasma cell carcinoma, multiple myeloma, cutaneous histiocytoma, and malignant histiocytosis.

Chemotherapy may also contribute to fever because of the potential of decreased WBCs and the release of cytokines. In addition to cancer cytokines, secondary infections may also cause a fever. Bacterial, viral, and fungal infections may be primary or secondary to neoplasia, chemotherapy (Harkin, 2016).

Additionally fevers may bee seen with septic joints, immune-mediated disease, pancreatitis, FIP, FELV, FIV, and urinary tract infections may also be seen in end-of-life patients (Harkin, 2016). Opioids may also cause hyperthermia. If presented an animal with a fever, consider the fever of unknown origin algorithm (Fig. 5.9).

Palliative management of fevers

Depending on the cause, fevers may be treated differently. With presumed or diagnosed canine cancer patients, veterinarians could consider utilizing acetaminophen/paracetamol at 10−15 mg/kg PO q 8−12 h. Start on the low end of the dose and

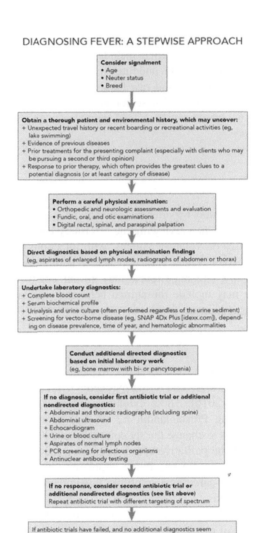

DIAGNOSING FEVER: A STEPWISE APPROACH

Consider signalment
• Age
• Neuter status
• Breed

Obtain a thorough patient and environmental history, which may uncover:
+ Unexpected travel history or recent boarding or recreational activities (eg, lake swimming)
+ Evidence of previous diseases
+ Prior treatments for the presenting complaint (especially with clients who may be pursuing a second or third opinion)
+ Response to prior therapy, which often provides the greatest clues to a potential diagnosis (or at least category of disease)

Perform a careful physical examination:
• Orthopedic and neurologic assessments and evaluation
• Fundic, oral, and otic examinations
• Digital rectal, spinal, and paraspinal palpation

Direct diagnostics based on physical examination findings
(eg, aspirates of enlarged lymph nodes, radiographs of abdomen or thorax)

Undertake laboratory diagnostics:
+ Complete blood count
+ Serum biochemical profile
+ Urinalysis and urine culture (often performed regardless of the urine sediment)
+ Screening for vector-borne disease (eg, SNAP 4Dx Plus [idexx.com]), depending on disease prevalence, time of year, and hematologic abnormalities

Conduct additional directed diagnostics based on initial laboratory work
(eg, bone marrow with bi- or pancytopenia)

If no diagnosis, consider first antibiotic trial or additional nondirected diagnostics:
+ Abdominal and thoracic radiographs (including spine)
+ Abdominal ultrasound
+ Echocardiogram
+ Urine or blood culture
+ Aspirates of normal lymph nodes
+ PCR screening for infectious organisms
+ Antinuclear antibody testing

If no response, consider second antibiotic trial or additional nondirected diagnostics (see list above)
Repeat antibiotic trial with different targeting of spectrum

If antibiotic trials have failed, and no additional diagnostics seem reasonable, **consider corticosteroid trial** for immune-mediated disease

FIGURE 5.9

An algorithm addressing fevers of unknown origin.

Created by Dr Keith Harkin ©2016. Original publication Today's Veterinary Practice. Used with permission from Dr. Keith Harkin, Harkin, K. Uncovering the cause of fever in dogs. Today's Veterinary Practice (July/August 2016).

timing and increase the dosing and timing as needed. Veterinarians may consider administering acetaminophen with an opioid for additional pain management if needed. Hydrocodone is more bioavailable orally than codeine. Never use Tylenol, acetaminophen, or paracetamol in cats as the LD50 is low. NSAIDs may be another option for fever management.

If there is an immune-mediated etiology in dogs, consider administering steroids ie: prednisone at 1−2 mg/kg PO q 12−24 h potentially for the rest of the life of the patient.

With cats if there is cancer or immune-mediated disease, you could consider using steroids such as prednisolone starting at a dose of 0.5−1 mg/kg q 12−24 h.

If there is a suspicion of sepsis or bacterial or fungal infections, then consider the proper antibiotic or antifungal. A fan may be useful to cool the animal with very high temperatures.

Crisis kit

As a fever is not necessarily a crisis, having information for clients and setting expectations can help them utilize the medication that they may need, or should contact a veterinarian if it is a concern.

Frailty

Frailty is not readily studied in veterinary medicine. Frailty is a syndrome in people defined by weight loss, muscle loss, and weakness, fatigue/lethargy, slow walking speed, low exercise but no identifiable disease (Cimons, 2013). Frailty and persistent pain are linked in humans (Guerriero, 2020). Additional studies are needed to evaluate the clinical signs of frailty and the relation to pain in the companion animal. There is a Frailty index developed in 2019 to understand frailty in the dog, which is thought to be a good model for human frailty (Banzato, 2019; Hua, 2016). This index is moderately predictive of death in dogs. Frailty may occur in dogs or cats.

Physical therapy and good pain management are utilized in human medicine and may be a crucial part of helping animals with frailty. More research needs to be done to learn more about this elusive disease process in dogs and cats with frailty.

Hydration/nutrition for the late-stage patient

"An animal who is eating is going to live longer than an animal who is not." This is a common maxum. Adequate nutrition and hydration may be a challenge for clients to maintain for their animals as they develop late-stage disease. There are many different etiologies that may cause Dysrexia (see Dysrexia section). Providing clients options for care after discussing their goals can help the veterinarian formulate a dietary plan. Consulting with a board-certified veterinary nutritionist may expand your tools for nutritional care of the end of life patient.

Although there are numerous studies related to appropriate health and disease-based animal nutrition, there is little research on how to provide adequate nutrition for late-stage animal patients that may be refusing their balanced diet. The authors reviewed human palliative nutritional studies to research novel ways to provide nutrition and hydration for palliative and hospice animal patients.

In addition, animals may have different nutritional and metabolic requirements at the end of life. Nutrition and hydration are essential for sustaining life; however, decreasing metabolic needs in late-stage patients may change their requirements as they approach death. Giving clients additional food options may help reduce family anxiety related to decision-making with late-stage disease.

Goals of care discussion

Humans are social creatures, and food and feeding are part of our social behavior with our animals. Clients may feel that they are not providing adequate care for their pet if the animal is not eating. Establishing the nutritional goals for the pet and then providing tools to clients will help the veterinarian create a nutritional plan. Giving clients a list of additional foods to try that may be more nutritionally sound, or if dysrexic and end stage, high, dense calorie foods to maintain nutrition can empower the client. In addition, helping clients find novel fluid administration that is comfortable for both the client and the animal, can establish a different social interaction with their beloved pet. Helping caregivers with their pet's nutritional needs will strengthen the bond between pet and caregiver. Force feeding an end-stage pet may not extend their life and may break the bond between beloved pet and person.

Managing the primary causes of dysphagia, dysrexia will also contribute to a feeding plan. See other sections on dysphagia and dysrexia for additional medical management.

Comfort feeding

The following list is adapted from a human nutritional toolkit with modifications for use in animals (McAnelly, 2015). Once the animal has stopped eating their balanced diet, the client may offer fresh, or cooked "human" foods. Providing calorically dense foods can help sustain the end-stage patient in the short term. Using dense callory foods allows the patient to receive a more considerable number of calories in smaller portions. In addition, feeding smaller portions q 3–4 h may help animals eat more over a 24 hour period. Clients should be informed that these foods (especially high-fat foods) may cause or exacerbate other adverse symptoms, including pancreatitis, nausea, diarrhea, or vomiting. These foods should only be used with the knowledge that the animal is in late-stage or end-stage disease and that all other options have been exhausted.

The following nutrition and fluid list is based upon our clinical experience. There may be other foods that are not on this list that may be included in the future. Additionally, the options listed below may not encourage an animal to eat. This list is a general guideline.

"Go home and feed him whatever he wants" is a common statement the authors have heard from clients regarding end stage disease and dysrexia. And while it may be true that we need to offer a wide variety of foods, giving the clients direction can help them prepare foods to sustain their animal.

Foods to try for animals who have stopped eating a balanced diet:

Dogs—Low fat/ high carbohydrate: sweet potato, carrots, apples, bananas, pudding. *Lower fat/higher protein foods:* white fish, chicken breast meat, turkey breast meat. *Higher fat/higher protein foods:* steak, hamburger, chicken, chicken soup (low to no sodium), turkey, deli meat (without nitrates is best), baby food (any flavor, meat only, without garlic or onion powder added, ice cream, cheesecake filling, eggs, salmon, crab, lobster, fried chicken, rotisserie chicken, and cat food, etc. *Use with added caution:* bacon (due to high fat content), and peanut butter (as some brands contain Xylitol).

Cats tend to be more interested in higher fat/higher protein foods though they may make them nauseous after eating, especially cats with CKD. For cats consider baby food (any flavor, meat only, without garlic or onion powder added), tuna or other fish, steak, hamburger, chicken, chicken soup (low sodium), blenderized, turkey, deli meat (no nitrates are better), ice cream, eggs, Fancy Feast, Fancy Feast Broths, Friskies other canned food (especially if it is smelly), Churu or Delectables and Iams Ocean Fish. May try the foods listed in the dog comfort food list. Texture can also matter to animals, especially cats. Try various textured food, such as gravy, slurry, and different shapes of dry kibble. It is also possible that trying different surfaces may help encourage appetite with some animals.

Warming foods may help encourage an animal to eat. Creating "gravy" by adding water or broth to kibble or canned food or baby food may encourage and animal to eat and drink. An animal may only eat with hand feeding.

The use of appetite stimulants and anti-nausea medications may be useful and are addressed in other sections. Please see the section on dysrexia for more information.

Supplementing hydration status with additional fluids

Hydration is an important aspect of care for with patients at any time and especially at the end-of-life. To assess hydration, the veterinarian or the client can evaluate skin turgor, mucus membrane moisture. For animals who are mildly dehydrated (5%) the skin turgor (or the ability of the skin to return to normal position after being pinched or pulled up at the scruff) is normal or minimally changed, mucus membranes in the mouth should be slightly tacky. For moderate dehydration (8%), there is a moderate change in skin turgor and mucus membranes are dry. Eyes may look somewhat sunken. For severe dehydration (10–12%), there is a significant change in skin turgor and mucus membranes are very dry. Eyes may appear very sunken (Scherk, 2018).

For the home care veterinarian, providing adequate hydration to animals who are dehydrated, either due to disease, or lack of intake may be challenging to handle. These animals may be generally painful, very thin, have oral ulcers, or other disease processes that make it difficult for them to take in oral fluids. IV fluid therapy is ideal, however, in the home, SQ fluids could be considered for supplementation. The client should be made aware of their options. There are many different formulas to calculate fluid requirements. Using a formula: for example, body weight (BW) in kilograms (KG) × 60 mL/day to calculate the daily requirement for a healthy animal and then multiplying that by the presumed additional need (i.e., 1.5–2 times for a dehydrated animal, or one that has a constant loss, such as in renal failure or diarrhea) will give the veterinarian an approximate daily fluid requirement for the animal. Supplementation of the daily requirement may be influenced by how much fluid the animal may be taking in orally daily, and then supplementing the loss. Monitoring both the body weight fluctuations and measuring the fluids daily may help more accurately maintain the hydration needs of the patient. Mild to moderately dehydrated patients may be able to be maintained in the home setting, severely dehydrated patients may require IV fluid therapy in a hospital setting, or the clients may consider euthanasia or palliative sedation if the client does not elect euthanasia.

Some animals will not tolerate having SQ fluids given and may need oral fluid supplementation. Utilizing a formula, oral supplementation can be divided into multiple supplementations over a 24 hour period and may include ice cubes/chips in water, slightly warmed water, water added to canned or dry food, commercial (no sodium added) or homemade broth, water based tuna juice, Fancy Feast Broths, or other dog or cat broths on the market. The client will have to be diligent in monitoring the ins and outs by measuring the fluids daily, and weight of the animal daily to help maintain hydration.

Giving medications in a novel way

In addition, having novel ways of giving medications to animals is an important tool for the house call veterinarian. Animals who are anorexic or hyporexic may not take their medications that have been given orally because the client has been giving them in food, which then increases the likelihood the animal will be in distress or have pain. Animals may also excel at spitting out pills, and many clients do not want to or are not able to place medication into the back of the throat of an animal. Tools for giving medications to an anorexic or hyporexic animal may include:

- *Creating novel forms of medications*: Compounding the current medications into different forms, liquids, transdermal, suppository, injectable.
- *Using highly palatable and malleable foods*: Pill pockets, shredded cheese or raw hamburger may help hide a pill or capsule. (Use raw foods with caution).
- *Sticky substances*: The client can mix the medication in Karo syrup or honey and rub it on their gums. This works best with medications that are not time released and can be crushed or powder removed from a capsule. This is a novel way to give crisis medications.
- *Peanut Butter*: The client can try mixing medications with a small amount of peanut or other nut butter and place it on the roof of their mouth, though they may be able to get it out of their mouth. Make sure the peanut butter or other nut butter does not contain xylitol. For dogs only.
- *Novel combinations of food*: The client can try one of the foods listed for the client and see if the pet is interested and will eat a novel food and then hide it in the novel food. They can also double up on novel foods, for example, placing medication in peanut butter on bread and hiding it with the bread, or place pill in cream cheese and then wrap cream cheese with raw bacon. These combinations

may have to change on occasion with very smart dogs to continue to give medications to dogs.

- *Gelatin Capsules*: The client can place the medication(s) in a gelatin capsule and hide it in food. Works well with bitter medications such as tramadol.

Hypercalcemia
Etiology/DDX

Hypercalcemia may occur due to one or more factors. A number of hormones, cytokines have been associated with the development of hypercalcemia and include osteoclast activating factor, parathyroid hormone-related protein parathyroid hormone (PTH), 1,25-dihydroxyvitamin D, humoral hypercalcemia of malignancy has cytokines such as interleukin-1 and tumor necrosis factor, prostaglandins, and humoral factors such as renal 1-alpha-hydroxylase. Hypercalcemia in the end-stage patient may result in the weakening of bone and can also have secondary clinical signs that may influence decision making.

Common differentials seen in late stage veterinary patients for hypercalcemia include lymphoma, anal gland adenocarcinoma, primary hyperparathyroidism, secondary hyperparathyroidism, CKD, carcinomas, such as mammary, squamous cell, nasal, multiple myeloma, primary bone neoplasia, or metastasis to the bone, granulomatous inflammation (i.e., fungal), Addison's disease (Nelson, 2010).

Clinical signs

Hypercalcemia may affect a number of systems including the neuromuscular, gastrointestinal (GI), kidney, and cardiac systems. Animals with hypercalcemia may develop neuromuscular signs such as tremors, cardiac arrhythmias, weakness, confusion, become stuporous, or become comatose. Animals who have hypercalcemia may develop delirium (Rothrock, K. S., 2020a,b). Pain may be seen in patients with hypercalcemia. Pain may present as generalized, referred or patients may have specific bone pain. GI signs can also occur with hypercalcemia, including nausea, gastrointestinal ulcers, and constipation. Animals may secondarily develop polyuria and polydipsia from tubular insensitivity to antidiuretic hormone (ADH) and secondary diabetes insipidus. Chronic hypercalcemia may have the sequalae of ischemic kidney damage, calcification, calciuria, and irreversible kidney damage, in addition to calcium deposits forming in other organs, skin (Rothrock, K. S., 2020a,b).

Palliative management

Manage the primary disease: Treating the underlying disease is the first step to treating hypercalcemia (see the appropriate section for management of specific disease or symptom).

Hydration of the animal: Hydration with SQ or preferably IV fluids may helps to treat the clinical signs of hypercalcemia. If symptomatic, consider hospitalization and IV fluids. If the patient is not movable, or the client elects to stay home providing SQ fluids, adding in a a loop diuretic such as furosemide and/or steroids can help to decrease calcium levels.

Diuretics and steroids: Furosemide 2—4 mg/kg q 8—12 h IV or SQ can help after the correction of dehydration (VIN staff, 2017). Steroids such as prednisone at 1—2 mg/kg q 12 h PO or SQ, may help (VIN staff, 2017). Steroids may decrease the reabsorption of calcium in the bowel, and they increase calciuresis (Bodtke, 2016).

Calcitonin and Bisphosphonates: Calcitonin can help decrease hypercalcemia, and bisphosphonates are now being utilized for hypercalcemia more in veterinary patients (Rothrock, K. S., 2020a,b). Calcitonin 4—8 U/kg SQ q 2—4 h for dogs and cats (VIN Staff, 2017). Bisphosphonates that may be used are pamidronate 1—2 mg/kg IV over 2 h, zoledronate 0.25 mg/kg IV over 15 min, alendronate 2—4 mg/kg q 7 days PO (Rothrock, K. S., 2020a,b). Zoledronate may be preferable in the home setting over the other two bisphosphonates because of the shortened time to give IV (when compared to pamidronate), and it is more bioavailable than alendronate.

Gabapentinoids: Gabapentin or pregabalin may decrease the clinical neurologic symptoms of hypercalcemia by inhibiting the Ca^{++} channels in the CNS (Sutton, 2002).

Gastrointestinal medications: Nausea may be alleviated with Cerenia or ondansetron. Constipation may be due to changes in motility or mechanical changes due to one or more tumors. Consider a stool softener such as, Miralax or Lactulose along with IV or SQ fluids if there is constipation. If phosphate binders are required, aluminum hydroxide should be considered instead of calcium salt-based medications.

Delirium: If the patient develops delirium, it may be a point to discuss euthanasia with a client or they may consider euthanasia. See section on Delirium for further treatment.

Hypertension

Senior, late-stage, and end-of-life patients may develop hypertension secondarily to an underlying disease. Primary hypertension in dogs and cats is rare. Situational hypertension may occur because of transient increase in the sympathetic nervous system. House call veterinarians are in a unique position to evaluate animals in their environment and may be able to assess hypertension in this population of animals better due to the decreased stress response in the home. Having a standard protocol for blood pressure measurements are essential and making sure the same individual and the same equipment and location is used and documented should be part of the protocol (Acierno et al., 2018; Acierno, 2018).

Etiology/DDX

Hypertension is defined as a sustained systolic pressure greater than 160. Primary idiopathic hypertension may seen in cats with no known disease though it is rare (Acierno et al., 2018). More commonly in cats, secondary hypertension is related to a disease such as chronic renal failure or hyperthyroidism. Less common causes in cats include primary hyperaldosteronism, diabetes melliatus, hyperadrenocorticism, and pheochromocytoma (Acierno et al., 2018). Differentials for secondary hypertension in dogs may include, chronic renal failure, diabetes mellitus, hyperthyroidism, hyperadrenocorticism, pheochromocytoma, and hyperaldosteronism are the most common diseases associated with hypertension (Dixon-Jimenez, 2020). Some medications may also elevate blood pressure, NSAIDs, glucocorticoids, phenylpropanolamine, ephedrine, erythropoietin, mineralocorticoids, and DDAVP (Acierno et al., 2018).

Long term hypertension can damage organs, including changes seen in the brain, heart, blood vessels, eyes, and kidney. Keeping hypertension stable can help ease clinical signs associated with hypertension.

Clinical signs of hypertension

There may be no clinical signs at the time of discovery of hypertension. However, as the animal has persistent hypertension, clinical signs may occur. Early clinical signs may include howling, or vocalizations, head pressing, sudden blindness, or abnormal behavior that may include ataxia, altered mentation, and disorientation (Acierno et al., 2018). Further examination may elucidate retinal hemorrhage or detached retinas, vestibular-like events, transient or fulminant strokes, seizures, epistaxis, and collapse (Ware, 1999; Acierno et al., 2018).

Palliative management

For dogs, consider starting with an ACE inhibitor, such as benazepril or and angiotensin II receptor antagonist, telmisartan. Benazepril dose Dogs: 0.5 mg/kg PO q 12−24 h, dose may be increased incrementally up to 2 mg/kg divided into twice a day dosing. Cats: 0.5 mg/kg q 24 h, Telmisartan dose Dogs/Cats: 0.5−1 mg/kg PO q 24 h (VIN staff, 2017). Dogs with pheochromocytoma may need a secondary therapeutic such as τ-(phenoxybenzamine) and β-blockers (atenolol) or surgical excision. Amlodipine and spironolactone may also be helpful to decrease hypertension in a dog (Acierno et al., 2018).

For cats, amlodipine is the primary hypertension medication in proteinuric cats with moderate-to-severe hypertension, Adding an ACE inhibitor, may be helpful, if amlodipine is not decreasing the hypertension. Semintra is a telmisartan (angiotensin II receptor antagonist), FDA approved drug for cats. Amlodipine dose: Cats: 0.625−1.25 mg per cat PO q 12−24 h, Dogs 0.1−0.5 mg/kg PO q 12−24 h (VIN staff, 2017).

In humans, as they become a late-stage to end-stage in their disease, medical doctors may remove, or minimize the patients hypertension medications, as the patient may become hypotensive on the medication and should be a consideration in veterinary patients. Regular monitoring of patients can help minimize this issue for veterinary patients. If the patient's hypertension is stable, monitor monthly and adjust medications as needed. If the patient's hypertenstion is unstable or they are symptomatic, monitor the blood pressure more frequently, daily, or weekly, until symptoms subside or the animal approaches death (Acierno et al., 2018).

Liver cancer and other late-stage liver diseases
Etiology/DDX

Providing palliatve care for patients with late-stage liver disease in the home is not as commonly seen as in the hospital setting. Most liver diseases treated in the home are neoplastic in origin, most commonly hepatocellular carcinoma. Acute hepatic failure may also occur because of infection such as canine adenovirus 1, leptospiroisis, toxoplasma, leishmania, inflammation, toxin, gall bladder diseases such as cholangiohepatitis, biliary mucocoele and hepatic lipidosis. Chronic liver failure may occur due to chronic hepatitis, copper storage disease, endocrine diseases, such as diabetes mellitus, Cushings and cirrhosis from chronic illness. This section is going to focus on hepatic neoplasia and the chronic symptoms arising from hepatic failure as these are more common with end stage patients and in the home setting and there are references available that go into more depth.

Types of liver cancer seen in dogs
Bile duct carcinoma
    Carcinoid or endocrine carcinoma
    Hemangiosarcoma and other sarcomas
    Hepatoma or hepatocellular carcinoma
    Mast cell tumors.
    Metastasis (VSSO Staff, 2021a,b).
Liver cancer seen in cats
Bile duct carcinoma
    Carcinoid or neuroendocrine carcinoma
    Hemangiosarcoma and other sarcomas hepatoma or hepatocellular carcinoma
    Myelolipoma
    Mast cell tumors
    Lymphoma
    Liver sarcoma (VSSO Staff, 2021a,b).

Clinical signs

Clinical signs and complications for hepatic neoplasia may include ascites, hepatic encephalopathy, thrombus, coagulopathies, or thrombocytopenia. Infections may also occur. Pain may increase in significance especially as tumors grow. Patients may develop visceral hypersensitivity as well (Christian-Miller, 2018). Visceral hypersensitivity occurs due to inflammation, tumor cytokines, and neuropathic changes in the CNS (Christian-Miller, 2018). In addition, hepatocellular carcinoma or other hepatic tumors may metastasize to bone and create bone pain (see the Osteosarcoma section for further information regarding pain management) (Christian-Miller, 2018; VSSO Staff, 2021a,b). Clinical signs for hepatic encephalopathy can include confusion, inappetence, dullness, irritability, lethargy, ataxia, personality changes, head pressing, sudden blindness, disorientation, incoordination, confusion, stupor, ptyalism, seizures, coma, and death (Salgado, 2013).

Cirrhosis may occur with chronic liver diseases. Cirrhosis of the liver may develop into portal hypertension and hepatorenal syndrome (the kidneys fail secondarily to liver failure). Cirrhotic liver patients may also develop coagulopathies such as disseminated intravascular coagulopathy (DIC). Cirrhosis may also alter the liver's ability to process medications, by changing the ability to absorb the bioavailability of some medications, altering the Cytochrome P450 metabolism, and changing hepatic and, therefore, renal clearance of the medication. Change in dosing of medication should be considered in animals with cirrhosis, or suspected liver failure.

Palliative management for late-stage liver disease

Early palliative care is beneficial for liver disease (Woodrell, 2018). Working with a general practitioner or specialist to get the patient access to timely palliative care can help improve their long-term quality of life and gives additional support to the caregivers.

Pain management: For hepatic neoplasia, pain management is complex. Patients may have pain that may include components of, nociceptive, inflammatory, and neuropathic pain and visceral hypersensitivity. In addition, hepatic neoplasia becomes more painful over time (Christian-Miller, 2018).

Nociceptive Pain: For acute or severe chronic pain, opioids should be considered. Tramadol, while having opioid properties in cats, should not be utilized as it needs to metabolize via the liver. Buprenorphine and morphine may be considered for use in cats due to glucuronidation metabolism. Fentanyl, methadone, and hydromorphone all utilize cytochrome P450 metabolism and may be less bioavailable but may be used for dogs and cats with hepatic disease. Codeine should be avoided (Soleimanpour, 2016). Acetaminophen/paracetamol may be used, but with caution. Dogs only: 10 mg/kg PO q 12 h (VIN staff, 2017).

Neuropathic pain: The neuropathic component of pain can be treated with gabapentin or pregabalin, or an antidepressant, such as amitriptyline. Gabapentin Dogs: 3–20 mg/kg PO 1–3 times per day. Cats: 3–10 mg/kg PO q 8–24 h (can go higher if needed, likely more sedative) Dogs: Pregabalin is administered at a dosage of 2–4 mg/kg orally three times a day (Kent, 2012). Cats: studies of pregabalin in cats are still limited, but the starting dose we are using for this species is 1–2 mg/kg q 12 h (Dewey, 2019). Amitriptyline: neuropathic pain: dogs: 1–2 mg/kg PO q12–24h, cats: 0.5–2 mg/kg PO SID may be helpful in addition to NSAIDs. Dosing should start on the lower end and increase as needed over time (Christian-Miller, 2018).

Inflammatory pain: Drugs to use with caution in patients with liver failure include NSAIDs especially with cirrhosis. See list of NSAIDs in pain management chapter.

Visceral hypersensitivity: Cerenia may be useful for serosal pain. Cerenia dosing: Dogs: 2 mg/kg PO q 24 h, 1 mg/kg SQ q 24 h, Cats: 1 mg/kg PO q 24 h, or 0.5 mg/kg SQ q24 h (VIN staff, 2017).

Palliative radiation therapy is provided for pain management in people and could be considered with animals, and clients should discuss this with an oncologist.

Treatment for other sequale of hepatic disease:

Hepatic encephalopathy: Hepatic encephalopathy may be treated with lactulose orally or via rectal administration to help lower the ammonia levels. Delirium may still occur without raised ammonia levels (see Delirium section of this chapter to rule out other causes). Lactulose 1−3 mL/10 kg PO q6-8 h, adjusted to produce 2−3 soft stools a day (Salgado, 2013). Although diarrhea may be a separate issue an antibiotic may be useful. (see Diarrhea section in this chapter for further information). Neomycin 20 mg/kg PO q 12 h for 3−5 days. Or Metronidazole 7.5 mg/kg PO q 8−12 h (Salgado, 2013). Seizures can be treated with Levetiracetam 20 mg/kg IV or PO q 8 h (Salgado, 2013).

Nutraceuticals, Vitamins, Antioxidants: Hepatoprotective nutraceuticals such as SAM-e, Milk Thistle or silibinin may be helpful with hepatic neoplasia, hepatic encephalopathy or liver failure. Vitamin E may help as an antioxidant. Liver diets are available that may contain antioxidants and vitamins (Webster et al., 2019).

Ascites: (see the Ascites section for additional information and treatments) may occur, and because of ascites, dyspnea can be a sequelae. Increased respiratory effort and rate may also occur because of pain and/or metabolic changes.

Hypoglycemia: Hypoglycemia resulting from liver failure may be treated in the home with an oral Karo syrup or honey, to effect (VIN Staff, 2017). In addition, feeding small meals, throughout the day may help keep the glucose more stable.

Clotting disorders: If there are coagulopathies resulting from end-stage hepatic disease, (see Bleeding section), fresh frozen plasma transfusions or vitamin K may be used to treat these. While fresh frozen plasma transfusions are rarely administered in the house call environment. vitamin K1 2.5−5 mg/kg PO q 24 h may be more easily added to the home treatment plan (VIN staff, 2017). This would be warranted if prothrombin (PT) is elevated due to vitamin K deficiency, malnutrition, cirrhosis, or cholestatic hepatic disease. Vitamin K supplementation can be provided for the rest of the life of the animal (both dogs and cats) if indicated.

Metastasis

The spread of neoplasia is a concern for the client. The progression of cancer may influence decision making and to be prepared to answer questions for clients, we will briefly review. Metastasis may initiate by extending into the local interstitial tissue, progressing to a nearby lymph node or blood vessel. The microenvironment contains proteins including, cytokines, collagen, fibrin, growth factors which may interact with the tumor cell, and the tumor cell genetics and epigenetics may play a role in metastasis. In addition, the immune system and the microbiome may also play a role. The tumor cells may prime the microenvironment of metastasis, sending out secretory factors and extracellular vesicles prior to sending invading tumor cells. Messenger RNA helps the tumor prime these new sites (Fares, Fares, Khachfe, Salhab, & Fares, 2020). Understanding the progression of metastasis is ongoing in studies in both human and veterinary medicine. Predicting sites of metastasis has been documented in human medicine to a greater extent as compared to in veterinary medicine. Literature on metastasis in humans may help veterinarians to predict the likelihood of spread, as well as the anatomic locations of spread, in the species we work with until further end-of-life studies in veterinary species become available (Fig. 5.10). The following figure indicates the progression of metastasis.

There are four primary sites that can become foci for metastases to occur: lung, bone, liver, and brain. There are also secondary sites of metastasis that include, kidneys, spleen, peritoneum and thoracic cavity, and skin. A review of the literature on human-based metastasis finds common areas of metastasis for specific cancers. Human mammary and prostate cancers have a high affinity to metastasize to bone, ovary, pancreas, and gallbladder (National Cancer Institute, 2017). Rectal/anal/colon/S.I./stomach cancers tend to metastasize to peritoneum, liver, and intra-abdominal lymph nodes (National Cancer Institute, 2017). The head and neck cancers tend to metastasize to the lymph nodes of the head, face, and neck and then to bone and lung (National Cancer Institute, 2017). The other cancers studied, lung, prostate, bone, kidney, liver, esophagus, uterus, and skin, tend to have a more randomized metastasis. This infographic shows anatomical proximity and connection to metastasis in people (Fig. 5.11).

Lung metastasis is the most common site of metastasis for most cancer types. Metastasis may be in the form of pulmonary nodules (most common) or pleural nodules and fluid in the pleural space, carcinomatosis, or endobronchial tumors (Herold, 1996). Metastasis to the lungs may develop bleeding (depending on the tumor type) or pulmonary edema (which tends to occur late or end stage), and occasionally a spontaneous pneumothorax or ventilation-perfusion (V/Q) mismatch (Popper, 2016). In humans, dyspnea secondary to pulmonary metastasis may be treated with opioids, bronchodilators, and anticholinergics for excessive bronchial secretions. Furosemide may help those with pulmonary edema, however, since pulmonary edema tends to be an end-stage sign, it may only used towards the very end of life. Nebulized opioids or inhaled nitrous oxide have also been used to treat dyspnea in those patients who cannot take medications orally. Oxygen therapy is also helpful for those with pulmonary metastasis who are dyspneic (Popper, 2016).

Brain metastasis: Primary lung cancer, mammary cancerand melanomas commonly metastasize to the brain in humans (Soffietti, 2002). For patients with a solitary brain mass, surgery may be recommended along with radiation (Soffietti, 2002). For those who have tumors refractory to radiation or have multiple masses, chemotherapy or stereotactic radiation is utilized (Lu-Emerson, 2012). People

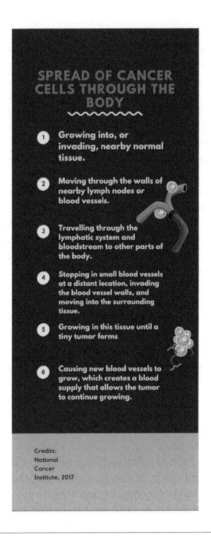

FIGURE 5.10

Metastasis.

Reproduced from the National Cancer Institute website 2017, used with permission from the National Cancer Institute© 2021. Created on Canva by Mina Weakley and Lynn Hendrix © 2021.

with brain metastasis have symptoms that include headaches, seizures, vomiting, ±nausea, changes in smell, behavior, and changes in their ability to breathe, swallow, hear, and move in addition to lethargy (Lu-Emerson, 2012). Humans with brain metastasis are prone to thromboembolic complications. Treatments involve controlling clinical signs. Palliative radiation may help. Gamma knife radio-surgery is used in humans for treatment or palliation. Treatment of pain includes opioids and acetaminophen and steroids. Seizures may occur with primary brain tumors and secondary metastasis and can be treated with anti-seizure medications;

TYPICAL SITES OF METASTASIS BASED ON CANCER TYPE IN HUMANS

Cancer Type	Main Sites of Metastasis (humans)
Bladder	bone, liver, lung
Breast	bone, brain, liver, lung
Colon	liver, lung, peritoneum
Kidney	adrenal gland, bone, brain, liver, lung
Lung	adrenal gland, bone, brain, liver, other lung tissue from primary tumor
Melanoma	bone, brain, liver, lung, skin, muscle
Ovary	liver, lung, peritoneum
Pancreas	liver, lung, peritoneum
Prostate	adrenal gland, bone, liver, lung
Rectal	liver, lung, peritoneum
Stomach	liver, lung, peritoneum
Thyroid	bone, liver, lung
Uterus	bone, liver, lung, peritoneum, vagina

FIGURE 5.11

Typical sites of metastasis in humans. Information from the National Cancer Institute.

Graphic created on Canva by Mina Weakley and Lynn Hendrix ©2021. Used with permission and with attribution from the National Cancer Institute 2021. Canva used in graphic creation.

refractive seizures may need multiple medications (see the Seizure section for drug dosing). Steroids may also be useful for primary brain tumors, metastasis. Nausea may also occur and may be treated with Cerenia or ondansetron or both (see Nausea section for drug dosing) (Steigleder, 2013).

Liver metastasis: The types of cancer that tend to spread to the liver include GI, lung, mammary, and pancreatic cancers. Patients with liver metastasis often form ascites, which can lead to nausea, discomfort, pain, and difficulty breathing. Treatment for humans is local palliative radiation (Yang, 2016). Palliative management for hepatic metastasis is located in the liver disease section.

Bone metastasis: Bone metastasis is painful and may occur with many tumor types. Clinical signs may include pain, swelling, fever, urinary or fecal incontinence, pathologic fractures, hypercalcemia. See Osteosarcoma and Hypercalcemia for additional palliative treatments.

Palliative management: For metastasis management, see individual areas suspected for more specific information on treating that organ system.

Some additional notes: Steroids are often used for a patient with a brain tumor, primary or metastatic. Prednisone or prednisolone 0.5–2 mg/kg PO SID-BID for the remaining life of the pet.

Opioids may be used with end-stage brain metastasis; however, it is best to avoid opioids, such as Fentanyl, that may raise intracranial pressure.

NSAIDs should be avoided in late-stage liver metastasis. Steroids may be used with caution and tylenol (acetaminophen dose for dogs only: 10–15 mg/kg PO q 8–12 h) should be used with caution in dogs with liver metastasis.

Nausea/vomiting

Nausea can be an insidious component of late-stage disease. The clinical signs of nausea may include decreased or absent appetite, licking of lips, or lip smacking, restlessness, excessive ptylism, swallowing, pica, borborygmi, lethargy, turning their head away from food when offered, retching, gagging, vomiting. However, nausea in people can have absent signs and clients may not recognize other nausea signs before animals become anorexic or start vomiting. If expected or anticipated, we can catch signs of nausea earlier in addition to preparing clients with medications in their crisis kits for nausea and vomiting.

Etiology/DDX: Nausea may be separate from vomiting. An animal can be nauseous without vomiting, however the vomiting animal is always nauseous. Nausea should be treated if the animal is not eating. There is an extensive list of the etiology of nausea/vomiting which may be found in other references. Listed here are the common differentials of vomiting seen at the end of life patient.

1. Neoplasia: primary gastrointestinal, renal, liver, splenic, brain, and metastasis/carcinomotosis
2. acute renal failure, renal neoplasia
3. Acute or chronic liver failure, hepatic lipidosis, hepatic neoplasia
4. Congestive heart failure
5. Inflammatory bowel disease
6. Medications, such as NSAIDs, chemotherapy, steroids, and antibiotics (Tams, 2003)
7. Radiation therapy may cause nausea and vomiting in cancer patients
8. Vestibular disease
9. Foreign bodies are not as common in the elderly, though it may happen. However, if a young animal has a terminal illness, it is more likely to occur secondarily to their terminal illness and contribute to vomiting.
10. Dehydration may also contribute to vomiting and nausea.

Palliative management of nausea and vomiting

If the client approves, identify and correct the source of the vomiting with appropriate testing and treatment.

Fluid therapy may be helpful if dehydrated or there is continued fluid loss.

Remove medications that are known to cause vomiting, at least temporarily.

Add an anti-emetic, or anti-nausea medication: Cerenia® (Maropitant)-Dogs 2 mg/kg PO, Cats 1 mg/kg (VIN Staff, 2017).

Ondansetron- Dogs 0.1−1 mg/kg PO, Cats 0.5−1 mg/kg PO (VIN Staff, 2017).

Consider a prokinetic, such as metoclopramide or erythromycin, if obstruction is not suspected. Metoclopramide 0.2−0.5 mg/kg q 8−12 h SQ, PO for dogs and cats (VIN Staff, 2017).

Crisis kit

It is good to include injectable Cerenia at 2 mg/kg for dogs or 1 mg/kg for cats given SQ or Ondansetron meltaway tablets at 1 mg/kg PO for dogs and cats (VIN staff, 2017). A bag of fluids, an IV set, and needles may also be included in the crisis kit in order to ameliorate dehydration in animals who are vomiting. Instructions on how to give SQ fluids should be included in the crisis kit.

Neuromuscular disease

Degenerative myelopathy

Etiology/DDX

Canine degenerative myelopathy (CDM) is a progressive neuromuscular disease affecting upper and lower motor neurons significantly with large and giant breed dogs, which tends to occur in middle age (Morgan, 2016; Story et al., 2020). Prembroke Welsh Corgi's also can develop CDM. Amyotrophic lateral sclerosis (ALS) is a degenerative disease affecting nerves in the motor cortex and spinal cord, mainly affecting both upper and lower motor neurons in humans (Story et al., 2020). There is a proliferation of microglia, astrocytes, and oligodendrocytes causing a neuroinflammatory response. Degenerative myelopathy is genetically related to ALS in humans. Both have a mutation in the super dioxide dismutase one gene (SOD-1), though it is a small percentage of people compared to dogs who present with this mutation (Nardone, 2016). Degenerative myelopathy initially has upper motor neuron signs and as the disease progresses also affects lower motor neurons. ALS is not generally diagnosed until upper and lower motor neurons are both affected. CDM is diagnosed postmortum with changes in the axons. Degeneration, and demylination of axons are noted as well as astroglia proliferation. The sensory degeneration does occur, generally before motor neuron degeneration and should be considered when treating (Nardone, 2016; Morgan, 2016). Additional clinical signs of sensory degeneration for ALS is included in the following section.

Canine degenerative myelpathy (CDM) is considered a good model of study for ALS. Differentials may include intravetebral disc disease, osteoarthritis, neoplasia, cruciate ruptures (Story et al., 2020).

Clinical signs

The clinical signs of ALS are similar to the clinical signs veterinarians observe with CDM. There are stages of ALS, early, mid, late, and end-stage, and like CDM, are progressive. A review of both the stages of ALS and corresponding observations in veterinary patients is warranted. The authors recognize translational medicine is not exact, however, since these two diseases share a genetic trait and phenotypic clinical signs a review seems appropriate.

Early stages of ALS may include fatigue, poor balance, and tripping when walking (the authors have had clients comment that their dog "is just slowing down or aging"). The clinical signs for the middle stage of ALS becomes more evident; muscles may twitch, lose muscle mass, muscle contracture is sometimes seen and have a hard time getting up without assistance, starting to see weakness in swallowing, choking, difficulty eating, and coughing (veterinarians might see concurrent laryngeal paralysis—GOLPP). People report ALS in this stage to be a painful condition, with paresthesia, "pins and needles type pain", shooting pain, and muscle fasciculations (Morgan, 2016; Nardone, 2016). Patients in the late stages of ALS, may need a wheelchair due to limited mobility, they may also experience fatigue, headaches, and susceptibility to pneumonia. End-stage ALS is associated with, Decreasing appetite and fluid intake, and finally, respiratory failure happens with most ALS patients, less common sequelae to death may be due to, pulmonary embolism, cardiac arrhythmias, and pneumonia from aspiration (Bodtke, 2016).

To continue until the end of a dogs CDM disease is a rare occurrence in the United States. The vast majority of dogs are euthanized as soon as they lose the ability to rise, or walk, in the author's experience. In the case of late-stage degenerative myelopathy, animals will need a wheelchair or wagon. If they get to end-stage disease, dogs may need assistance eating and drinking and are prone to develop aspiration pneumonia. ALS patients will eventually lose the ability to speak, eat, and breathe. They die of respiratory failure, with humans, researchers looked at suffocation and found 90% of patients hypoventilate, become hypercapnic, and lose consciousness before respiratory failure (van Leeuwen, 2013). There is a grading scale developed by Morgan, et.al. available for CDM. Most dogs are euthanized prior to Grade 4. Grade 1 starts with paraparesis and general proprioceptive ataxia which may include progressive general proprioceptive ataxia with corresponding conscious proprioceptive deficits, asymmetric and spastic paraparesis, and intact spinal reflexes. Grade 2 adds nonambulatory paraparesis to paraplegia in pelvic limbs with mild to moderate muscle loss in the pelvic limbs, decreased to absent spinal reflexes in pelvic limbs and urinary and fecal incontinence may occur at this stage. Grade 3 develops when there is thoracic limb weakness and flaccid pelvic limbs with an absence of reflexes and severe muscle loss in pelvic limbs. Dogs with Grade 3

CDM have developed urinary and fecal incontinence. Grade 4 occurs when all 4 limbs are flaccid and develop brain stem signs, such as difficulty swallowing, dyspnea. The brain stem signs will progress to respiratory failure and death (Morgan, 2016).

Palliative management

Rehabilitation: Physical rehabilitation and underwater treadmill therapy can help strengthen muscles and help animals maintain their balance for as long as possible (Staff of MSU, 2021). Adding a certified canine rehabilitation practitioner to the end-of-life team may help the quality of life of the degenerative myelopathy patient. Physical therapy techniques clients may be able to perform at home can include back stepping, side stepping, sit/down/stand, Cavaletti's with 5 poles to walk across (clients can use large dowels, ladders, or broomsticks many examples of DIY tools are available on YouTube videos), weight shifting, and walking on uneven surfaces, spins, and stairs (Staff of MSU, 2021).

Physical support aids: Having a Help 'em Up Harness (or equivalent) with a harness for the front limbs and a harness for the hind limbs can help clients to assist animals with mobility and also with getting up from the ground. Orthotics, booties, toe-up wraps and other devices to increase traction may help with mobility. Keeping the patient's nails short can also help the animal get up and down and maintain stability. More information on wheelchairs and other aids in the Physical Support chapter.

Acupuncture: Acupuncture may be a therapeutic that has been proposed to slow the progression of CDM (Silva, 2017). More research needs to be done to evaluate the efficacy of acupuncture in the progression of the disease.

Pain management: NSAIDs and acetaminophen may be a good first-line pain therapy for CDM. In addition to an anti-inflammatory, antidepressants such as amitriptyline may also be considered as a first line pain medication.

Gabapentin or pregabalin may be useful; however, it has been reported that some dogs get weaker while taking gabapentin. Gabapentin dose for neuropathic pain: dogs: 3–5 mg/kg PO q12–24h to start, increasing up to 10–20 mg/kg PO q 8–12 hours as needed (VIN staff, 2017).

NMDA antagonists may be neuroprotective and may be beneficial for CDM. Subanesthetic ketamine SQ 0.5–1 mg/kg SQ PRN (anecdotal. May need to be given monthly or more frequently. Studies need to be done to assess the efficacy) Amantadine dogs, cats: 2–5 mg/kg PO q 12–24 h (VIN staff, 2017). Start on the lower end of the dosing and timing and increase as needed.

If patients have severe, unrelenting, or acute pain, opioids would be appropriate to use and should be included in a crisis kit for degenerative myelopathy.

Antioxidants: Antioxiants may be useful in the treatment of CDM, however, have not been shown to slow or stop the progression. Consider a diet change to one of the diets for cognitive dysfunction for additional antioxidants. Vitamin B12 may be useful in slowing the progression of CDM (Story et al., 2020).

Laryngeal paralysis/Geriatric Onset Laryngeal Paralysis and Polyneuropathy (GOLPP)

Etiology/DDX

Dogs may develop laryngeal paralysis that may be congenital or acquired via trauma, neoplasia, endocrinopathy, or idiopathic, and moreover may also develop polyneuropathy. In a recent study, a gene that may be associated with GOLPP, contactin-associated protein 1 CNTNAP1, was found in Labs, Leonbergers, and Saint Bernards (Letko, 2020). In addition, there are other genes that have been identified that may be contributing to the GOLPP, *ARHGEF10* and *GJA9* and a mutation in *RAPGEF6 gene* (Hadji Rasouliha, 2019). Further studies may elucidate whether these genes that may contribute to degenerative myelopathy. GOLPP is most commonly diagnosed in geriatric, large breed dogs 8–13 yrs of age.

Clinical signs—The clinical signs of laryngeal paralysis may include harsh upper airway stridor, a change in the tone of vocalizations and bark, throat clearing, and non-productive cough. The patient may have additional polyneuropathy signs which may include, signs similar to degenerative myelopathy such as paresis in pelvic limbs initially, moving to thoracic limbs in later stages, sarcopenia, and difficulty rising from a sit or laying position or laying down from a standing position, pain.

Emergency clinical signs of laryngeal paralysis: stridor, dyspnea especially in hot weather, heatstroke, and aspiration pneumonia.

Palliative management

Clients may consider surgery a significant decision that they may struggle with. However, the surgery Unilateral Arytenoid Lateralization may be palliative and can extend the life of the dog. One possible complication is that this surgery may predispose patients to is aspiration pneumonia.

Rehabilitation may help patients with GOLPP. Having a veterinarian trained in rehabilitation on the veterinary team can provide additional support for the patient and may help extend the quality of life. The underwater treadmill can help improve strength and stablity in the limbs and improve range of motion. A Transcutaneous Electrical Nerve Stimulation (TENS) unit may help stimulate muscles which may help with pai. See the list of rehabilitation exercises that a client may be able to do at home in the degenerative myelopathy section. Another therapy that has been utilized is acupuncture. Some studies suggest that acupuncture may help improve their quality of life (Silva, 2017).

Other non-medical strategies to consider for a dog with GOLPP may include, keeping the dog in a cooled indoor area and only walking in the early morning or late evening hours especially during hot months. Xanthan gum can thicken water to help swallow it and feeding meatballs can also help to prevent aspiration pneumonia.

Passive air flow on the face helps with breathlessness. A fan, especially at night for white noise, helps keep cool, increases passive airflow, and may help the dog sleep at night. Directing air on the dog's face may be most effective; however, moving the fan every time the animal moves may not be practical.

Crisis kit

The crisis kit should include an opioid, acepromazine, or gabapentin to calm a patient that becomes anxious (leading to increased stridor or dyspnea). Placing a fan and nebulization and cooling of the room may help the animal with breathlessness. The disease trajectory for laryngeal paralysis or GOLPP can fluctuate with periods of normalcy and periods of emergency respiratory distress.

Musculoskeletal issues
Osteoarthritis

Osteoarthritis is one of the most common geriatric diseases for both dogs and cats. Osteoarthritis (OA) is also known as degenerative joint disease. There may be many risk factors that lead to OA, genetics, age, sex, obesity, previous joint trauma, or cruciate ligament tear (Anderson, 2020). Genetics is the most influential risk factor with conformation of joints playing a large role. It is reported that 20% of dogs over one year of age have radiographic signs of OA in North America (Anderson, 2020). Up to 65% have radiographic changes consistent with OA (Morgan, 2016). For cats, the clinical signs of OA may not be recognised until late stages and may be underdiagnosed. In one retrospective study, 22% of 491 cats ages one and older, had radiographic changes (Godfrey, 2005). Changes in joints may be more subtle radiographically, clinical signs may also be subtle. Around 40% of cats show signs of osteoarthritis in their lifetime and 90% of cats have radiographic changes by age 12 (FDA staff, 2021; Hazewinkel, Meij, Picavet, & Voorhout, 2011; Lascelles et al., 2012).

Etiology/DDX: Primary OA develops because of changes with cartilage homeostasis linked with aging and obesity (Morgan, 2016). In healthy tissue, cartilage consists of a matrix of proteoglycan macromolecules and type 1 collagen. With OA, there are shifts toward catabolism from matrixins in the matrix. As the amount of proteoglycans decrease, there is a loss of both chondroitin sulfate and water. The wear and tear in the movement in the joint makes additional microscopic damage to the matrix that progresses to macroscopic damage and results in cartilage loss. As the severity of the loss of cartilage increases, the synovial fluid also decreases. It becomes cyclic damage (Morgan, 2016). Secondary OA may occur because of genetic risk factors, such as joint dysplasia, or luxating patella disease processes, such as a joint infection or osteochondritis dissecans injuries such as cruciate ligament rupture that a animal may endure in their lifetime

(Anderson, Zulch, O'Neill, Meeson, & Collins, 2020). Secondary OA may occur in a single joint and may be due to subchondral bone trauma (Morgan, 2016). Breeds that have a higher incidence of cruciate tears include Rottweilers, Golden, and Labrador Retrievers (Anderson, 2020). Hip or elbow dysplasia occurs more commonly in Mastiffs, Boxers, German Shepherds, Golden or Labrador retrievers, and Bernese mountain dogs (Anderson, 2020). Breeds that are predisposed to experiencing luxating patellas include chihuahuas, Pomeranians, Yorkshire Terriers, and French Bulldogs (Anderson, 2020).

Clinical signs

Clients may first notice periodic lameness or that the animal is "just slowing down" or declining walks. Clients may notice their pets being stiff upon rising and may "warm out of it" as they have additional movement. Additional clinical signs in dogs can include, stiff gait, decreased range of motion, crepitus in the joint, thickening of joint, lethargy, pain, weight gain, weight shifting while standing, limping, difficulty jumping onto furniture or going up or down stairs, falling, exercise intolerance (Lascelles, 2019). Joint fluid may contain increased cell counts compared to healthy joint fluid (Morgan, 2016). In cats, changes may be subtle. The clinical signs for cats may include changes in behavior such as, decreased mobility, hesitating before jump or not jumping onto furniture, weight loss, decreased appetite, decreased to absent grooming, inappropriate elimination, aggression, withdrawal from family or hiding, (FDA staff, 2021).

Monitoring with a validated pain survey/scale for canine or feline osteoarthrititis can help with home assessment. See pain management section for additional pain scales for both dogs and cats. Radiographs are recommended, however changes may not be evident in early OA.

Palliative management

Patients who develop OA are supported with many different types of therapies. Weight management, first and foremost, has been found to be a key component to maintaining healthy joints and minimizing the development of signs of OA.

Omega 3 Fatty Acids are recommended to reduce inflammation.

Glucosamine/chondroitin sulfate may be found in supplement form, chewables, joint formulas, and diets. Adequan is an injectable polysulfated glycosaminoglycan that can be given in the home setting. The dose for Adequan in dogs is 4.44 mg/kg IM or SQ (VIN staff, 2017).

NSAIDs—Carprofen for dogs 2—4 mg/kg q 12 h for cats 12.5 mg per adult cat PO q 7 days (use with caution in cats, off label use), meloxicam for dogs, 0.2 mg/kg PO once then 0.1 mg/kg q 24 h, for cats 0.1 mg/kg once, then 0.05 mg/kg/day, then reduce the dose to 0.02 mg/kg/day or go to every other day at the 0.05 mg/kg dose, Deracoxib—Dogs 1—4 mg/kg q 24 h can start on the higher end and decrease dose after 7 days to 1—2 mg/kg q 24 h, robenacoxib for dogs and cats 1—2 mg/kg PO q 24 h (VIN staff, 2017).

Gallaprant (Grapiprant): For dogs only 2 mg/kg PO q 24 h. Calculate to the nearest ½ tablet. Change to different pain medication if no improvement in 14 days (VIN staff, 2017).

Gabapentin—Dogs: 3—20 mg/kg PO 1—3 times per day. Cats: 3—10 mg/kg PO q 8—24 h (can go higher if needed, likely more sedative) (VIN staff, 2017).

Amantadine—dogs, cats: 2—5 mg/kg PO q 12—24 h. Start on the lower end and increase as needed (VIN staff, 2017).

Acetaminophen/Paracetamol 10—15 mg/kg PO q 8—12 h (VIN staff, 2017). It is recommended to start on the low end and increase over time with need. This can be given with NSAIDs or steroids (use with caution with CKD and liver failure patients, however). It can also come in formulations with codeine or hydrocodone. Codeine is not very bioavailable in dogs when given orally, approximately 4% with one study (KuKanich, 2016). Hydrocodone metabolizes to hydromorphone and is more bioavailable orally than other oral opioids, approximately 40%—80% (KuKanich, 2013). Both are metabolized in the liver with cytochrome P450.

This text would not be complete without the mention of the new Anti-Nerve Growth Factor monoclonal antibodies (Anti-NGF mAb). This up and coming therapeutic may change the equation of the treatment of OA. It is currently available in Europe under the name Librela® for dogs and Solensia® for cats. Solensia has been approved in the US, though it has not been released as of this writing.

The underwater treadmill and other rehabilitation techniques can help strengthen musculature, maintain balance longer (Staff of MSU, 2021). Adding a veterinarian trained in rehabilitation to the veterinary team may add to the quality of life of the OA patient. Rehabilitation techniques clients may be able to perform at home can include back stepping, side stepping, sit/down/stand, Cavaletti's with 5 poles to walk across (clients can use large dowels, broomsticks), weight shifting, and walking on uneven surfaces, spins, and stairs (Staff of MSU, 2021). Clients can view videos on various rehabilitation techinques on YouTube.

The use of CBD in OA appears to be effective for pain management in OA at 2 mg/kg PO q 12 h (Gamble, 2018). Additional research should continue to evaluate the efficacy of CBD use for OA. The addtional challenge for the use of CBD are the unregulated products having effective labeling, consistant dosing of CBD. A search of the FDA warning letters list for CBD will show many products that received warning letters for labeling/content issues. https://www.fda.gov/news-events/public-health-focus/warning-letters-and-test-results-cannabidiol-related-products. There are issues of legality of use as well, as the laws around cannabis are changing quickly.

Crisis kit

The most common crisis issue with chronic OA is acute pain. An acute flare-up of pain can keep an animal down and potentially stimulate a euthanasia decision, which may be appropriate. Opioids should be in the crisis kit for acute pain along with an adjunct, such as gabapentin, and a tranquilizer to help patients sleep until you can get there for a consultation or euthanasia (or they can get them to an ER).

Osteosarcoma

Etiology/DDX: Osteosarcoma is a common cancer seen by palliative and hospice veterinarians. The dogs who develop osteosarcoma tend to be large and giant breed dogs, however osteosarcoma can be seen in small dogs and cats. Osteosarcoma in cats tends to be rare. Osteosarcoma primarily affects the appendicular skeleton, though patients can develop it in their axial skeleton. Differentials include chondrosarcoma, lymphoma, hemangiosarcoma, fibrosarcoma, giant cell tumor, histiocytic sarcoma, melanoma, multiple myeloma, multilobular osteochondrosarcoma, spindle cell sarcoma, squamous cell carcinoma, synovial sarcoma, and bone metastasis from other tumor types (Curran, 2015).

Clinical signs

Dogs with osteosarcoma have varying degrees of lameness that tend to increase over time as the tumor grows and pain increases, and patients may present with non-weight bearing lameness. People with pain from cancer in the bone report the pain as significantly painful, whether the cancer is from a primary tumor or metastasis (Jimenez-Andrade, 2010). The pain may occur due to an number of factors including significant remodeling of the bone, microfractures in the cortex, and occasionally can develop a cortex-to-cortex pathologic fracture. In addition, osteosarcoma can have other clinical signs sucha as hypercalcemia and anemia. Lab work may show and increase in Alkaline Phosphatase (Curran, 2015). The dog may also develop other clinical signs associated with chronic, and moderate-to-severe pain, such as anxious or irritable behavior, decreased or absent appetite, resistance to walk, play, get up or down, weight loss, and disturbances in the sleep/wake cycle (Hardy, 2020). Clinical signs that may occur in the axial skeleton include, exophthalmos, dysphagia, anorexia, nasal discharge, paresis, and swelling (Curran, 2015).

As pain is a contributing factor to the palliation of osteosarcoma, a brief review on possible causes of pain is included. Pain may start with osteoclast proliferation in osteosarcoma and the remodeling of osteosarcoma bone and the production of an osteoclast local acidosis (Jimenez-Andrade, 2010). Pain has also been associated with two acid-sensing channels: transient receptor potential vanilloid 1 (TRPV1) and acid-sensing ion channel-3 (ASIC-3). TRPV1 receptors are affected by heat as well as acid. In addition with humans, blocking the receptor for nuclear factor κB ligand (RANKL) is used to help with bone pain. Denosumab (under proprietary name XGEVA) has shown to be effective in deceleration of growth, decreasing pain and reducing metastasis. As of this writing, however, it is not cost-effective for most (approximately 3500 USD) for one vial (Fig. 5.12).

Furthermore, the tumor cells and tumor stromal cells, including neutrophils and macrophages, also produce cytokines that contribute to the production of pain with osteosarcoma. Osteosarcoma cells and tumor stromal cells commonly produce TNF, IL-1, IL-6, PGE2, and NGF (Jimenez-Andrade, 2010). Inflammatory pain mediators may be responsive to Cox 2 inhibitors, such as meloxicam (Naruse, 2006).

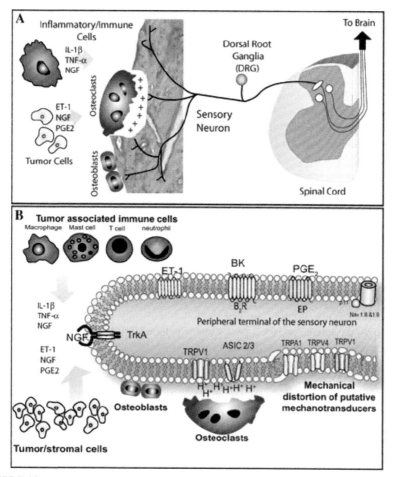

FIGURE 5.12

Osteoclast involvement in tumor-associated bone pain. Schematic showing factors in bone (A) and receptors/channels expressed by nociceptors that innervate the skeleton (B) that drive bone cancer pain. A variety of cells (tumor cells and stromal cells including inflammatory/immune cells, osteoclasts, and osteoblasts) drive bone cancer pain (A). Nociceptors that innervate the bone use several different types of receptors to detect and transmit noxious stimuli that are produced by cancer cells (yellow), tumor-associated immune cells (blue), or other aspects of the tumor microenvironment. There are multiple factors that may contribute to the pain associated with cancer (B). The transient receptor potential vanilloid receptor-1 (TRPV1) and acid-sensing ion channels (ASICs) detect extracellular protons produced by tumor-induced tissue damage or abnormal osteoclast-mediated bone resorption. Tumor cells and associated inflammatory (immune) cells produce a variety of chemical mediators including prostaglandins (PGE2), nerve growth factor (NGF), endothelins (ET-1), and bradykinin (BK). Several of these proinflammatory

NGF has been of particular interest in osteoarthritis pain management (Enomoto, 2019). NGF is also expressed by osteosarcoma cells and contributes to pain, and an anti-NGF drug may help decrease pain. The research in people indicates that it decreases pain for both osteosarcoma and bone metastasis patients (Sevcik, 2005). More research needs to be done to examine the efficacy of pain management of the new anti-NFG monoclonal antibody drug for osteosarcoma or bone metastasis. Zoetus has a new anti-NGF monoclonal antibody drug, bedinvetmab or Liberla® and frunevetmab or Solensia®, available in Europe. The United States is still awaiting the Zoetis product for dogs and cats as of this writing.

There is also a neuropathic component to the pain caused by osteosarcoma. The tumor invades the sensory nerves, upregulates glial fibrillary acidic proteins, galanin and creates hypertrophy of satellite cells. Similar changes have been proposed with other neuropathic pain (Jimenez-Andrade, 2010). Using gabapentin or pregabalin is useful as an adjunct for a multimodal approach to pain management with osteosarcoma.

Palliative management

The current standard of curative treatment for osteosarcoma is amputation of the limb or a limb spare surgery followed by radiation therapy. Regardless of if the client elects to do palliative care for a post surgery patient or in leu of surgery, pain management needs to be multimodal.

Gabapentin: Dogs/Cats: 10—20 mg/kg to start (this differs from other sections of this chapter). Anecdotally, higher dosing is needed. And go up to what they need, without making them too sleepy (some dogs are more sensitive than others).

Pregabalin: Dogs 2—4 mg/kg PO q 12 hours, Cats 1—2 mg/kg PO q 12 hours (VIN staff, 2017).

NSAID or steroids: Choosing between an NSAID and steroids may be difficult in some cases. NSAIDs may slow the progression of the disease, steroids can help with appetite, and decrease inflammation but may not slow the progression. There are some *in vitro* studies looking at NSAIDs and osteosarcoma cells. It is shown in other cell lines that NSAIDs seem to have a cytotoxic effect (Zuckerman, 2019). See the Pain Mangement chapter for more information.

---

mediators have receptors on peripheral terminals and can directly activate or sensitize nociceptors. It is suggested that movement-evoked breakthrough pain in cancer patients is partially due to the tumor-induced loss of the mechanical strength and stability of the tumor-bearing bone so that normally innocuous mechanical stress can now produce distortion of the putative mechanotransducers (TRPV1, TRPV4, and TRPA1) that innervate the bone.

Graphic and caption by Used with permission from Naruse, T. N. (2006). Meloxicam inhibits osteosarcoma growth, invasiveness and metastasis by COX-2-dependent and independent routes. Carcinogenesis, 584—592; Jimenez-Andrade, J. M. (2010). Bone cancer pain. Annals of the New York Academy of Sciences, 173—181.

Carprofen 2−4 mg/kg PO BID for the rest of the dog's life, unless they cause GI upset, bleeding (VIN Staff, 2017).

Meloxicam 0.1 mg/kg PO q 24 h for dogs, 0.02−0.1 mg/kg for cats. (The FDA does have a warning for use in cats, that it can cause renal failure and death so use with caution and with discussing the side effects with the client) (VIN Staff, 2017).

Prednisone 0.5−1 mg/kg BID to start for 3−5 days, then q 24 h. If need be, move back up. The goal is to give enough for clinical signs but minimize the side effects of the steroids.

Bisphosphonates—can help with pain and reabsorption of bone and hypercalcemia.

Zoledronate 0.1 mg/kg IV in 60 mL 0.9% NaCl given over 15 min as a CRI. (Zoledronate is 100× more potent than pamidronate in decreasing reabsorption). Administer every 28 days (VIN Staff, 2017).

Pamidronate 1−2 mg/kg IV in 250 mL of 0.9% NaCl given over 2 h as a CRI. (Not as useful in the home setting) (VIN staff, 2017).

Alendronate 10−20 mg *per dog* PO q 24 hours. Administer on an empty stomach with water, then a small meal 30−60 minutes post adminstration. Alendronate may not be highly bioavailable orally and the parenterals are recommended over Alendronate (VIN staff, 2017).

NMDA antagonist—are useful in preventing windup pain.

Amantadine 2−5 mg/kg PO q 12−24 h. Start on the lower end and increase as needed (VIN staff, 2017).

Subanesthetic ketamine SQ 0.5−1 mg/kg SQ PRN (anecdotal. May need to be given monthly or more frequently. Studies need to be done to assess the efficacy) (VIN staff, 2017).

Subanesthetic ketamine in CRI 0.5 mg/kg bolus then CRI of 10 mcg/kg/minute for about 2 h. There are subcutaneous drip pumps that may be utilized for a CRI. RX Actuator makes a subcutaneous pump. https://www.rxactuator.net/.

Memantine 0.3−0.5 mg/kg q 12−24 h (Wright, 2017).

Opioids Opioids left in the home in crisis kits should be a last resort, due to a high concern for diversion to humans. There should be an exceptionally good paper trail and documentation with signatures of costs, and side effects, and potential harm to humans. In human medicine, opioids for end-of-life patients are distributed through a pharmacy only. Hospice and palliative care doctors and nurses do not carry opioids to the home, nor do they take them away. They will leave disposal information for hospice patients. The author employs this strategy to have a solid paper trail. The other drawback to oral opioids is the degree of bioavailability in dogs (which varies by opioid) and cats due to the first-pass metabolism in the liver.

Mu agonists Methadone (schedule II): Dogs: 0.25−0.5 mg/kg SQ q 3−4 h. Cats: 0.1−0.25 mg/kg SQ q 3−4 h. Has some NMDA antagonist properties (VIN Staff, 2017).

Morphine (schedule II): Dogs: 0.25−1 mg SQ or 0.2−0.5 mg/kg q 6−8 h for liquid formulations. Cats 0.1−0.25 mg/kg SQ q 2−4 h or 0.2−0.5 mg/kg q 6−8 h of oral liquid (can cause anaphylaxis, vomiting, dysphoria, constipation). Should have naloxone (reversal agent) in case of side effects (VIN Staff, 2017).

Hydromorphone (schedule II): Dogs/cats 0.05—0.1 mg/kg SQ q 2—4 h (can cause hyperthermia in some patients). Use with caution in MDR-1 mutation patients as they may be predisposed to toxicity (VIN Staff, 2017). Can cause vomiting, diarrhea, panting. Can be partially reversed with butorphanol and naloxone.

Fentanyl patches may not be ideal due to variable uptake and the need for changing every 3 days and cost. However, they can help if that is the only option available to you.

Partial mu agonists Buprenorphine (schedule III): Dogs 0.01—0.05 mg/kg SQ or TM q 8—12 h. Cats 0.01—0.02 mg/kg SQ or TM q 4—12 h. 0.12 mg/kg sustained-release SQ every 72 h, 0.24 mg/kg Simbadol only SQ q 24 h up to 3 days (this dose can cause profound sedation with other buprenorphine formulations). Use with caution in MDR-1 mutation patients as they may be predisposed to toxicity from norbuprenorphine—the metabolite of buprenorphine (VIN Staff, 2017).

K-agonist/μ-antagonist Butorphanol: Dogs: 0.1—0.5 mg/kg SQ q 1—4 h, 0.55 mg/kg PO q 6—12 h, though it may be more sedating than analgesic, not ideal for bone cancer patients. First pass metabolism makes oral butorphanol ineffective for analgesia. Cats: 0.2—0.4 mg/kg q 1—4 h (VIN Staff, 2017). Can be used in a crisis kit with other medications such as gabapentin and acepromazine or an α2-2agonist.

Local anesthetics Lidocaine patches may also be useful near a healed surgery site for phantom pain, or over the tumor for local pain relief.

Anti-NGF monoclonal antibodies—when they are available (Enomoto, 2019).

Nonmedical therapies
Cold therapy

Cold therapy may be useful in the bone cancer patient, as TPRV1 receptors are involved in the local acidosis and are initiated by acid and heat. A cold compress in the location of cancer may temporarily decrease the pain sensation. Cold compresses should last about 5—10 min and be done 2—3 times a day. Refrigerated pack of ice packs or a bag of frozen peas can be a useful cold pack.

Crisis kit

Acute Pain: Should include a μ-agonist for pain. If clients are preparing the animal for euthanasia, then doubling the dose to address breakthrough pain, and adding other medications can relieve the animal's immediate discomfort and help to get them to sleep or relax. It is possible to inadvertently induce dysphoria in a patient by giving opioids, and clients should be educated about this possibility.

The kit should also contain a tranquilizer that can work in conjunction with the μ-agonist to calm the animal. Gabapentin and Trazadone may also be helpful.

One could also consider acepromazine (a phenothiazine which provides no analgesic properties) or dormosedan 0.1 mL/10 lbs on gums. (α2-agonists do provide some pain relief, but may cause vomiting).

A fitted splint or an expandable splint might be useful to consider having on hand in case an animal experiences a pathological fracture https://www.therapaw.com/.

Oral care for diseases of the head and neck

Patients with late stage disease may also have oral disease that may affect their quality of life. Elder veterinary patients may have severe dental disease, and animals may not get proper dental care as they age. They may subsequently be euthanized for not eating or having other problems such as dysphagia. Patients may develop neoplasia in the oropharynx that may cause dysphagia or anorexia. Oral ulcers may occur with CKD patients or cancer patients. And if clients choose to palliate their animal until the end of their disease, oral care will be important aspect of care, especially in their last days to keep them comfortable. This section discusses the issues that may arise in the oral cavity with late-stage patients. Dysphagia, and dysrexia are discussed in other sections.

Etiology/DDX for disease of the head and neck

Oral ulcers or pain in the oral cavity are commonly seen in the end-stage patient. Oral ulcers or oral pain may occur as a result of renal failure, head or neck neoplasia, moderate to severe dental disease, acutely broken or chronically worn teeth, viral or bacterial disease, or stomatitis/mucositis.

Head and neck tumors may originate from different locations in the head or neck. This section focuses on oropharyngeal tumors. Cats with oropharyngeal tumors are predominately squamous cell carcinomas (SCC), though they may also develop, though more rare, melanomas, fibrosarcoma, osteosarcoma, odontoma, osteoma. Dogs with oropharyngeal neoplasia may develop, melanomas, followed by SCC, fibrosarcoma, and dental tumors such as epulides. Pain is the predominant concern for oropharyngeal neoplasia, along with decreasing appetite, ptyalism, bleeding from tumor or from a loss of teeth, and secondary infection or abscess development. Thyroid tumors may be seen, though less common than oral tumors and concerns may include pain, the ability to breathe or swallow and how aggressive it may be.

Oral mucositis/stomatitis occurs predominantly in cats, though dogs can also be affected as well. Chemotherapy and radiation may contribute to stomatitis/mucositis. Bacterial infections may occur; *Pasteurella multocida* is the predominant species seen with stomatitis (Lee, 2020). Cats with immune-mediated stomatitis may also have different oral microflora that may contribute to there stomatitis. Viruses may contribute to feline stomatitis with calicivirus and herpesvirus may be involved in the development of stomatitis (Lee, 2020). Stomatitis in cats may also be due to immune-mediated disease with lymphocytic-plasmacytic infiltrates found (Rothrock K., Stomatitis, 2020c).

Clinical signs

Pain is a primary concern with diseases of the head and neck. Clinical signs that may be noted with pain of the oral cavity, include: anorexia or hyporexia, adypsia or hypodypsia, ptyalism, pawing, rubbing or scratching repeatedly at the face, licking the air or bed or floor or thoracic limbs, depression, and lethargy. Licking something other than the area that hurts may be a sign of referred pain or pain they are unable to reach. It can also be a sign of nausea.

Palliative management of disease of the head and neck

The current standard of care for stomatitis is full dental extraction. However, patients may be medically managed, if the client opts out of full dental extraction. Stomatitis may need antibiotics for secondary infections. Corticosteroids may help decrease inflammation methylprednisolone acetate (7.5–20 mg per cat SC q 3–4 weeks) or prednisolone (0.5–2 mg/kg PO q 12–48 h), cyclosporine has been used to some success (5 mg/kg PO q 24 h) (Rothrock K., Stomatitis, 2020c).

Pain management for stomatitis, oral ulcers, dental disease should include an opioid along with adjunctive therapy. Buprenorphine (schedule III): dogs 0.01–0.05 mg/kg SQ or TM q 8–12 h, cats: 0.01–0.02 mg/kg SQ or TM q 4–12 h 0.12 mg/kg sustained release SQ every 72 h. Simbadol® only-0.24 mg/kg SQ q 24 h using up to 3 days (this dose can cause profound sedation with other buprenorphine formulations). Use with caution in MDR-1 mutation patients as they may be predisposed to toxicity from norbuprenorphine—the metabolite of buprenorphine (VIN staff, 2017). Gabapentin, used as an adjunct, 3–5 mg/kg to start and increase with need up to 10–20 mg/kg PO q 8–12 hours (VIN staff, 2017).

Stem cell therapy is currently being studied and may be a future treatment for stomatitis (Lee, 2020).

For stomatitis, ulcers from other causes, or oral tumors, pain management may also include oral antibiotics, and "magic mouthwash." The "Magic Mouthwash" that is prepared for use in humans contains equal parts oral 2% viscous lidocaine (a local anesthetic), Benadryl (which is used as a local anesthetic and drying agent), and Maalox (an antacid used as a coating agent). Other formulations could include an antibiotic, steroid, agents for bleeding, other coating agents, such as sucralfate, and other pain medications, such as buprenorphine. Create the formulation with the assistance of a compounding pharmacy for your individual patient needs based on the disease process. Compounding pharmacies can also formulate: "magic mouthwash" as a spray-on, a liquid, or a gel and with flavoring to make it more palatable.

Pancreatic disease, late-stage

Dogs and cats have some common pancreatic diseases seen at the end of life and they include diabetes mellitus, pancreatitis, and pancreatic carcinoma (Lidbury, 2016). This section will review Diabetes Mellitus and pancreatic carcinoma as those are more commonly seen end of life disease. Pancreatitis may also occur with late stage patients, however, treatment for pancreatitis is covered in other texts and end-of-life care does not deviate from standard care and so will not be reviewed in this section. There may be challenges for the client caring for an animal with pancreatic disease. An animal with chronic pancreatitis or diabetes can be financially, emotionally and sometimes physically challenging for the client to treat. Supporting clients treating their pets with diabetes in the home may improve the quality of life, both for pet and client. Palliative care for pancreatic carcinoma may strengthen the bond between pet and their caregivers. This section will start with diabetes and then follow with pancreatic neoplasias.

Etiology/DDX of diabetes

Diabetes mellitus is a commonly seen geriatric disease in both dogs and cats. It may be an end-of-life disease that the client chooses to do a combination of management and palliation. It is more likely, in the author's experience, that a general practitioner or a specialist will diagnose and start treatment for diabetes before the home end-of-life care veterinarian examines the pet. Considering this, the author will provide a brief review, and then a discuss current palliative care considerations for the diabetic patient.

The pancreas has two types of cells involved in glucose metabolism, β-cells that secrete insulin, and the α-cells that secrete glucagon. Insulin manages the glucose in the body, driving it into the cells or into storage in the muscles or liver. Glucagon helps with the release of glucose from muscle and liver stored glycogen (Rothrock, 2020a). Diabetes mellitus is either type I, insulin-dependent diabetes due to immune-mediated destruction of the beta cells in dogs or chronic pancreatitis in cats, type II, which may be due to decreases of insulin production caused by beta cell dysfunction or peripheral insulin resistance, or type III hormone-induced insulin resistance (progesterone, cortisol, epinephrine, growth hormone, glucagon) (sometimes called gestational diabetes in people). Dogs more commonly develop type I diabetes, and cats more typically develop type II, up to 80%−95% in cats (Rothrock K., Diabetes Mellitus, 2020a). Type III has been reported in cats and dogs (Rothrock K., Diabetes Mellitus, 2020a). Cats with type II diabetes may go into remission with weight loss (Nelson, 2014). Factors that may be involved in the etiology of diabetes mellitus is represented in the following graphic (Fig. 5.13) (Nelson, 2014).

Clinical signs of diabetes

The first clinical signs clients may notice cats or dogs experiencing may include, polyuria, polydipsia, polyphagia with weight loss, and/or lethargy when initially diagnosed. Cataracts and diabetic polyneuropathy may also be symptoms client may notice. Diabetic polyneuropathy may present as hindlimb weakness, difficulty jumping, and plantigrade posture of pelvic limbs. Animals can also have a generalized weakness with ventroflexion, other rule outs may include hypokalemia, and thiamine deficiency. Other less specific clinical signs may be unkempt haircoat, dehydration, and abdominal distention from hepatomegaly. Pets with diabetes mellitus may also have comorbidities such as pancreatitis, acromegaly, and hyperadrenocorticism (Rothrock K., Diabetes Mellitus, 2020a). Complications of diabetes

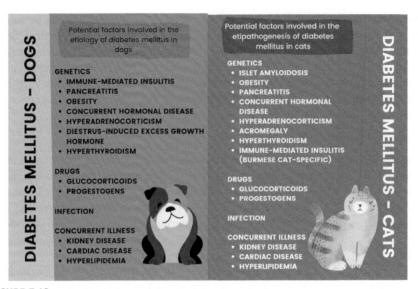

FIGURE 5.13

Diabetes mellitus.

Graphic created on Canva by Mina Weakley and Lynn Hendrix © 2021. Nelson, R. W. (2014). Animal models of disease: Classification and etiology of diabetes in dogs and cats. The Journal of Endocrinology, T1–9.

may include hypo or hyperglycemia, or diabetic ketoacidosis, or hyperosmolar hyperglycemia if their diabetes is not well controlled (Nelson R. W., 2014).

The animal may have potentially distressing diabetic signs may include pain, diabetic neuropathy, loss of sight from cataracts, thirst, pressure sores, ischemia of limbs, brain (stroke), dehydration, constipation, lethargy, seizures from hypoglycemia or hyperosmotic, nonketotic diabetes (Nelson R. W., 2014).

Potentially distressing clinical signs for the caregiver to monitor for can include the animal not eating seizures due to hypoglycemia, urinating frequently, especially if urinating inappropriately, urinary tract infections, diabetic neuropathy. Administering insulin and providing extensive nursing care may also become stressful for the caregiver.

Palliative management

Late-stage diabetic animals need higher levels of veterinary and nursing attention. The client should be made aware of the addition level of care and advised of the cost and time involved.

Blood Glucose monitoring—As the general practitioner or emergency veterinarian is more likely to diagnose and prescribe insulin, we will not go into the initial dosing for insulin. However, home monitoring of blood glucose (BG) and adjustment of insulin can be achieved with home care. The client/caregiver could be taught to use a standard BG monitor at home or a Freestyle Libre, a new type of BG monitor could be placed in the clinical setting. The Freestyle Libre has liberated animals from going into the clinic for further testing. The client can download an app onto their phone and is able to obtain multiple blood glucose readings throughout the day and minimizing stress on the animal.

Hypoglycemia—Cats can be at particular risk of hypoglycemia. Their insulin needs can change with weight loss, vomiting, lack of appetite, erratic eating, renal disease (concurrent), liver impairment, liver carcinoma, and pancreatic cancer. Creating a palliative plan is essential before a hypoglycemia crisis. Other crises may include hyperglycemia, uncontrolled diabetes, and difficulty in medicating. Any of these episodes may become a decision-making point for people regarding euthanasia.

The palliative management plan may include the current standard of curative care for diabetics (Diehl, 2021). The palliative plan could also include developing an advanced directive and having a plan in place for crises, in addition to a daily plan and check in times. Pain management is recommended early in the disease for diabetic neuropathy.

Animals with diabetes have microvascular changes which includes diabetic neuropathy (Cade, 2008). Other microvascular changes include retinopathy and nephropathy. The mechanism for microvascular pathology may include an increase and accumulation of Advanced Glycation End Products (AGE), and increase in free radicals, changes in signaling, and the RAS system (Cade, 2008). Patients with diabetic neuropathy develop demyelination and axonal degeneration of the mylenated neurons and regeneration of unmyelinated fibers and changes of the microangiopathy (Boucek, 2006). Nerve damage is induced by accumulation of intracellular glucose and glycating sugar, enhanced oxidative damage, protein kinase C activation, and ischemia in addition to the changes in the microvascular blood flow (Boucek, 2006).

There are 5 stages of diabetic neuropathy in people:

1. Numbness and pain intermittently—mild chronic pain
2. More regular pain and numbness—moderate chronic pain
3. Severity increases—Severe chronic pain
4. Constant numbness—nerve damage in permanent by this stage.
5. Total loss of feeling—this is when humans may need amputation. (Boucek, 2006)

Early treatment of diabetes and continued monitoring to maintain adequate control is optimal for the prevention or treatment of early diabetic neuropathy. Pets with clinical signs of diabetic neuropathy may benefit from treatment with gabapentin early in the course of their disease. Start gabapentin at a low dose. For cats, start at 3–5 mg/kg and increase to 10 mg/cat PO q12-24 h PRN. For dogs, start between 3 and 5 mg/kg PO every 12–24 h and increase over time. Doses of 10–20 mg/kg PO q 8 h are routinely used, and they can go even higher if needed (VIN staff, 2017). Use of a validated Diabetic Neuropathy scale would be useful however, there are currently no validated scales that assess diabetic neuropathy in animals

(Mythili, 2010). Further reading on Human Diabetic Neuropathy scales can be found here: https://www.ncbi.nlm.nih.gov/pmc/articles/PMC6513667/.

In addition to gabapentin, other supplements may also help slow progression of diabetic neuropathy. α-lipoic acid, acetylcysteine and α-tocopherol, γ-linolenic acid-containing oils or acetyl-L-carnitine have been shown to help diabetic neuropathy in rat models (Boucek, 2006). Additional studies in companion animals would be needed to evaluate the efficacy of additional supplements for use in diabetic neuropathy. Monitoring of kidney values and changes in the retina may also be useful to evaluate early microvascular changes and as they progress with their disease.

Crisis kit for diabetes

Emergencies for animals with diabetes mellitus may include hypoglycemia from insulin overdose, diabetic ketoacidosis, vomiting, acute pain, weakness, profound dehydration. The crisis kit should include: An opioid for acute pain, adjuncts for additional pain management, a sugar for hypoglycemia, SQ fluids, anti-emetic for vomiting, dehydration.

μ-agonists for acute pain

Methadone (schedule II): Dogs: 0.25–0.5 mg/kg SQ q 3–4 h. Cats: 0.1–0.25 mg/kg SQ q 3–4 h. Has some NMDA antagonist properties (VIN staff, 2017).

Morphine (schedule II): Dogs: 0.25–1 mg SQ or 0.2–0.5 mg/kg q 6–8 h for liquid formulations. Cats: 0.1–0.25 mg/kg SQ q 2–4 h or 0.2–0.5 mg/kg q 6–8 h of oral liquid (can cause anaphylaxis, vomiting, dysphoria, constipation). Should have naloxone (reversal agent) in case of side effects (VIN staff, 2017).

Hydromorphone (schedule II): Dogs/cats: 0.05–0.1 mg/kg SQ q 2–4 h (can cause hyperthermia in some patients). Use with caution in MDR-1 mutation patients as they may be predisposed to toxicity (VIN staff, 2017). Can cause vomiting, diarrhea, and panting. Can be partially reversed with butorphanol and naloxone.

Partial μ-agonists

Buprenorphine (schedule III): Dogs: 0.01–0.05 mg/kg SQ or TM q 8–12 h. Cats: 0.01–0.02 mg/kg SQ or TM q 4–12 h 0.12 mg/kg sustained release SQ every 72 h, 0.24 mg/kg Simbadol only SQ q 24 h up to 3 days (this dose can cause profound sedation with other buprenorphine formulations). Use with caution in MDR-1 mutation patients as they may be predisposed to toxicity from norbuprenorphine—the metabolite of buprenorphine (VIN staff, 2017).

K-agonist/μ-antagonist

Butorphanol: Dogs: 0.1–0.5 mg/kg SQ q 1–4 h, 0.55 mg/kg PO q 6–12 h, though it may be more sedating than analgesic, not ideal for bone cancer patients. First pass metabolism makes oral butorphanol ineffective for analgesia. Cats: 0.2—0.4 mg/kg q 1—4 h (VIN staff, 2017). Can be used in a crisis kit with other medications such as gabapentin and acepromazine or an alpha 2 agonist.

For additional pain management: Gabapentin: 3—20 mg/kg PO q 8—12 h. Can also be used as an adjunct for seizures (VIN staff, 2017).

Pregabalin: Dogs: Pregabalin is administered at a dosage of 4 mg/kg orally three times a day (Kent, 2012). Cats: studies of pregabalin in cats is still limited, but the starting dose we are using for this species is 1—2 mg/kg q 12 h (Dewey C., 2013).

For Seizures: Midazolam: 0.5 mg/kg intranasally (VIN staff, 2017)

Diazepam: 0.5—1 mg/kg intranasally or rectally (VIN staff, 2017).

For Vomiting: Ondansetron: dissolvable tablet 0.5 mg/kg on gums, or in buccal surface. Or Cerenia injectable. For dogs: 1mg/kg SQ q 24 h , For cats 0.5 mg/kg SQ q 24 h (VIN staff, 2017).

For hypoglycemia: Karo syrup or honey

For dehydration: Fluids: 0.9% NaCl SQ (IV is perferable, however in the home setting, this may be easier to provide to clients and easier for them to perform at home in a crisis)

Pancreatic cancer

Pancreatic cancer is not as commonly seen in companion animals as diabetes. Pancreatic cancer can be managed in the home while monitoring for the clinical signs that may arise. Pancreatic cancer is reported to be moderately to severely painful with humans and is likely equally as painful in companion animals. Pancreatic neoplasia may be managed in the home setting prior to euthanasia. Types of pancreatic cancer seen in dogs, insulinoma-islet cell carcinoma, glucagonoma, and gastrinoma. Cats tend to develop exocrine pancreatic adenocarcinoma. Patients with pancreatic neoplasm may develop paraneoplastic syndrome. While pancreatic cancer is rare, and some are very rare in companion animals, we have included them for client education.

Insulinoma

Etiology/DDX

Insulinomas are β-Cell neoplasias of the pancreas. Identified after the primary hormone excreted, the β-Cell neoplasia secrete insulin, somatostatin, glucagon, gastrin, pancreatic polypeptide, insulin-like growth factor 1 (somatomedin), and serotonin (Rothrock K., Insulinoma, 2018). The hormonally active tumor releases insulin which drives hypoglycemia. The hypoglycemia primarily affects the brain, which has an increased need for glucose as a primary energy source. If the hypoglycemia continues, there may be ischemic, irreversible neuronal damage. Insulinomas are most commonly reported in dogs, and are rare in cats (Rothrock K., Insulinoma, 2018).

Metastatic sites for insulinomas may include: liver, small intestine, and lungs and mesenteric lymph nodes, mesentery ± skull, and vertebrae in dogs (VSSO Staff, 2021a,b).

Clinical signs

The initial clinical presentation may be weakness or collapse secondary to hypoglycemia. Weakness, tripping/falling over/lameness, seeming to fall asleep easily, or being lethargic are common clinical sign. Patients may also have unexplained weight loss, anorexia, and vomiting in their history (Rothrock K. S., 2020a,b).

Treatment

The primary treatment for an insulinoma is surgery. Specific post op complications that may arise are pancreatitis, or persistent hypoglycemia.

Glucagon CRI's have been used as emergency management of the hypoglycemic—hyperinsulinemic crisis by achieving and maintaining normoglycemia despite intractable hyperinsulinemia. Glucagon physiologically opposes the actions of insulin by increasing hepatic glycogenolysis and gluconeogenesis.

Alloxan (65 mg/kg IV) is a derivative of uric acid, which alters the permeability of pancreatic β-cells and causes permanent β-cell destruction resulting in prolonged hyperglycemia or normoglycemia. Alloxan is toxic to renal tubular epithelial cells and causes renal failure in 10% of dogs. Streptozotocin may also be considered however it is unlikely to be utilized in the home setting as it is an IV drug that nneds to be given over time (Rothrock, Rishniw, & Shell, 2018).

While these may not be the palliative treatments a home vet might use being versed in them may help communicating all treatment options to the client for an informed decision. As palliatve veterinarians, we are more likely to be focused on making dietary adjustments and treating cancer pain.

Palliative management

Concerns for palliative management include, persisitant hypoglycemia and increasing pain. Vomiting, anorexia may also arise and be of concern with palliated patients. Palladia and prednisone can be utilized for the palliative management of insulinomas. Prednisone antagonizes insulin and stimulates hepatic gluconeogenesis and glycogenolysis. The dose for dogs with insulinoma is, prednisone is 0.25—0.5 mg/kg PO q 24 h (VIN staff, 2017). Palladia dose (needs further review and evaluation), however, in one study 2.5 mg/kg q 48 h. Discussion with an oncologist may help support the continued use of Palladia (Flesner, 2019). Octreotide inhibits synthesis and secretion and the dose in dogs is 2—4 mcg/kg q 8—12 h (Rothrock K., Insulinoma, 2018; VIN staff, 2017).

A recommended diet for insulinoma includes: high protein, higher fat, complex carbohydrates. Having low glycemic index for carbohydrates in the diet tends to work best for animals with insulinoma. Consultation with a veterinary nutritionist is recommended to obtain a balanced diet. Frequent smaller meals every 3—4 h may benefit the patient.

For pain management, patients may also benefit from gabapentin, opioids as the pain increases with growth and metastasis. The crisis kit information for pancreatic neoplasm is at the end of this section.

Glucagonoma

Glucagonomas are rare in veterinary patients. The alpha cells of the islets of Langerhans are the cells involved in the release of glucagon and glucagonomas arise in the alpha cells.

Etiology/DDX

Glucagonomas are associated with a characteristic dermatitis of the footpads, and superficial necrolytic dermatitis. Survival times range from 3 days to 9 months. Differentials can include pemphigus foliaceus, Systemic Lupus Erythematosus, generic dog food dermatosis, and zinc-responsive dermatosis. Disease progression may include: multiple diffuse hypoechogenic foci in the liver (= honeycomb pattern) is present in 50% (4/8) dogs with glucagonoma and is consistent with hepatic metastases (VSSO Staff, 2021a,b).

Palliative management

Palliative management of glucagonma may include steroids and octreotide. Amino acid supplementation, eggs, high protein diets may help with clinical signs. Prognosis is poor (Keller, Gastrointestinal Endocrine Tumors, 2014a,b). Prednisone in dogs and prednisalone in cats can be given 0.5—1 mg/kg PO q 12—24 h in a tapering dose. Octreotide for dogs 2—3 mcg/kg SC q 12 h (VIN staff, 2017).

Gastrinoma
Etiology/DDX

Gastrinomas are primarily a functional endocrine, pancreatic tumor involving the G-cells, the neuroendocrine cells responsible for the release of gastrin. These cells can be found in the duodenum, pyloric antrum and the pancreas. These tumors are rarely found in cats and dogs (Rothrock K., Gastrinoma, 2020b). There is a report of one dog with an extra pancreatic gastrinoma has been reported in the root of the mesentery (Rothrock K., Gastrinoma, 2020b). (Also known as Zollinger—Ellison syndrome gastrinomas may develop excess peptic acid in the stomach and intestine).

Gastrinomas are usually solitary neoplasms, with 60% showing up in the right lobe, 40% in the pancreatic body, and the left lobe rarely involved. Metastasis is common with 76%—85% at presentation and may occur in: liver (65%), regional lymph nodes (30%), and 25% to spleen, peritoneum, and mesentery (VSSO Staff, 2021a,b).

Clinical signs

Gastrointestinal ulceration is a common clinical sign occuring in 95% of cats and dogs with gastrinoma. Locations where ulcerations may be seen, are as follows: esophageal ulceration in 20%, gastric ulceration in 45%, duodenal ulceration in 78%, jejunal ulceration in 6%, and GI perforation in 25% (VSSO Staff, 2021a,b). Other clinical signs with gastrinomas may include are vomiting, anorexia, weight loss lethargy, hematemesis, melena, and abdominal pain (Keller, Gastrointestinal Endocrine Tumors, 2014a,b).

Palliative management

Octreotide: 5 mcg/kg IV may help stabilize a gastrinoma patient (Lane, 2016). For dogs, it can also be given 8—60 mcg per dog up to q 8 hr. For cats, c2 mcg/kg SC q 8 hr × 2 doses, then 4 mcg/kg q 8 hr for 2 doses, then 10 mcg/kg SC q 8 hr. In combination with q 12 hr proton-pump inhibitor therapy (VIN staff, 2017).

Palladia may be useful for gastrinoma, however, in one case report the cat became anorexic with the use of Palladia (Lane, 2016). Discuss use of palladia for gastrinoma with a veterinary oncologist.

Pain management should include management for neuropathic and inflammatory pain. Gabapentin or pregabalin may be considered for mild to moderate pain, opioids may be useful in severe pain. Treatment for gastrointestinal ulcerations may include, sucralfate 0.5—1 grams PO given in a slurry per dog q 8—12 hours, 100—250 mg per cat, PO given in a slurry q 8—12 hours. In addition, famotidine 0.5—2 mg/kg PO q 12—24 hours (VIN staff, 2017).

Crisis kit for pancreatic tumors

μ-agonists

Methadone (schedule II): Dogs: 0.25—0.5 mg/kg SQ q 3—4 h. Cats: 0.1—0.25 mg/kg SQ q 3—4 h. Has some NMDA antagonist properties (VIN staff, 2017).

Morphine (schedule II): Dogs: 0.25—1 mg SQ or 0.2—0.5 mg/kg q 6—8 h for liquid formulations. Cats: 0.1—0.25 mg/kg SQ q 2—4 h or 0.2—0.5 mg/kg q 6—8 h of oral liquid (can cause anaphylaxis, vomiting, dysphoria, constipation). Should have naloxone (reversal agent) in case of side effects (VIN staff, 2017).

Hydromorphone (schedule II): Dogs/cats: 0.05—0.1 mg/kg SQ q 2—4 h (can cause hyperthermia in some patients). Use with caution in MDR-1 mutation patients as they may be predisposed to toxicity (VIN staff, 2017). Can cause vomiting, diarrhea, and panting. Can be partially reversed with butorphanol and naloxone.

Partial μ-agonists

Buprenorphine (schedule III): Dogs: 0.01–0.05 mg/kg SQ or TM q 8–12 h, Cats: 0.01–0.02 mg/kg SQ or TM q 4–12 h 0.12 mg/kg sustained release SQ every 72 h, 0.24 mg/kg Simbadol only SQ q 24 h up to 3 days (this dose can cause profound sedation with other buprenorphine formulations). Use with caution in MDR-1 mutation patients as they may be predisposed to toxicity from norbuprenorphine—the metabolite of buprenorphine (VIN staff, 2017).

K-agonist/μ-antagonist

Butorphanol: Dogs: 0.1–0.5 mg/kg SQ q 1–4 h, 0.55 mg/kg PO q 6–12 h, though it may be more sedating than analgesic, not ideal for bone cancer patients. First pass metabolism makes oral butorphanol ineffective for analgesia. Cats: 0.2–0.4 mg/kg q 1–4 h (VIN staff, 2017).

Opioids can be used in a crisis kit with other adjunct medications such as gabapentin and acepromazine or an α2-agonist.

For additional pain management: Gabapentin: 3–20 mg/kg PO q 8–12 h (VIN staff, 2017).

Pregabalin: Dogs: Pregabalin is administered at a dosage of 4 mg/kg orally three times a day (Kent, 2012). Cats: studies of pregabalin in cats is still limited, but the starting dose we are using for this species is 1–2 mg/kg q 12 h (Dewey C., 2013).

For Seizures: Midazolam: 0.5 mg/kg intranasally (VIN staff, 2017).

Diazepam: 0.5–1 mg/kg intranasally or rectally (VIN staff, 2017).

For Vomiting: Ondansetron: dissolvable tablet 0.5 mg/kg on gums, or in buccal surface. Or Cerenia injectable. For dogs: 1mg/kg SQ q 24h, For cats 0.5 mg/kg SQ q 24 h (VIN staff, 2017)

For hypoglycemia: Karo syrup or honey for insulinoma patient.

Seizures

Seizures may occur with late stage palliative patients. Management of seizures may be challenging in late-onset, late-stage seizure patients, and may be a consideration for euthanasia for clients.

Etiology/DDX of common old age seizures

Seizures first occuring late in life can have different etiologies than the seizures that occur in earlier years. The common differentials of late-in-life, first-time seizures include intracranial neoplasia, metastasis, hepatic encephalopathy, hypertension, and dementia (seizures are reported in people with dementia, though rare (Mendez & Lim, 2003)), LS-CKD-azotemia, electrolyte disturbances, stroke, either infarcts or hemorrhage, and hypoglycemia in diabetic animals or those with insulinomas.

Less commonly seen by house call veterinarians are the inflammatory diseases, granulomatous meningoencephalopathy and pug dog encephalitis. MRI remains the standard of diagnosis for the intracranial disease after ruling out extracranial disease with other testing (Dewey, 2013).

If MRI is not available, or the client chooses to do palliative care instead of curative care, the presentation of the clinical seizure signs may help identify location of the seizure in the brain based on human medicine studies (Mangano, 2004). Further research in veterinary medicine is needed to evaluate location of the seizure based on the presentation of the seizure.

With people when both hemispheres are involved they will have generalized seizures. The seizure can also present as an absent seizures. Examples of absent type seizures in animals may include, the dog or cat who looks off into space or at a wall, fly biting, tail chasing. The seizure may also present as tonic—clonic seizures, atonic seizures, tonic seizures or clonic seizures, myoclonic seizures, or status epilepticus (Yennurajalingam, 2016). Tonic seizures present as the stiffening of body, and clonic seizures present with muscle twitching. Myoclonic seizures are a brief spasming of muscle or muscle groups, appearing similar to the reflexive jerk of the body that can happen when you fall asleep (Mangano, 2004).

When both hemispheres are involved, the seizures may be short, cerebral frontal lobe seizures may occur multiple times in a day and tend to be tonic/clonic seizures (Mangano, 2004).

Occipital lobe seizures may be more focal, appearing as facial twitches, eyelid twitches, may be on the contralateral side, and may have visual changes in people, which may or may not be apparent in animals. Occipital lobe seizures may also present as generalized tonic clonic seizures (Mangano, 2004).

Parietal lobe seizures may present as partial/focal or generalized seizures. In humans, loss of language occurs, and they can develop paresthesia (Mangano, 2004).

Temporal lobe seizures tend to present as a focal seizure. People can have auditory, olfactory, or epigastric sensations or hallucinations. Temporal lobe seizures may cause vomiting, alterations in consciousness, and postictal confusion (Mangano, 2004). More research needs to be done to evaluate the accuracy of seizure location generation and type of seizure in companion animals.

Palliative Management and anticonvulsant therapy

Seizure management: Phenobarbital is still the "gold standard" for treatment of seizures in veterinary patients. Dogs: 1—2.5 mg/kg PO q 12 h. Steady-state serum concentrations of phenobarbital are not reached until 1—2 weeks after treatment is initiated and dosing should be minimally changed during this time. If seizures are not being controlled, dosage may be increased by 20% at a time, with associated monitoring of serum phenobarbital levels. Phenobarbital serum concentration may be checked after steady state has been achieved; if it is less than 15 mcg/mL the dose may be adjusted accordingly. If seizures recur the dose may be raised up to a maximum serum concentration of 45 mcg/mL. High plasma concentrations may be associated with hepatotoxicity. For more accurate dosing, dogs <12 kg should be dosed using oral solution without xylitol (VIN staff, 2017).

Cats: 1.5−2.5 mg/kg PO q 12 h (VIN Staff, 2017).

Levetiracetam (Keppra®): Dogs: 7−25 mg/kg PO q 8 h for maintenance. Cats: 20 mg/kg PO q 8 h for maintenance, can increase the dose to 40 mg/kg (titrated up) (VIN staff, 2017).

Zonisamide—Dogs: 5−10 mg/kg PO q 12 h. Cats: 5−10 mg/kg PO q 24 h (VIN Staff, 2017).

Gabapentin/pregabalin—can be used as an adjunct medication for animals that may develop seizures with their disease. Gabapentin: Dogs: 3−20 mg/kg PO 1−3 times per day. Cats: 3−10 mg/kg PO q 8−24 h (can go higher if needed, likely more sedative) (VIN Staff, 2017).

Pregabalin: Dogs: pregabalin is administered at a dosage of 4 mg/kg orally three times a day (Kent, 2012). Cats: studies of pregabalin in cats is still limited, but the starting dose we are using for this species is 1−2 mg/kg q 12 h (Dewey, 2013).

CBD-May be useful as an adjunct for seizures; however, more research needs to be done with veterinary patients. A 2019 study did show a reduction in seizure activity in about 30% of cases compared to the control group. However, it is a small study, and the dogs who had >50% reduction of seizures were statistically the same for both groups (McGrath, 2020).

Anti-inflammatory: Animals who have either have diagnosed or presumed brain neoplasia should have corticosteroids as part of their palliative plan. Prednisolone or prednisone in addition to anticonvulsant therapy. Dose: 0.5−2 mg/kg PO q 12−24 h (the goal is the lowest possible dose to control the clinical signs, while minimizing side effects) (VIN staff, 2017).

Animals with seizures may also experience headaches. Consider NSAIDs or acetaminophen or paracetamol if the animal is not currently on a steroid. Acetaminophen can be given with NSAIDs or steroids but it is not recommended to give NSAIDs and steroids concurrently. Clients may decide that seizures are an endpoint in a euthanasia decision.

Crisis kit

Benzodiazepines: Midazolam: 0.2−0.5 mg/kg intranasally can give rectally as well, during a seizure.

CBD: Hemp-based CBD dosing 1−2 mg/kg q 12 h. Seems to be more bioavailable in dogs than cats (Deabold, 2019).

Gabapentin: 3−20 mg/kg PO 1−3 times per day. Cats: 3−10 mg/kg PO q 8−24 h (can go higher if needed, likely more sedative).

Pregabalin: Dogs: pregabalin is administered at a dosage of 4 mg/kg orally three times a day (Kent, 2012). Cats: studies of pregabalin in cats is still limited, but the starting dose we are using for this species is 1−2 mg/kg q 12 h (Dewey, 2013).

Sleep/wake disturbances

Sleep/wake disturbances can affect a wide variety of patients in palliative medicine and many etiologies which have already been discussed in other areas of this chapter. Sleep disorders are a problem for people at the end of life, and this may also be an issue with veterinary patients as they age. For people, obesity, decreased exercise, diabetes, apnea, and pain can contribute to sleep loss and sleep–wake disturbances (Institute of Medicine (US) Committee on Sleep Medicine and Research; Colten HR, Altevogt BM, editors, 2006). These clinical signs should also be considered with the veterinary patient who may be having sleep/wake disturbances.

Sleep/wake disturbances are most often associated with cognitive dysfunction. However, normal aging changes may also be responsible for disruptions in the sleep cycle for dogs. Exercise can decrease with age, pain may increase, daily tasks may change (Takeuchi, 2002). In the authors experience, a common cause of a sleep/wake disturbance is pain. Chronic pain should be treated in addition to any other treatments for specific disease and may require multimodal therapy before there is a change in sleep behavior.

Palliative management

There is a combination of pharmaceuticals and nonpharmaceuticals when dealing with sleep–wake disturbances. Pharmaceutical therapy of sleep/wake disturbances can include medications for anxiety (benzodiazapines, antidepressants), pain management (opioids, gabapentinoids), hormonal management (melatonin), and tranquilizers (acepromazine). (see other sections for additional dosing information.) Nonpharmaceuticals therapies may include a fan, white noise generator, massage, and changing lighting during evening hours (ie: not keeping lights on overnight.).

Skin care, end-of-life

The end-of-life veterinary patient may have a primary dermatologic disease, such as dermal tumors or some late-stage disease can develop secondary skin problems, such as hygromas, peripheral edema. Animals with end-stage disease are often recumbent, or struggle to get up, show preference for sleeping outside, or on hard surfaces as a response to pain. Mobility issues may predispose patients to insect infestation, matting, and elongated nails, in addition to decubitus ulcers, and hygroma issues.

Disease related: Peripheral edema may be secondarily associated with diseases such as, heart or renal failure, cancer. Palliative management for peripheral edema can include short term use of diuretics, short-term pressure wraps, massage of the limb, and alternating cool and warm compresses. Peripheral edema may be a clinical sign that the clients may consider for euthanasia. Dermal tumors such as soft tissue sarcomas, mast cell tumors may ulcerate and cause pain, discharge, or bleeding and can become secondarily infected or develop maggot infestation.

Palliative management of ulcerated dermal tumors should include pain management, bleeding treatment, cool therapy, and oral antibiotics. Pain may be two-fold, with both acute and chronic pain. It is important to treat acute ruptures/ulcers with opioids, +/− and NMDA antagonist and they work synergistically. The chronic pain from the growing cancer should also be addressed for both inflammatory and neuropathic pain. It is possible to use Tegaderm dressing and hydrogel sheets for dermal tumors that are ulcerated and bleeding. Other treatments to try could include honey treatment, wet to dry wraps. Oral antifibrinolytics, sucha as aminocaproic acid or tranexamic acid may help decrease or arrest bleeding. Other treatment may include Yunnan Baiyao, orally or in an areosol spray for direct use. Oozing or bleeding tumors are often an end point for clients. Ulcerated dermal tumors can be challenging to treat for the end-of-life patient and may be a point at which owners may want to consider euthanasia.

Fragile skin of the elderly animal

Elderly humans develop fragile skin and though we do not see it as often in elder veterinary patients, the potential for fragile skin should be considered when handling elderly animals. Fragile skin in elderly animals has been associated with increased steroid hormones that inhibit collagen synthesis. Cushing's, iatrogenic steroid treatment, diabetes, hepatic lipidosis, and neoplastic or paraneoplastic disease, such as a progesterone secreting adrenal tumor or cholangiocarcinoma (Kunder, 2013). Use of megestrol acetate (progesterone) may also contribute (Kunder, 2013). There is also a report of cats developing cachexia and fragile skin syndrome without concomitantly having increased corticosteroids or hormones (Furiani, 2017). Diagnosis of the underlying disease may help adjust treatment plan. Lacerations or tears in skin can be sutured, however the skin may continue to tear despite repair, and these can be frustrating and difficult to treat. Care should be taken to not scruff elderly cats, to be very gentle with elderly dogs, using medication and other gentle, stress reducing techniques to handle them if they are a challenging to work with. Fragile skin damage may be an unfortunate and uncomfortable end for a beloved pet.

Recumbent skin problems: Decubitus or decubital ulcers—aka "Bedsores" are difficult late-stage complications in skin management. Decubitus ulcers occur due to pressure, decreased circulation, and changes in sensory input leading to ischemia and then necrosis. They may occur more frequently in sarcopenic, cachexic patients. Predisposed patients may have neurologic disease, cardiovascular disease, dehydration, malnutrition, and hypotension (Zaidi, 2021). Decubitus ulcers can be a poor prognostic indicator. Similarly to decubital ulcers, hygromas can also become a problem with recumbent animals.

Palliative management may include soft bedding or a pressure-relieving pillow placed under the animal, and treatment of the open ulcer with Tegaderm dressing and hydrogel sheets can help heal open wounds on the skin. If those are not readily available, then utilizing antibacterial ointment, cream, or silver sulfadiazine with prestick bandaging material may be a quick solution. Opioids can be used to treat acute pain, and an NSAID can be used for chronic pain management. Within 3–7 days, changing the opioids for gabapentin and continuing the NSAID can continue the pain management as they heal. If pain is more complex, adding an NDMA antagonist, either subanesthetic ketamine 0.5 mg/kg SQ PRN or amantadine 2–5 mg/kg PO SID to BID, may be useful. Oral antibiotics may also be useful. Hygromas may be treated with elbow covers, in addition to other treatments.

Grooming related: Matting can be a source of pain for animals. Small mats may not be painful; however, once they start coalescing and becoming more significant on the body, they do cause pain. Mats can also harbor insects, such as fleas or maggots.

Palliative management could include sedation or anesthesia and removal of mats. Employing a groomer who understands handling fragile elderly patients can remove concerns about tearing skin, manhandling, clipper burn (which may be more significant for an elderly or frail pet).

Elongated nails may make it more difficult for the animal to move or get up or lay down, especially on slippery flooring. Excessively long nails may put additional torque or pressure on joints of the feet and limbs, resulting in added chronic pain and mobility issues.

Palliative management may include sedating, if needed and trimming nails on a regular basis. Adding nail grips can help with slippage on hardwood, tile, linoleum floors.

Insects: fleas, flies, maggots, and ticks. As much as we hope to not see additional insects on pets, we occasionally see an animal who lives outside or is in a location to have many fleas, or flies creating fly strike or laying eggs and creating maggots. They may have a burden of ticks, depending on where they are located.

Palliative management for fly strike or maggots includes treating with the latest insecticide available. Add pain management for patients who may be recumbent and have maggots or fly strike. Consider treating with opioids for a few days for the acute pain and NSAIDs for the inflammatory pain. Treat the affected skin with a topical antibiotic or oral antibiotic depending on the location of the affected area.

For ticks or fleas, remove those seen and start the patient on an insecticide for ticks and fleas. Remove mats if needed.

Finding maggots on an animal may be a point at which clients may consider euthanasia.

Interventional therapies

Interventional therapies are practiced in palliative medicine for human patients, but these would be rare for in-home veterinary end-of-life patients. Interventional therapies will be discussed briefly to help clients know all of their options so that they may make informed decisions. The following are interventional therapies that may be considered.

Interventional therapies could include nerve blocks for pain management, steroid injections epidurally, or in a joint.

Spinal cord or peripheral nerve stimulation (may help with phantom pain) with the use of the TENS unit (transcutaneous electrical nerve stimulation).

Use of urinary catheters for animals who might not be able to urinate on their own.

Chest tubes being placed for animals with pleural effusion.

SQ or IV Port placement (for SQ or IV fluid therapy or other medications that may be given SQ or IV frequently). SQ port placement is more common for home use, however, with human palliative ppatients IV ports are placed for home use and could be considered for veterinary patients.

Feeding tube placement, either nasoesophageal in the short term or esophageal feeding tubes or a PEG tube for longer term feeding anorexic or dysphagic patients.

Placing an animal on a ventilator in the home setting may not be done but could be sent to a referral center for ventilator support. This would not be a common practice in palliative medicine, for people or animals.

Integrative care

As mentioned in the early part of the chapter, integrative therapy is beyond the scope of this book; this book has been meant to build a foundation for evidence-based veterinary palliative medicine. This author believes any therapy utilized for an end-of-life patient should be evaluated with a critical. Clients may be interested in using integrative care, and whether the house call vet uses in practice or not, they should consider having a basic understanding of integrative care so they may educate clients appropriately. There are many books on integrative veterinary care available for those who are interested in learning more. Acupuncture, laser therapy, and the Assisi loop, are examples of integrative therapy that have been utilized for pain management. Herbal therapies may also be utilized for various diseases. Nonmedical therapies are used in human palliative care, such as massage, heat or cold therapy and music therapy. There is a short review in the pain management section.

Conclusion

Palliative management of clinical signs may include the same medications and therapies that general practitioners and specialists utilize; however, they may be utilized in different ways. In-home providers of palliative veterinary care tend to incorporate outside-the-box, thinking and innovative problem solving for our patients. This chapter has explored different ways of thinking outside the box and has also touched upon where we would benefit from additional studies in our profession. Veterinary palliative medicine is bridging the potential gap of care from a terminal diagnosis to euthanasia. As a result, we can partner with our clients to provide a greater standard of care for our patients. We like to thank Dr. Eve Harrison for her contributions to this chapter.

Disclaimer

This chapter will examine veterinary palliatve medicine in light of the evidence-base in human palliative medicine. Lists of differentials in this chapter will be limited to diseases seen in end-of-life patients. For this chapter, both human and animal texts and studies have been drawn from, and the authors have noted when the content reflects human-based information. When we can, we will extrapolate from the standard of care in human palliative medicine and evaluate the possibility of using similar treatments in veterinary medicine. More research may be needed to evaluate the efficacy of different medications and approaches in companion animals. The authors also recognize that human medicine has differences than veterinary medicine, and treatments, medications, and efficacy may vary between species. Veterinary specialists have been consulted about the use and efficacy of particular human medications, and the authors will not include contraindicated medications in the text. The authors may suggest new uses for medications or novel medications if there has been no contraindication found.

This text is meant to be practical, and as such, the review is limited and the drugs suggested are limited to palliative therapies, though we may include standard dosing in addition to a more palliative approach. We recognize that veterinary palliative patients may be seen by general practitioners and specialists, and we hope to expand upon what is currently offered for these patients. We hope looking at cases from a different and shfited perspective, including the client perspective in palliating their pets and bridging a potential gap between client and veterinarian, terminal diagnosis, and euthanasia can help improve the lives of both your clients and their beloved pets and improve your practice.

Integrative therapies are not specifically included in this text, though the authors recommend learning more by consulting integrative resources. Whether you utilize them or not, you will find clients who will have questions and want to utilize alternative or integrative therapies, or the animal will already be on those therapies and it would benefit the client and patient to have knowledge about those therapies. Additional information and references on integrative therapies are at the end of the pain management chapter.

This chapter is arranged alphabetically for ease of look up.

References

Acierno, M. J., Brown, S., Coleman, A. E., Jepson, R. E., Papich, M., Stepien, R. L., & Syme, H. M. (2018). ACVIM consensus statement: Guidelines for the identification, evaluation, and management of systemic hypertension in dogs and cats. *Journal of veterinary internal medicine, 32*(6), 1803–1822. https://doi.org/10.1111/jvim.15331

Acierno, M. J. (2018). ACVIM consensus statement: Guidelines for the identification, evaluation, and management of systemic hypertension in dogs and cats. *Journal of Veterinary Internal Medicine*, 1803–1822.

Al-Khatib, S. M. (2018). Guideline for Management of patients with ventricular arrhythmias and the prevention of sudden cardiac death. *Circulation*, e272–e391.

Ajith Kumar, A. K., & Mantri, S. N. (2021). Lymphangitic Carcinomatosis. *StatPearls (1)*. Treasure Island, FL: StatPearls Publishing. https://www.ncbi.nlm.nih.gov/books/NBK560921/.

Ali, S. G. (2014). Sarcopenia, cachexia and aging: Diagnosis, mechanisms and therapeutic options - a mini-review. *Gerontology*, 294–305.

Alves, J. C., Santos, A., Jorge, P., & Pitães, A. (2021). The use of soluble fibre for the management of chronic idiopathic large-bowel diarrhoea in police working dogs. *BMC veterinary research, 17*(1), 100–101. https://doi.org/10.1186/s12917-021-02809-w

Ammouri, L. (2010). Palliative treatment of malignant ascites: Profile of catumaxomab. *Biologics*, 103–110.

Anderson, K. L., Zulch, H., O'Neill, D. G., Meeson, R. L., & Collins, L. M. (2020). Risk Factors for Canine Osteoarthritis and Its Predisposing Arthropathies: A Systematic Review. *Frontiers in veterinary science, 7*, 220. https://doi.org/10.3389/fvets.2020.00220

Anderson, K. L. (2020). Risk factors for canine osteoarthritis and its predisposing arthropathies: A systematic review. *Frontiers in Veterinary Science*, 220.

Azhar, G. W. (2013). New approaches to treating cardiac cachexia in the older patient. *Current Cardiovascular Risk Reports*, 480–484.

Bailiff, N. L. (2002). Clinical signs, clinicopathological findings, etiology, and outcome associated with hemoptysis in dogs: 36 cases. *Journal of the American Animal Hospital Association*, 125–133.

Baker Rogers, J. M. (2020). *Dyspnea in palliative care*. StatPearls Publishing.

Banzato, T. F. (2019). A frailty Index based on clinical data to quantify mortality risk in dogs. *Science Reports*, 16749.

Barnette, C. (July 20, 2020). *Diagnosing canine cognitive dysfunction: Symptoms and treatment*. From Dispomed: https://www.dispomed.com/diagnosing-canine-cognitive-dysfunction-symptoms-and-treatment/.

Bartges, J. (2012). Chronic kidney disease in dogs and cats. *Veterinary Clinics of North America: Small Animal Practice*, 669–692.

Barzegari, H. K. (2021). Intravenous furosemide vs nebulized furosemide in patients with pulmonary edema: A randomized controlled trial. *Health Science Reports*, e235.

Berger, E. P. (2018). Retrospective evaluation of toceranib phosphate (Palladia) use in cats with mast cell neoplasia. *Journal of Feline Medicine and Surgery*, 95–102.

van Beusekom, CD, v. d. (2015). Feline hepatic biotransformation of diazepam: Differences between cats and dogs. *Research in Veterinary Science*, 119–125.

Bissett, S. A. (2007). Prevalence, clinical features, and causes of epistaxis in dogs. *Journal of the American Veterinary Medical Association*, 1843–1850.

Biswas, A. K. (2020). Cancer-associated cachexia: A systemic consequence of cancer progression. *Annual Review of Cancer Biology*, 391–411.

Bodtke, S. L. (2016). *Hospice and palliative medicine handbook: A clnical guide* (1st ed.) (Self published).

Booth, D. Y. (2019a). Nebulized tranexamic acid for the use of epistaxis: A case report. *The Journal of Emergency Medicine*, 30934–30935.

Booth, S. J. (2019b). Improving the quality of life of people with advanced respiratory disease and severe breathlessness. *Breathe*, 198–215.

Boucek, P. (2006). Advanced diabetic neuropathy: A point of no return? *Journal of the Society for Biomedical Diabetes Research*, 143–150.

Brown, C. E. (2016). Chronic kidney disease in aged cats: Clinical features, morphology, and proposed pathogeneses. *Veterinary Pathology*, 309–326.

Brown, J. C. (2016). Effect of aminocaproic acid on clot strength and clot lysis of canine blood determined by use of an in vitro model of hyperfibrinolysis. *American Journal of Veterinary Research*, 1258–1265.

Bush, S. H. (2009). The assessment and management of delirium in cancer patients. *The Oncologist*, 1039–1049.

Cade, W. T. (2008). Diabetes-Related Microvascular and Macrovascular Disease in the Physical Therapy Setting. *Journal of the American Physical Therapy Association, 88*(11), 1322–1335. https://doi.org/10.2522/ptj.20080008

Campbell, B. G. (2006). Dressings, bandages, and splints for wound management in dogs and cats. *The Veterinary Clinics of North America. Small Animal Practice*, 759–791.

Candellone, A., Cerquetella, M., Girolami, F., Badino, P., & Odore, R. (2020). Acute Diarrhea in Dogs: Current Management and Potential Role of Dietary Polyphenols Supplementation. Antioxidants (Basel, Switzerland)*, 9*(8), 725. https://doi.org/10.3390/antiox9080725

Cardinali, D. P. (2010). Clinical aspects of melatonin intervention in Alzheimer's disease progression. *Current Neuropharmacology*, 218–227.

Casamian-Sorrosal, D.,W. S. (2010). The use of mirtazapine as an appetite stimulant in dogs and cats: A prospective observational study. In *British small animal veterinary association 2010 proceedings online*. Birmingham: British Small Animal Veterinary Association.

Center, S. (2004). Fluid accumulation disorders. *Small Animal Clinical Diagnosis by Laboratory Methods*, 247–269.

Chaitman, J.,G. F. (2021). Fecal microbiota transplantation in dogs. *Veterinary Clinics of North America*, 219–233.

Chapman, R. (2008). Canine models of asthma and COPD. *Pulmonary Pharmacology & Therapeutics*, 731–742.

Chilukuri, P. O. (2018). Dysphagia. *Missouri Medicine*, 206–210.

Christian-Miller, N. (2018). Hepatocellular cancer pain: Impact and management challenges. *Journal of Hepatocellular Carcinoma*, 75–80.

Cimons, M. (November 29, 2013). *Frailty is a medical condition, not an inevitable result of aging (Op-Ed)*. From Live Science https://www.livescience.com/41602-frailty-is-medical-condition.html.

Cook, A. (2018). Dealing With Dysrexia in Dogs and Cats. *Today's Veterinary Practice*. https://todaysveterinarypractice.com/dysrexia-dogs-cats/.

Cook, A. (2020). Dealing with dysrexia in dogs and cats. *Today's Veterinary Practice*.

Cooper, R. L. (2011). Peritoneal dialysis in veterinary medicine. *Veterinary Clinics: Small Animal Practice*, 91–113.

Cornell CVM Staff. (June 18, 2020). *Ascites is a serious symptom* (Cat Watch).

Couto, G. (2002). *Disseminated intravascular coagulation* (WSAVA. WSAVA/VIN).

Curran, K. S. (January 12, 2015). *Bone neoplasia*. From VIN https://www.vin.com/Members/Associate/Associate.plx?from=GetDzInfo&DiseaseId=464&pid=607.

Davey, C. H. (2020). Fatigue in individuals with end stage renal disease. *Nephrology Nursing Journal: Journal of the American Nephrology Nurses' Association*, 497–508.

Deabold, K. A. (2019). Single-dose pharmacokinetics and preliminary safety assessment with use of CBD-rich Hemp nutraceutical in healthy dogs and cats. *Animals: An Open Access Journal from MDPI*, 832.

Desai, J. P.,M. F. (2021). *Peritoneal metastasis*. StatPearls. Retrieved from https://www.ncbi.nlm.nih.gov/books/NBK541114/.

Dev, R. W. (2017). The evolving approach to management of cancer cachexia. *Oncology/Cancer Network, 31*.

Dewey, C. (2013). Practical seizure management in dogs and cats. In *World small animal veterinary association world congress proceedings, 2013*. Ithica, NY: WSAVA.

Dewey, C. W. (2019). Canine cognitive dysfunction. In K. Goldberg (Ed.), *Advances in palliative medicine* (pp. 476−499). Philadelphia: Elsevier.

Diehl, S. (2021). *Palliative conversations with Dr Diehl. (L. Hendrix, interviewer)*.

Dixon-Jimenez, A. R. (2020). *Systemic hypertension in dogs and cats*. From Today's Veterinary Practice https://todaysveterinarypractice.com/systemic-hypertension-in-dogs-cats/.

Duong, S., Patel, T., & Chang, F. (2017). Dementia: What pharmacists need to know. *Canadian pharmacists journal : CPJ = Revue des pharmaciens du Canada : RPC, 150*(2), 118−129. https://doi.org/10.1177/1715163517690745

Dzierżanowski, T. (2018). The occurrence and risk factors of constipation in inpatient palliative care unit patients vs. nursing home residents. *Gastroenterology Review/Przegląd Gastroenterologiczny*, 299−304.

Enomoto, M. M. (2019). Anti-nerve growth factor monoclonal antibodies for the control of pain in dogs and cats. *The Veterinary Record*, 23.

Farbicka, P. (2013). Palliative care in patients with lung cancer. *Contemporary Oncology*, 238−245.

Fares, J., Fares, M. Y., Khachfe, H. H., Salhab, H. A., & Fares, Y. (2020). Molecular principles of metastasis: a hallmark of cancer revisited. *Signal transduction and targeted therapy, 5*(1), 28. https://doi.org/10.1038/s41392-020-0134-x

FDA staff. (2021). Osteoarthritis in Cats: More Common Than You Think. *FDA website*. https://www.fda.gov/animal-veterinary/animal-health-literacy/osteoarthritis-cats-more-common-you-think.

Feliciano, J. L. (2021). Pharmacologic interventions for breathlessness in patients with advanced cancer. *Journal of the American Medical Association*, e2037632.

Finney, L. J. (2019). Is it safe to prescribe benzodiazepines or opioids for dyspnoea in interstitial lung disease? *Breathe, 15*, 137−139. https://doi.org/10.1183/20734735.0015-2019

Flesner, B. K. (2019). Long-term survival and glycemic control with toceranib phosphate and prednisone for a metastatic canine insulinoma. *Journal of the American Animal Hospital Association*, e55105.

Fournier, Q.,S. J. (2021). Chemotherapy-induced diarrhoea in dogs and its management with smectite: Results of a monocentric open-label randomized clinical trial. *Veterinary and Comparative Oncology*, 25−33.

Freeman, L. M. (2012). Cachexia and sarcopenia: Emerging syndromes of importance in dogs and cats. *Journal of Veterinary Internal Medicine*, 3−17.

Furiani, N.,P. I. (2017). Reversible and cachexia-associated feline skin fragility syndrome in three cats. *Veterinary Dermatology*, e121.

Gamble, L. J. (2018). Pharmacokinetics, safety, and clinical efficacy of cannabidiol treatment in osteoarthritic dogs. *Frontiers in Veterinary*, 165.

Gautam, C. S. (2020). Repurposing potential of ketamine: Opportunities and challenges. *Indian Journal of Psychological Medicine*, 22−29.

Germain, M. J. (2011). Palliative care in CKD: The earlier the better. *American Journal of Kidney Diseases*, 378−380.

Girol, A. M.-T.-B. (2019). Use of tranexamic acid in cats with cavitary hemorrhage due to high-rise syndrome. In *European veterinary emergency and critical care congress*.

Glińska, K. N. (2007). Use of a variety of biochemical parameters in distinguishing non-malignant from malignant ascites. In *17th ECVIM-CA congress, 2007. ECVIM congress.*

Godfrey, D. R. (2005). Osteoarthritis in cats: a retrospective radiological study. *The Journal of small animal practice, 46*(9), 425−429. https://doi.org/10.1111/j.1748-5827.2005.tb003 40.x

Goldstein, N. M. (2013). *Evidence-based practice of palliative medicine.* Philadelphia: Elsiever.

Grobman, M. R. (2016a). Investigation of neurokinin-1 receptor antagonism as a novel treatment for chronic bronchitis in dogs. *Journal of Veterinary Internal Medicine*, 847−852.

Grobman, M. R. (2016b). Maropitant as s a novel treatment for chronic bronchitis in dogs. *Journal of Veterinary Internal Medicine*, 847−852.

Gruen, M. E. (2014). Use of trazodone to facilitate postsurgical confinement in dogs. *Journal of the American Veterinary Medical Association*, 296−301.

Guerriero, F. (2020). Linking persistent pain and frailty in older adults. *Pain Medicine*, 61−66.

Gurney, M., & Bradbrook, C. (2020). Subcutaneous ketamine for analgesia. *Blog-Zero Pain Philosophy.* https://www.zeropainphilosophy.com/post/subcutaneous-ketamine-for-analgesia.

Hadji Rasouliha, S. B. (2019). A RAPGEF6 variant constitutes a major risk factor for laryngeal paralysis in dogs. *Genetics, 15.*

Hamnilrat, T., Lekcharoensuk, C., Choochalermpporn, P., & Thayananuphat, A. (2015). Flash Visual Evoked Potentials in Normal Pomeranian Dogs and Those with Canine Cognitive Dysfunction. *The Thai Journal of Veterinary Medicine, 45*(3), 323−329. https://he01.tci-thaijo.org/index.php/tjvm/article/view/39800.

Hardy, C. (July 9, 2020). *Bone cancers in dogs.* From Colorado State University/Flint Animal Cancer Center https://www.csuanimalcancercenter.org/2020/07/09/bone-cancer-in-dogs/.

Harkin, K. (July/August 2016). Uncovering the cause of fever in dogs. *Today's Veterinary Practice.*

Hawkins, E. D. (2021). *Coughing dogs: Determining why.* From Clinicians Brief https://www.cliniciansbrief.com/column/category/column/capsules/coughing-dogs-determining-why#:~:text=Differential%20diagnoses%20include%20pulmonary%20edema,disease%2C%20and%20severe%20fungal%20pneumonia.

Hazewinkel, H. A., Meij, B. P., Picavet, P., & Voorhout, G. (2011). Cross-sectional study of the prevalence and clinical features of osteoarthritis in 100 cats. *Veterinary journal (London, England : 1997), 187*(3), 304−309. https://doi.org/10.1016/j.tvjl.2009.12.014

Herman, J. P. (2016). Regulation of the hypothalamic-pituitary-adrenocortical stress response. *Comprehensive Physiology*, 603−621.

Herold, C. B. (1996). Lung metastasis. *European Radiology*, 596−606.

Hill, N. E. (2017). Impact of ghrelin on body composition and muscle function in a long-term rodent model of critical illness. *PLoS One.* https://doi.org/10.1371/journal.pone.0182659.

Hofmann, S. H. (2017). Patients in palliative care-Development of a predictive model for anxiety using routine data. *PLoS One*, e0179415.

Hoshino, T. T. (2009). Pharmacological treatment in asthma and COPD. *Allergology International: Official Journal of the Japanese Society of Allergology*, 341−346.

Hristov, T. (2019). Vascular endothelial growth factor (VEGF) in abdominal fluid in dogs with oncological and non-oncological diseases. *Macedonian Veterinary Review*, i−iv.

Hua, J. H. (2016). Assessment of frailty in aged dogs. *American Journal of Veterinary Research*, 1357−1365.

Huang, S.,R. J. (2000). Blockade of nuclear factor-kappaB signaling inhibits angiogenesis and tumorigenicity of human ovarian cancer cells by suppressing expression of vascular endothelial growth factor and interleukin 8. *Cancer Research*, 5334–5339.

Hunt, G. (2002). *Abdominal conditions of the dog and cat*. WSAVA 2002. WSAVA/VIN.

Institute of Medicine (US) Committee on Sleep Medicine and Research, Colten, H. R., & Altevogt, B. M. (2006). Extent and health consequences of chronic sleep loss and sleep disorders. In H. R. (Ed.), *Sleep disorders and sleep deprivation: An unmet public health problem* (pp. 55–136). Washington DC: National Academies Press.

Jensen AP, B. C. (2019). Clinical effect of probiotics in prevention or treatment of gastrointestinal disease in dogs: A systematic review. *Journal of Veterinary Internal Medicine*, 1849–1864.

Jimenez-Andrade, J. M. (2010). Bone cancer pain. *Annals of the New York Academy of Sciences*, 173–181.

Johannes, C. M. (2021). The use of capromorelin for the clinical problem of inappetence. *Today's Veterinary Practice*.

Johnson, M. (2007). Management of end stage cardiac failure. *Postgraduate Medical Journal*, 395–401.

Kaseer, H. S. (2021). *Aminocaproic acid*. StatPearls.

Kasvis, P. V. (2019). Health-related quality of life across cancer cachexia stages. *Annuls of Palliative Medicine*, 33–42.

Keller, N. (2014a). *Gastrointestinal endocrine tumours*. WSAVA 2014. QLD, AU: WSAVA.

Keller, N. (2014b). *Gastrointestinal endocrine tumours*. WSAVA 2014 proceedings. WSAVA/VIN.

Kent, M. (2012). Newer anticonvulsant agents. In *NAVC conference 2012 small animal*. Orlando: NAVC.

Keuhn, N. (2018). Cancers and tumors of the lung and airway in dogs. In *MSD manual, veterinary manual*. Kenilworth, NJ: Merek and Co., Inc.

Koga, K.,D. G.-G.-G.-K. (2015). Coexistence of two forms of LTP in ACC provides a synaptic mechanism for the interactions between anxiety and chronic pain. *Neuron*, 377–389.

Koppe, L. F.-Z. (2019). Kidney cachexia or protein-energy wasting in chronic kidney disease: Facts and numbers. *Journal of Cachexia, Sarcopenia and Muscle*, 479–484.

Kottusch, P. T. (2009). Oberlebenszeit bei Nahrungs- und Flüssigkeitskarenz [Survival time without food and drink]. *Archiv für Kriminologie*, 184–191.

Kowalska, J. M. (2019). Effectiveness of physiotherapy in elderly patients with dementia: A prospective, comparative analysis. *Disability and Rehabilitation*, 815–819.

KuKanich, B.,S. J. (2013). Pharmacokinetics of hydrocodone and hydromorphone after oral hydrocodone in healthy Greyhound dogs. *The Veterinary Journal*, 266–268.

KuKanich, B. (2016). Pharmacokinetics and pharmacodynamics of oral acetaminophen in combination with codeine in healthy Greyhound dogs. *Journal of Veterinary Pharmacology and Therapeutics*, 514–517.

Kunder, D. M. (February 28, 2013). A diagnostic approach to skin disease in geriatric cats. In *DVM 360*.

Lambert, L. H. (2018). Palliative management of advanced peritoneal carcinomatosis. *Surgical Oncology Clinics of North America*, 585–602.

Lane, M. L. (2016). Medical management of gastrinoma in a cat. *Journal of Feline Medicine and Surgery Open Reports, 2*, 2055116916646389.

Larsson, L. D. (2019). Sarcopenia: Aging-related loss of muscle mass and function. *Physiological Reviews*, 427–511.

Lascelles, B. (2019). Managing OA with anti-NGF therapy. *Today's Veterinary Practice.*

Lascelles, B. D. X., Dong, Y. H., Marcellin-Little, D. J., Thomson, A., Wheeler, S, & Correa, M. (2012). Relationship of orthopedic examination, goniometric measurements, and radiographic signs of degenerative joint disease in cats. *BMC Veterinary Research, 8*, 10. https://doi.org/10.1186/1746-6148-8-10

Lee, D. B. (2020). An update on feline chronic gingivostomatitis. *Veterinary Clinics of North America: Small Animal Practice*, 973−982.

van Leeuwen, PW, v. d. (2013). De terminale fase bij amyotrofische laterale sclerose [Terminal care in patients with amyotrophic lateral sclerosis]. *Nederlandsch Tijdschrift voor Geneeskunde*, A6295.

Lena, A. E. (2019). Cardiac cachexia. *European Heart Journal Supplements: Journal of the European Society of Cardiology*, L24−L27.

Letko, A. M.-J. (2020). A CNTNAP1 missense variant is associated with canine laryngeal paralysis and polyneuropathy. *Genes*, 1426−1440.

Levenson, J. W. (2000). The last six months of life for patients with congestive heart failure. *Journal of the American Geriatrics Society*, S101−S109.

Li, B. F.-H.-H.-C.-X. (2019). Adverse drug reactions of Yunnan Baiyao capsule: A multicenter intensive monitoring study in China. *Annals of Translational Medicine, 118.*

Liao, P., Johnstone, C., & Rich, S. (2021). Bleeding Management in Hospice Care Settings. *Palliative Care Network of Wisconsin.* https://www.mypcnow.org/fast-fact/bleeding-management-in-hospice-care-settings/.

Lidbury, J. A. (2016). New advances in the diagnosis of canine and feline liver and pancreatic disease. *The Veterinary Journal*, 87−95.

Lu-Emerson, C. E. (2012). Brain metastases. *Continuum*, 295−311.

Madari, A. F. (2015). Assessment of severity and progression of canine cognitive dysfunction syndrome using the CAnine DEmentia Scale (CADES). *Applied Animal Behaviour Science*, 138−145.

Mahler, D. A. (2013). Opioids for refractory dyspnea. *Expert Review of Respiratory Medicine*, 123−134.

Mangano, F. M. (2004). Clues to anatomic location. *Epilepsy Foundation.* From Epilepsy Foundation https://www.epilepsy.com/living-epilepsy/epilepsy-and/professional-health-care-providers/co-existing-disorders/brain-tumors/clues-anatomic-location.

Marks, S. L. (2013). Diarrhea. *Canine and Feline Gastroenterology*, 99−108.

Marks, J. M. (December 15, 2017). *Bronchorrhea?.* From healthline.com https://www.healthline.com/health/bronchorrhea.

Martin, E. I. (2009). The neurobiology of anxiety disorders: Brain imaging, genetics, and psychoneuroendocrinology. *Psychiatric Clinics of North America*, 549−575.

May, K. L. (2019). Nutrition and the aging brain of dogs and cats. *Journal of the American Veterinary Medical Association*, 1245−1254.

McAnelly, K. (2015). *A palliative care approach to nutrition and hydration.* From Care Research.com.au https://www.caresearch.com.au/Caresearch/Portals/0/PA-Tookit/Clinical%20Newsletter%20Issue4.pdf.

McGrath, S. B. (2020). Randomized blinded controlled clinical trial to assess the effect of oral cannabidiol administration in addition to conventional antiepileptic treatment on seizure frequency in dogs with intractable idiopathic epilepsy. *Journal of the American Veterinary Medical Association*, 1301−1308.

McKenzie, B. (December 11, 2017). Yunnan baiyao for patients with hemorrhage, neoplasia. *Veterinary Practice News.*

Megna, J. L. (2002). Gabapentin's effect on agitation in severely and persistently mentally ill patients. *The Annals of Pharmacotherapy*, 12−16.

Mendez, M., & Lim, G. (2003). Seizures in elderly patients with dementia: epidemiology and management. *Drugs & aging, 20*(11), 791−803. https://doi.org/10.2165/00002512-200320110-00001

Mills, D. D.-B. (2020). Pain and problem behavior in cats and dogs. *Animals*, 318.

Mills, D. M. (2020). Development and psychometric validation of the canine anxiety scale. *Frontiers in Veterinary Science*.

Mondino, A.,D. L.-G. (2021). Disorders in dogs: A pathophysiological and clinical review. *Topics in Companion Animal Medicine*, 100516.

Monteiro, B., Steagall, P., Lascelles, B., Robertson, S., Murrell, J. C., Kronen, P. W., … Yamashita, K. (2019). Long-term use of non-steroidal anti-inflammatory drugs in cats with chronic kidney disease: from controversy to optimism. *The Journal of small animal practice, 60*(8), 459−462. https://doi.org/10.1111/jsap.13012

Morgan, R. S. (2016). Degenerative joint disease. *VINcyclopedia of Diseases*.

Moulton, J. E., von Tscharner, C., & Schneider, R. (1981). Classification of lung carcinomas in the dog and cat. *Veterinary pathology, 18*(4), 513−528. https://doi.org/10.1177/030098588101800409

Mythili, A. K. (2010). A Comparative study of examination scores and quantitative sensory testing in diagnosis of diabetic polyneuropathy. *International Journal of Diabetes in Developing Countries*, 43−48.

Nardone, R. H. (2016). Canine degenerative myelopathy: A model of human amyotrophic lateral sclerosis. *Zoology*, 64−73.

Naruse, T. N. (2006). Meloxicam inhibits osteosarcoma growth, invasiveness and metastasis by COX-2-dependent and independent routes. *Carcinogenesis*, 584−592.

National Cancer Institute. (February 6, 2017). *Metastatic cancer*. From National Cancer Institute https://www.cancer.gov/types/metastatic-cancer.

Nelson, R. W. (2010). *Hypercalcemia in dogs and cats: Etiology and diagnostic approach [proceedings]*. WSAVA 2010. WSAVA.

Nelson, R. W. (2014). Animal models of disease: Classification and etiology of diabetes in dogs and cats. *The Journal of Endocrinology, T1−9*.

Nenadović, K. V.-D. (2017). Cortisol concentration, pain and sedation scale in free roaming dogs treated with carprofen after ovariohysterectomy. *Veterinary World*, 888−894.

de Oliveira, P. (2020). Palliative care in pulmonary medicine. *Jornal Brasilerio de Pneumologia*, e20190280.

Ogilvie, G. K. (1998). Interventional nutrition for the cancer patient. *Clinical Techniques in Small Animal Practice, 13*(4), 224−231. https://doi.org/10.1016/S1096-2867(98)80007-8

Osekavage, K. E. (2018). Pharmacokinetics of tranexamic acid in healthy dogs and assessment of its antifibrinolytic properties in canine blood. *American Journal of Veterinary Research*, 1057−1063.

Ozawa, M., Chambers, J. K., Uchida, K., & Nakayama, H. (2016). The Relation between canine cognitive dysfunction and age-related brain lesions. *The Journal of veterinary medical science, 78*(6), 997−1006. https://doi.org/10.1292/jvms.15-0624

Palaia, I. T. (2020). Immunotherapy for ovarian cancer: Recent advances and combination therapeutic approaches. *OncoTargets and Therapy*, 6109−6129.

Pan, Y. L. (2018). Efficacy of a therapeutic diet on dogs with signs of cognitive dysfunction syndrome (CDS): A prospective double blinded placebo controlled clinical study. *Frontiers in Nutrition*, 127.

Penet, M. F. (2015). Cancer cachexia, recent advances, and future directions. *Cancer Journal (Sudbury, Mass.)*, 117–122.

Plumb, D. (2002). *Veterinary drug handbook* (4th ed.). Pharmavet Publishing.

Popper, H. (2016). Progression and metastasis of lung cancer. *Cancer Metastasis Reviews*, 75–91.

Powers, S. K. (2016). Disease-induced skeletal muscle atrophy and fatigue. *Medicine and Science in Sports and Exercise*, 2307–2319.

Prpar Mihevc, S. (2019). Canine cognitive dysfunction and Alzheimer's disease - two facets of the same disease? *Frontiers in Neuroscience*, 604.

Quimby, J. (2018). Mirtazapine in cats: Dosage, side effects, and efficacy. *Phamacology and Medications*.

Raouf, M. A. (2017). Rational dosing of gabapentin and pregabalin in chronic kidney disease. *Journal of Pain Research*, 275–278.

Rebar, A. H. (2009). Cytology of effusions (proceedings). In *Proceedings of DVM 360*.

Rhodes, L. Z. (2017). Capromorelin: A ghrelin receptor agonist and novel therapy for stimulation of appetite in dogs. *Veterinary Medicine and Science*, 3–16.

Rishniw, M., Sammarco, J., Glass, Eric N., & Cerroni, B. (2021). Effect of doxepin on quality of life in Labradors with laryngeal paralysis: A double-blinded, randomized, placebo-controlled trial. *Journal of Veterinary Internal Medicine, 35*(4), 1943–1949.

Rochon, P. A. (2017). The harms of benzodiazepines for patients with dementia. *Canadian Medical Association journal = journal de l'Association medicale canadienne*, E517–E518.

Rothrock, K. (January 25, 2018). *Insulinoma*. From Vincyclopedia of diseases https://www.vin.com/Members/Associate/Associate.plx?from=GetDzInfo&DiseaseId=5871&pid=607.

Rothrock, K. (July 30, 2020a). *Diabetes mellitus*. From VIN.com https://www.vin.com/Members/Associate/Associate.plx?from=GetDzInfo&DiseaseId=901&pid=607.

Rothrock, K. (April 15, 2020b). *Gastrinoma*. From VIN.com https://www.vin.com/Members/Associate/Associate.plx?DiseaseId=728.

Rothrock, K. (July 3, 2020c). *Stomatitis*. From VIN.com https://www.vin.com/Members/Associate/Associate.plx?from=GetDzInfo&DiseaseId=674&pid=607.

Rothrock, K., Rishniw, M., & Shell, L. (2018). Insulinoma (Canine). *VINcyclopedia*. https://www.vin.com/members/cms/project/defaultadv1.aspx?pid=607&id=4953260.

Rothrock, K. S. (June 8, 2020a). *Pancreatic neoplasia*. From VIN.com https://www.vin.com/Members/Associate/Associate.plx?from=GetDzInfo&DiseaseId=727&pid=607.

Rothrock, K. S. (March 19, 2020b). *Hypercalcemia of malignancy*. From VIN.com https://www.vin.com/Members/Associate/Associate.plx?from=GetDzInfo&DiseaseId=2041&pid=607.

Rozanski, R. (2009). Pulmonary edema (proceedings). In *Proceedings of DVM 360*.

Rozanski, E. (2020). Canine chronic bronchitis: An update. *The Veterinary Clinics of North America. Small Animal Practice*, 393–404.

Ryan, N. (2012). Gabapentin for refractory chronic cough: A randomised, double-blind placebo-controlled study. *The Lancet*, 1583–1589.

Salgado, M. C. (June 2013). *Hepatic encephalopathy*. From VetFolio/Compendium https://www.vetfolio.com/learn/article/hepatic-encephalopathy-diagnosis-and-treatment.

Salvin, H. E. (2011). The canine cognitive dysfunction rating scale (CCDR): A data-driven and ecologically relevant assessment tool. *The Veterinary Journal*, 331–336.

Sangisetty, S. L. (2012). Malignant ascites: A review of prognostic factors, pathophysiology and therapeutic measures. *World Journal of Gastrointestinal Surgery*, 87−95.

Scheidner, B. D. (2009). Use of memantine in treatment of canine compulsive disorders. *Journal of Veterinary Behavior: Clinical Applications and Research*, 118−126.

Scherk, M. (2018). Managing Feline Constipation - Relieving a Hard Problem. *Chicagoland Veterinary Conference, 1*.

Sevcik, M. A. (2005). Anti-NGF therapy profoundly reduces bone cancer pain and the accompanying increase in markers of peripheral and central sensitization. *Pain*, 128−141.

Sharp, C. (2011). *Managing pulmonary fibrosis in dogs*. DVM360.

Shmalberg, J. (2013). *Beyond Yunnan Baiyao: The safety, nutritional considerations, and efficacy of Chinese herbal products*. Orlando, FL: VMX.

Silva, N. L. (2017). Effect of acupuncture on pain and quality of life in canine neurological and musculoskeletal diseases. *The Canadian Veterinary Journal = La revue veterinaire canadienne*, 941−951.

Skribek, M. R. (2021). Effect of corticosteroids on the outcome of patients with advanced non-small cell lung cancer treated with immune-checkpoint inhibitors. *European Journal of Cancer*, 245−254.

Soffietti, R. R. (2002). Management of brain metastases. *Journal of Neurology*, 1357−1369.

Soleimanpour, H. S. (2016). Opioid drugs in patients with liver disease: A systematic review. *Hepatitis Monthly*, e32636.

Sood, A., Dobbie, K., & Wilson Tang, W. H. (2018). Palliative Care in Heart Failure. *Current treatment options in cardiovascular medicine, 20*(5), 43. https://doi.org/10.1007/s11936-018-0634-y

Sordo, L. (2021). Cognitive dysfunction in cats: Update on neuropathological and behavioural changes plus clinical management. *The Veterinary Record*.

Staff of Alzheimer's association. (2021). *Stages of Alzheimer's*. From Alzheimer's Association https://www.alz.org/alzheimers-dementia/stages.

Staff of Animal Surgical and Orthopedic Center. (June 24, 2020). *Signs of anxiety in dogs(and what to do about it!)*. From Animalsurgical.com https://www.animalsurgical.com/anxiety-in-dogs/.

Staff of IRIS. (2021). *IRIS treatment recommendations for CKD*. From Iris-kidney.com http://www.iris-kidney.com/guidelines/recommendations.html.

Staff of MSU. (2021). *Rehabilitation therapy*. From Michigan State University/Veterinary Medicine https://cvm.msu.edu/scs/research-initiatives/golpp/rehabilitation-therapy.

Staff of VetEducation. (2021). *Clinical use of tranexamic acid in the dog*. From VetEducation.com. https://veteducation.com.au/clinical-use-of-tranexamic-acid-in-the-dog/

Steigleder, T. S. (2013). Dying of brain tumours: Specific aspects of care. *Current Opinion in Supportive and Palliative Care*, 417−423.

Story, B. D., Miller, M. E., Bradbury, A. M., Million, E. D., Duan, D., Taghian, T., … Gray-Edwards, H. L. (2020). Canine Models of Inherited Musculoskeletal and Neurodegenerative Diseases. *Frontiers in veterinary science, 7*, 80. https://doi.org/10.3389/fvets.2020.00080

Sutton, K. G. (2002). Gabapentin inhibis high-threshold calcium channel currents in cultured rat dorsla root ganglion neurons. *British Journal of Phamacology*, 257−265.

Suzuki, M. N. (2012). Sensation of abdominal pain induced by peritoneal carcinomatosis is accompanied by changes in the expression of substance P and μ-opioid receptors in the spinal cord of mice. *Anesthesiology*, 847−856.

Takeuchi, T. (2002). Age-related changes in sleep-wake rhythm in dog. *Behavioural Brain Research*, 193−199.

Tams, T. R. (2003). The vomiting dog—diagnosis. In *WSAVA 2003 Proceedings*. WSAVA/VIN.

Taylor, M. K., Swerdlow, R. H., & Sullivan, D. K. (2019). Dietary Neuroketotherapeutics for Alzheimer's Disease: An Evidence Update and the Potential Role for Diet Quality. *Nutrients, 11*(8), 1910. https://doi.org/10.3390/nu11081910

Thomas, S. B. (2011). Breathlessness in cancer patients − implications, management and challenges. *European Journal of Oncology Nursing*, 459−469.

Thomas, D. R. (April 4, 2019). *Nutritional support for people who are dying or severely demented*. From Merek Manual Consumer Version https://www.merckmanuals.com/home/disorders-of-nutrition/nutritional-support/nutritional-support-for-people-who-are-dying-or-severely-demented.

Treggiari, E. P.-M. (2017). A descriptive review of cardiac tumours in dogs and cats. *Veterinary and Comparative Oncology*, 273−288.

Venugopal, A. (2014). Disseminated intravascular coagulopathy. *Indian Journal of Anesthesia*, 603−608.

Vetbook Staff. (November 8, 2012). *Octreotide*. From Vetbook.com http://www.vetbook.org/wiki/dog/index.php?title=Octreotide&oldid=5825.

Vilkovyskiy, I. F. (2020). Influence of hepatic neoplasia on life expectancy in dogs. *Veterinary World*, 413−418.

VIN Staff. (2017). *VIN veterinary drug handbook*. From VIN.com https://www.vin.com.

VSSO Staff. (2021a). *Cancer by location*. From VSSO.org https://vsso.org/dog-cancer-location.

VSSO Staff. (2021b). *Tumor site by location*. From VSSO.org https://vsso.org/cat-cancer-location.

Wang, Y. P. (2013). Mechanisms for fiber-type specificity of skeletal muscle atrophy. *Current Opinion in Clinical Nutrition and Metabolic Care*, 243−250.

Wang, R. R. (2017). Role of glutamate and NMDA receptors in Alzheimer's disease. *Journal of Alzheimer's Disease*, 1041−1048.

Ware, W. (1999). Systemic arterial hypertension. In R. C. Nelson (Ed.), *Manual of small animal internal medicine* (pp. 114−124). St. Louis: Mosby.

Webster, C., Center, S. A., Cullen, J. M., Penninck, D. G., Richter, K. P., Twedt, D. C., & Watson, P. J. (2019). ACVIM consensus statement on the diagnosis and treatment of chronic hepatitis in dogs. *Journal of veterinary internal medicine, 33*(3), 1173−1200. https://doi.org/10.1111/jvim.15467

Weisshaar, E. S. (2012). European guideline on chronic pruritus. *Acta Dermato-Venereologica*, 563−581.

Whelan, M. (2021). *Yunnan Baiyao, to use or not to use?* From MSPCA.org https://www.mspca.org/angell_services/yunnan-baiyao-to-use-or-not-to-use/.

Willard, M. (2011). *GI tract ulceration/erosion/GI bleeding*. WSAVA 2011. WSAVA/VIN.

Woodrell, C. D. (2018). Palliative care for people with hepatocellular carcinoma, and specific benefits for older adults. *Clinical Therapeutics*, 512−525.

Wrede-Seaman, L. (2019). *Symptom management algorithms: A handbook for palliative care* (4th ed.). Yakima, Washington: Intellicard, Inc.

Wright, B. (2017). Clinical advantages of ketamine and NMDA antagonist drugs. In *World small animal veterinary association congress proceedings*. WSAVA.

Wright, S. (2020). Limited utility for benzodiazepines in chronic pain management: A narrative review. *Advances in Therapy*, 2604–2619.

Xu, L., Y. J. (2000). Inhibition of malignant ascites and growth of human ovarian carcinoma by oral administration of a potent inhibitor of the vascular endothelial growth factor receptor tyrosine kinases. *International Journal of Oncology*, 445–454.

Yancey, M. F. (2010). Pharmacokinetic properties of toceranib phosphate (Palladia, SU11654), a novel tyrosine kinase inhibitor, in laboratory dogs and dogs with mast cell tumors. *Journal of Veterinary Pharmacology and Therapeutics*, 162–171.

Yang, Q. E. (2016). Long term effects of palliative local treatment of incurable metastatc lesions in colorectal cancer patients. *Oncotarget*, 21034–21045.

Yennurajalingam, S. B. (2016). *Oxford American handbook of hospice and palliative medicine and supportive care*. New York: Oxford University Press.

Yu, C.-C. D.-J.-Q.-B.-F.-H. (2020). Experimental evidence of the benefits of acupuncture for Alzheimer's disease: An updated review. *Frontiers of Neuroscience*, 549772.

Zaidi, S. R. H., S. S. (2021). *Decubitus ulcer*. StatPearls. Retrieved from https://www.ncbi.nlm.nih.gov/books/NBK553107/.

Zhou, H. X. (2015). Advanced chronic obstructive pulmonary disease: Innovative and integrated management approaches. *Chinese Medical Journal*, 2952–2959.

Zuckerman, L. M.-C. (2019). The effect of non-steroidal anti-inflammatory drugs on osteosarcoma cells. *European Review for Medical and Pharmacological Sciences*, 2681–2690.

Further reading

Abdallah, S. J. (2019). Updates in opioid and nonopioid treatment for chronic breathlessness. *Current Opinion in Supportive and Palliative Care*, 167–173.

Chronic pain management in the home setting

Lynn Hendrix, AA, BA, DVM, CHPV [1,2,3,4,8], **Eve Harrison, VMD, CVA, CCFP** [5,6,7,8]

[1]*Owner, Veterinarian, Beloved Pet Mobile Vet, Davis, CA, United States;* [2]*Former Board of Directors, IAAHPC, Chicago, IL, United States;* [3]*Consultant, Hospice, Palliative Medicine, End of Life, VIN, Davis, CA, United States;* [4]*President, Founder, World Veterinary Palliative Medicine Organization, Davis, CA, United States;* [5]*Founder, The House Call Vet Academy, Los Angeles, CA, United States;* [6]*Owner, Veterinarian, Marigold Veterinary, Los Angeles, CA, United States;* [7]*Consultant, House Call and Mobile Practice, Ask Jan For Help LLC, Kansas City, MO, United States;* [8]*Co-Founder, House Call and Mobile Vet Virtual Conference, Los Angeles, CA, United States e-mail address: dreveharrison@gmail.com*

Pain management is the backbone of veterinary palliative medicine. This chapter will summarize the pathophysiology of chronic pain and acute pain, as well as the different pain medications that can be used to create a multimodal approach to pain. This chapter aims to overview pain management for the house call veterinarian. Other books and resources are suggested at the end of the chapter. In addition, this chapter will also review the human experience of pain with specific diseases and how it may relate to animal patients. We recognize that the human experience may differ from the animal perception of pain; however, where possible, we will discuss the molecular, biochemical changes in the disease and relate it to the need for additional research that may need to be done to evaluate the animal patient. Finally, there will be a brief review of nonpharmaceutical pain therapies, recognizing that some may not have a sound basis of evidence beyond anecdotal experience. Also of note, pain management in the home setting may be limited by equipment, time, team members' abilities, as well as the client/caregiver capabilities, concerns, and needs of the caregiver. For example, placing an epidural may be a gold standard for clinical pain management for a particular disease, and yet it may be impractical in the home setting. It also may be appropriate to discuss euthanasia for those animals who may need more invasive pain management.

Recognizing chronic pain

The International Association for the Study of Pain (IASP) describes pain as "an unpleasant sensory and emotional experience associated with, or resembling that associated with, actual or potential tissue damage." (Staff of IASP, 2017). Human physicians have a saying "Pain is what the patient says it is." Physicians struggle when dealing with nonverbal patients who may be experiencing pain, utilizing behavioral clues, such as facial grimace to determine pain. Acute pain, such as surgical pain, is easy to recognize due to physiological changes including increased heart rate and respiratory rate, as well as dilated pupils. However, chronic pain is more challenging to recognize in people who can not verbalize their experience. Likewise, chronic pain has often gone unrecognized in our veterinary patients until more recent times. Veterinarians have special challenges when assessing pain as compared to our human physicians since each species may have different behaviors that may be expressions of pain. However, as veterinarians, we are trained to regularly observe behavior and watch body language, which gives us a distinct advantage over our physician colleagues.

Recognition of chronic pain by clients can be another challenge. Clients may not recognize behavioral changes, that would alert a veterinarian to chronic pain. Clients are often looking for signs of acute pain, such as vocalization or decreases in appetite. They may mistake pain for the idea that their animal may just be getting old and slowing down. Veterinarians can help clients understand the signs to watch for as well as how to interpret the signs they may already be seeing.

Veterinarians who work on a house call basis have a distinct advantage in terms of recognizing behavioral changes associated with pain, by seeing animals in their homes in a more relaxed state. Adrenalized animals may not show subtle signs of chronic pain after riding in a car and going into a vet hospital. People with chronic pain have mild behavioral changes when their pain becomes moderate, and significant behavioral changes when pain becomes severe (Arbuck, 2021). Mild-to-moderate chronic pain signs may go unnoticed by an observer. Veterinarians should be cognizant that companion animals may also follow this pattern. However, more studies may need to be done to verify this hypothesis in animals.

Although chronic pain may not be as easily recognized as acute pain, it should certainly be treated to prevent our veterinary patients from suffering unnecessarily.

The physiology of pain

There are four aspects of the ascending pain perception pathway: transduction, transmission, modulation, and perception. There are also descending pathways; however, their participation in the pain response is minimally understood. Transduction begins in the nociceptors, which are sensitive to mechanical, thermal, or chemical changes. Transduction initiates an electrical impulse through ion channels that stimulate the voltage-gated channels (Self, 2019).

Transmission ensues in the afferent fibers, which may be fast action myelinated A-delta (A-δ) fibers or slower action, unmyelinated C fibers that travel up the dorsal horn and then up to the brain (Self, 2019). A-δ fibers transmit thermal and mechanical information, while C fibers transmit from chemical, mechanical, and thermal receptors (Fox, 2012). Both types of fibers are found in the skin, periosteum, subchondral bone, joint capsule, blood vessels, muscle, tendons, peritoneum, pleura, and viscera (Tranquilli, 2004). A-δ fibers are linked with proprioception, A-β fibers conduct touch, and A-δ fibers convey pain and temperature, and C fibers are associated with pain, temperature and itch. (He, 2020).

Modulation occurs primarily in the dorsal horn of the spinal cord (Self, 2019). Modulation affects the signal going to the brain thus the perception of pain and can be modified with medication. The ascending pathway in the dorsal horn contains inhibitory and excitatory neurons that modify the pain signal and increase or decrease the signal going to the brain. Central sensitization occurs in the dorsal horn with upregulation of neurotransmitters and receptors that sensitizes the CNS, changing the membrane sensitivity and synaptic efficacy by modifying the excitability of the nerve (Latremoliere, 2009). Central sensitization can have additional effects on the experience of pain, creating allodynia and hyperalgesia. Allodynia is an increased sensitivity to touch. Hyperalgesia is an increased sensitivity to pain (Tranquilli, 2004).

The central descending pathways begin in the cortex, thalamus, amygdala, and periaqueductal gray matter in the midbrain, the nucleus raphe magnus in the pons, rostral ventral medulla, medulla oblongata, and down the spinal cord (Ossipov, 2010; Self, 2019). The central descending pathways inhibit or amplify pain and both effect and are affected by emotion. Depression and anxiety play a role in the modulation of pain with people, we do not know the role emotions play in animals (Ossipov, 2010). See the symptom management chapter for more on how anxiety plays a role in chronic pain.

Finally, the perception of pain occurs in the brain and may also be influenced by memory and emotions (Self, 2019). Anxiety and depression change people's perception of pain, and anxiety may change the perception of pain in animals. More research needs to be done with companion animals on emotions and perception of pain. The pathways of pain are illustrated in the following figure which also includes medications that can affect the various locations of pain transmission (Fig. 6.1).

Types of pain
Nociceptive pain

Nociceptive pain is initiated in nociceptors, specialized nerve endings that respond to mechanical, thermal, and chemical damage (Fox, 2012). Nociceptors have fast-acting, myelinated Aδ fibers or the slower unmyelinated C fibers and initiate transduction. Nociceptive pain tends to be acute. The nociceptive receptors initiate a release of cytokines and stimulate the fibers to depolarize and introduce an inflammatory response (Tranquilli, 2004). Behaviors seen with acute nociception may be vocalization, avoidance behavior, agitation, and sympathetic activation, such as increased heart rate, respiratory rate, and blood pressure (Tranquilli, 2004).

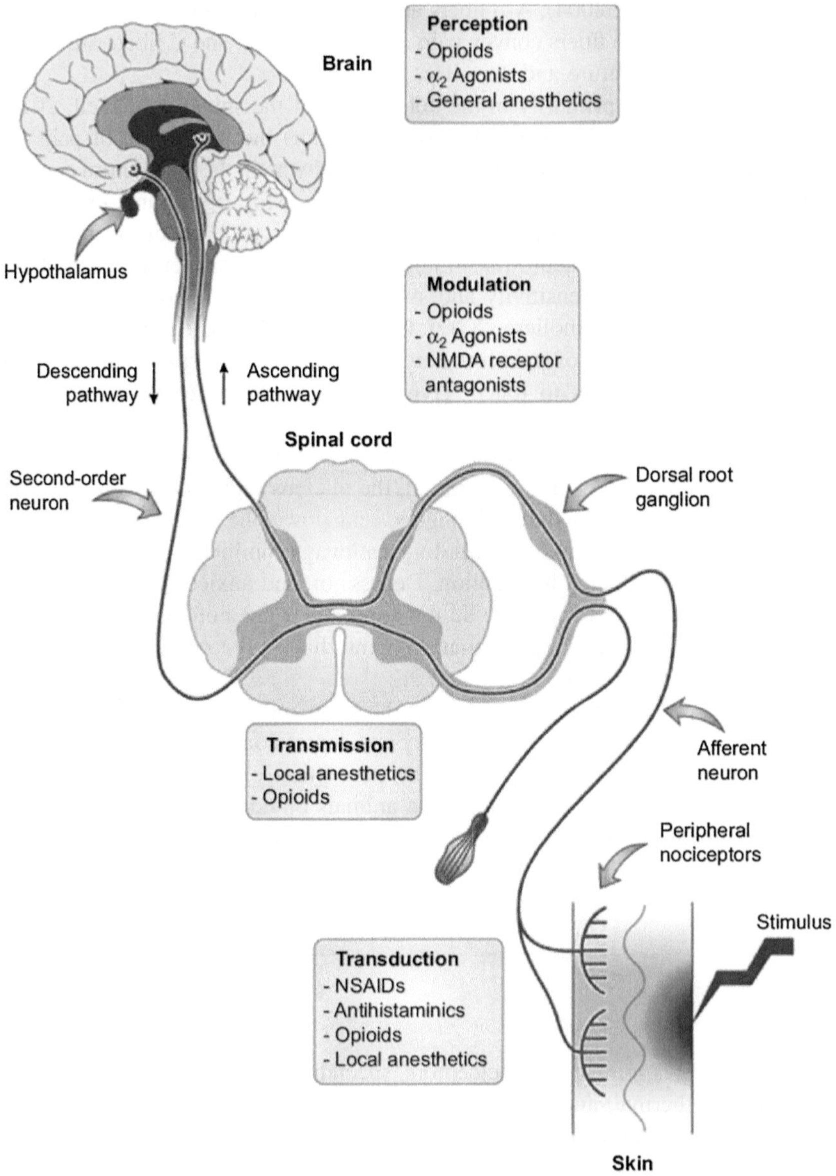

FIGURE 6.1

Pathways of transduction, transmission, modulation, and perception with therapeutics.

Used with permission from Dureja, G. I. (2017). Evidence and consensus recommendations for the pharma-logical management of pain in India. Journal of Pain Research, *709–736.*

Neuropathic pain

Although clients are typically good at identifying signs and watch for acute pain, chronic pain is more likely to be evaluated, identified and managed by the house call palliative veterinarian. The path to chronic pain begins with an acute pain insult that develops into an inflammatory process followed by a prolonged, maladaptive strategy that develops into neuropathic pain. Neuropathic pain can be acute because of a direct insult to nerves or a disease process occurring within the somatosensory nerves (Self, 2019). However, neuropathic pain is often a more chronic process transpiring when the acute nociceptive pain has lasted longer than expected from the initial insult and increased due to either peripheral or central sensitization (Fox, 2012).

Chronic neuropathic pain occurs due to alterations to the processing in the nerve via central or peripheral sensitization (Wessmann, 2019). Chronic neuropathic pain may be intermittent, with behaviors that may not be thought of as consistent with pain, such as scratching one spot, yelping for no clear cause, exaggerated responses to nonnoxious stimuli, such as petting (Wessmann, 2019). Some diseases have mixed nociceptive and neuropathic pain, such as cancer (Edwards, 2019).

Allodynia and hyperalgesia are both related to central sensitization. Allodynia is the sensation of pain with a stimulus that would not usually cause pain (e.g., a feather touching the skin is not usually painful, animals with allodynia would find it painful). Peripheral sensitization may also contribute to allodynia (Tranquilli, 2004). Allodynia occurs in the A-β fibers, low threshold Aδ or C fibers (Sandkühler, 2009). Hyperalgesia is an increased sensitivity to stimulation from a noxious stimulus. Hyperalgesia may also have modified CNS processing as well as central sensitization (Sandkühler, 2009). Allodynia appears to lower the pain threshold; hyperalgesia seems to be an amplified response to a painful stimulus (He, 2020). Allodynia may be associated in people with trigeminal neuralgia, postradiation pain, phantom pain, chronic postsurgical pain, Vitamin D and B deficiencies, chemotherapy, or complex regional pain syndrome (He, 2020). In humans, central sensitization is also related to increased emotional sensitivity and anxiety (He, 2020).

Inflammatory pain

Acute inflammatory pain results from a multifaceted cascade of mediators and cytokines and is a type of nociceptive pain. Inflammation is characterized by redness, swelling, heat, loss of function, and pain (Fox, 2012). Acute inflammation develops to protect the body from pathogens and promote healing of the area of damage (Muley, 2016). Acute inflammatory pain involves mediators and cytokines released locally that initiate an inflammatory response (Fox, 2012). The cells involved in acute inflammatory pain are mast cells, neutrophils, macrophages, T cells, and Schwann cells. Mast cells can release histamine, tumor necrosis factor (TNF), Interleukin-1 (IL-1), and prostaglandins (PGs). Neutrophils release PG, serine, and proteases. Macrophages release PGE2, TNF, IL-1β, nitric oxide, and nerve growth factor (NGF) to the local tissues (Self, 2019). In addition, direct heat (which can also be in capsaicin and other "heat" producing chemicals) and cold (menthol and other "cold" producing chemicals) can be inflammatory, with "heat" stimulating TRPV1 receptors and "cold" stimulating TRPM8 receptors contributing to inflammatory pain (Fox, 2012). These mediators cause a local acidosis that sensitizes the peripheral receptors (Varrassi, 2019).

Chronic inflammation, on the other hand, is maladaptive and occurs with peripheral and central sensitization (Varrassi, 2019). There can also be a neurogenic component to inflammatory pain, which may contribute to chronic inflammation. C fiber nociceptors cause vasodilation and edema in the skin as a response to heat or chemical stimuli (Schmelz, 2000). The vasodilation and edema then can activate immunomodulating cells and neuropeptides, including substance P, responsible for peripheral sensitization and neurogenic inflammation (Varrassi, 2019). Skin, joints, and the gastrointestinal system can be sensitive to inflammatory pain (Varrassi, 2019).

Visceral pain

The house call veterinarian is more likely to evaluate the end-of-life pet with visceral pain because of a chronic disease process. People describe visceral pain in different areas of their abdomen or locations that may not be associated with the organ causing pain. For example, a heart attack can cause pain radiating into a limb. Visceral pain in animals may be difficult for the veterinarian to localize, and referred pain may occur as well in animals (Fox, 2012).

Visceral pain involves a convergence of pathways into multiple dorsal horns, in addition to the vagal, pelvic, and splanchnic nerves, which may explain the diverse experience of pain (Fox, 2012). The gastrointestinal afferent innervation is through the vagus and pelvic nerve afferent fibers, which also have fibers from the splanchnic nerves. These may modulate nociception processing in the brain and spinal cord. Visceral afferents are made up primarily of A-δ fibers and C fibers. The figure below shows the various visceral pathways (Fig. 6.2) (Sikandar, 2012).

Visceral pain models suggest that pain occurs with distention of hollow organs or damage to an organ either chemically, such as inflammation, or due to ischemia, tumor growth, infection (Fox, 2012). Continued noxious stimuli, such as a tumor or inflammation, can create visceral hyperalgesia via central sensitization (Varrassi, 2019).

Phantom pain complex

Phantom pain complex may be encountered at a home visit with a patient receiving end-of-life care and is infrequently discussed in the veterinary literature. Phantom pain complex may occur with human amputees and involves a sensation of pain in the area of the missing limb or amputation stump (Pendergrass, 2018). With

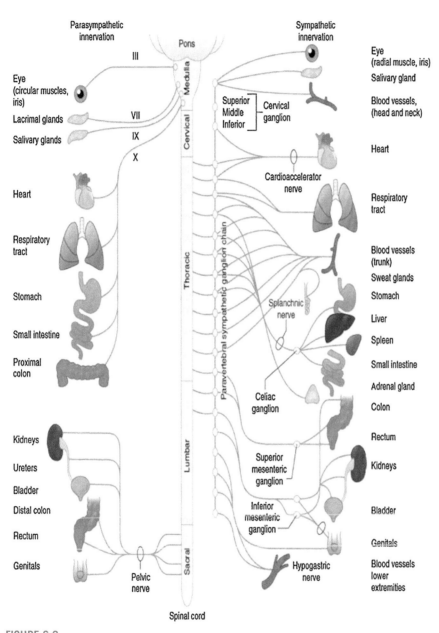

FIGURE 6.2

Visceral innervation.

From Miller's Anesthesia review, used with permission from Elsevier. Katz, B. V. (2021). Neuroantomay and visceral pain. In D. Y. Pak (Ed.), Interventional management of chronic visceral pain syndromes *(pp. 5–15):* Elsevier.

people, significant surgeries can also cause a phantom pain complex, such as following mastectomy or other organ removals (Kaur, 2018). Phantom pain has been found in 60%—80% of people postamputation, and has been found to persist chronically in up to 10% of human patients. The literature in veterinary medicine show numbers consistant with the human literature. Studies have also found that pre-amputation pain is a risk factor for postamputation pain (Pendergrass, 2018). Phantom pain complex may occur in animals with amputations of limbs, tails, and claws in cats. However, pain may also persist in other organ removals as it does in humans, and further studies are needed in order to examine this phenomenon in animals.

It has been hypothesized that the dorsal horn develops central sensitization after a peripheral nerve has been cut. There are measurable increases in glutamate concentrations and N-methyl D-aspartate (NMDA) in the central nervous system postamputation/surgery (Koga, 2016). In addition, there may be an upregulation of norepinephrine that potentiates the sympathetic nervous system and is involved in regulating pain sensitivity. Neural plasticity, the nervous system's ability to adapt and reroute nerve tissue, may also play a role (Latremoliere, 2009).

Pharmacological treatment for people with phantom pain can include amitriptyline, opioids and NSAIDs, as well as adjunct therapies such as treatment with a TENS unit, acupuncture, and massage (Kaur, 2018).

Summary of pain terminology

- Allodynia is an increased sensitivity to touch where pain occurs from a normally nonpainful stimulus (ex. feather on skin being painful).
- Analgesia is decreased to absent pain to a typically painful stimulus due to endogenous or exogenous influences.
- Central sensitization is enhanced excitability and responsiveness of spinal neurons.
- Hyperesthesia is a increased sensitivity to painful sensory input due to an amplification in the CNS.
- Hypoesthesia is a decreased sensitivity to sensory input and may have an number of etiologies.
- Neuralgia—pain from nerves or nerve pathways
- Neuropathy is a pathologic change to the nerve or nerve pathways.
- Paresthesia is numbness or tingling (AKA "pins and needles").
- Peripheral sensitization is a lowered threshold for nociceptor activation and increased the frequency of nerve impulse firing.
- Phantom pain complex is a term used in human and veterinary medicine for amputees who experience pain from a limb removed. Consider when developing a plan regarding pain in animals who have had a limb or large organ removed.
- Referred pain is pain that occurs in a different location than the cause of the pain.

Evaluating chronic and cancer pain in the late-stage patient
Changes in behavior

"She is just getting old, Doc" or "He has been slowing down for a while" are often-heard statements that a client may say to veterinarians about their older pets. Clients may not recognize behaviors that are expressions of chronic pain, as they are often only looking for signs of acute pain such as crying or inappetence. As a result, chronic pain in companion animals may go unrecognized by people for a long time. Veterinarians can educate clients to recognize changes in their pet's behavior in terms of chronic pain, however subtle, which will support those animals in acquiring proper pain management much more quickly. Humans show significant changes in behavior when they are approaching moderate or severe levels of chronic pain (Dueñas, 2016). In an animal, any significant behavioral change may be an indication of severe chronic pain.

Dog-specific chronic pain behavior

1. Pacing or restless behavior, especially at night
2. Inability or unwillingness to jump up, into out of the car, onto curbs or furniture they previously could get onto or go up or down stairs.
3. Other behaviors noted in dogs with chronic pain include panting, yawning, body stretching, body shaking, scratching, decreased play behavior, and squeezing into small spaces (Mills, 2020).

Cat-specific chronic pain behavior

1. Night waking and/or howling (although, these may be signs of other disease processes, such as cognitive dysfunction or hypertension).
2. Inability or unwillingness get into or out of their litter boxes, hesitation or inability to jump on the bed, couch, cat tree, or other furniture they used to be able to jump onto.
3. Other behaviors noted in cats with chronic pain-panting, yawning, body stretching, body shaking, scratching, decreased play behavior, squeezing into small spaces (Mills, 2020).
4. Cats may have changes in their facial expression and body language with chronic pain. Grimace scales are utilized in non-verbal people at the end of life. There is a validated grimace scale for cats. It is validated for acute pain and is being evaluated for chronic pain as of this writing. See Feline Grimace Scale (Stegall, 2020). Dogs may also have facial and body language changes; however, there is not currently a validated grimace scale in dogs. There are validated grimace scales for mice, rats, horses, rabbits, ferrets, pigs, donkeys, sheep.

Common pain-related behavior for dogs or cats

1. Defensive behavior—becoming more aggressive, especially when they were not aggressive animals prior, anticipating touch, withdrawal from family.
2. Fear/anxiety—animals who were not previously anxious can indicate pain or had a history of anxiety may have increased pain. See more in the symptom management chapter.
3. Attention-seeking or avoidance behavior with an increase in either behavior indicating increased pain.
4. Weight shifting (especially in larger dogs) to nonweight bearing on one or more limbs. Changes in gait, such as bunny hopping, stilted gait.
5. Inappropriate urination or defecation—it is often too painful for dogs to get up and go outside, or they try to but do not make it out and go by a door. Or they go where they lay because it is too painful to get up. For cats, going outside of the box can be because the box is too difficult to get into, too tall, litter is too deep.
6. Changes in grooming habits, overgrooming or absent grooming, and changes in coat appearance or hair loss can be indicative or associated with pain.
7. Licking surfaces such as dog/cat beds, floors, even other animals may be due to GI or other body pain (may also be due to other reasons such as gastrointestinal nausea) (Mills, 2020).
8. Changes in appetite and water intake can be due to pain. For example, neck, spinal, limb pain, dental or facial pain may significantly influence eating or drinking.
9. Pica may be indicative of gastrointestinal pain (Mills, 2020).
10. "Stargazing" and "fly-biting" have been hypothesized to be potential signs of gastrointestinal pain (Mills, 2020).

Assessing chronic pain

Recognizing pain behavior is the first step in the assessment of chronic pain in companion animals. From the initial veterinary evaluation, continued monitoring of the patient receiving palliative care requires reliable scales to gauge changes over time. Utilizing algorithms and validated pain scales can be a step forward in assessing the physical quality of life for these animals. The World Health Organization Cancer Pain Ladder is one example of a system used to assess chronic pain in humans (Anekar, 2021). This algorithm is a tool that we can use in palliative pain management for veterinary patients as well (Fig. 6.3).

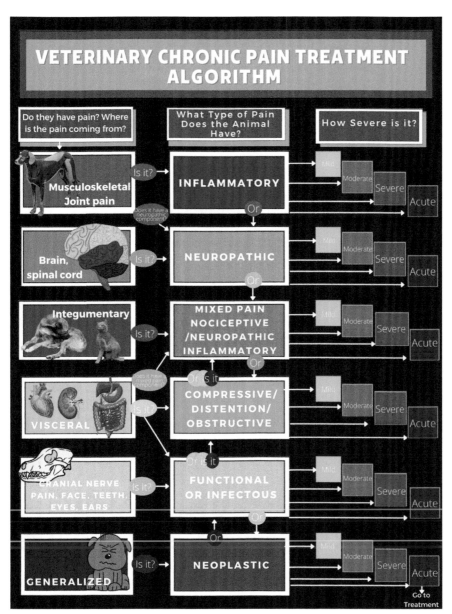

FIGURE 6.3

Algorithm for assessing chronic pain.

Created on Canva by Lynn Hendrix© 2021, Park, J. K. (2010). Current pharmacological management of chronic pain. Journal of the Korean Medical Association, 815–823.

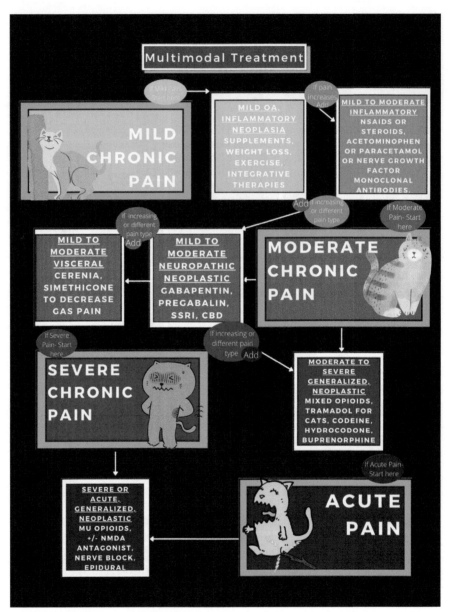

FIGURE 6.3 cont'd.

Validated chronic pain scales

Acute pain has been studied extensively, and a multitude of acute pain scales can be found in the human and veterinary literature. Chronic pain, however, can be more challenging to assess. In addition, assessing chronic pain can be more difficult because there may not be physiologic changes evident, and the changes in behavior that do exist may be subtle. Nevertheless, there are still a few validated chronic pain scales that may be beneficial to support clients in assessing their animal's chronic pain. The primary limitation of these chronic pain scales is that most of them relate specifically to osteoarthritis (OA). There are several quality-of-life scales that exist for other disease processes, which are included below, but these are not specific to the assessment of chronic pain.

Here are acute and chronic validated pain scales that are currently available:

1. Helsinki Chronic Pain Index was first validated in 2009 for OA (Epstein, 2013). It is client driven and has 11 questions, with a simple descriptive scale (SDS) for demeanor, behavior, locomotion, and a visual analog scale for pain and locomotion (Epstein, 2013).
2. Canine Brief Pain Inventory developed by the University of Pennsylvania is a short form with 11 questions describing pain by severity and interference with life. It is based on a human pain inventory scale and is also driven by client observation. This scale includes a description of pain in terms of the general function of the dog, enjoyment of life, ability to rise, walk, stand, and run, and overall function for the past 7 days (Epstein, 2013).
3. Liverpool osteoarthritis in dogs (LOAD) was first validated in 2009 for OA and is an SDS scale. It has 13 questions including five general questions and eight specific questions regarding exercise and movement (Gaynor, 2015).
4. Cincinnati Orthopedic Disability Index differs from other scales by using client-specific outcome measures (Epstein, 2013).
5. Canine osteoarthritis staging tool is not currently a validated tool (as of this writing); however, it may be a helpful staging tool for OA. The scale does correspond to the LOAD scale (Cachon, 2018).
6. Feline musculoskeletal pain index was validated for OA in cats and evaluates pain, mobility, activity, affect, and cognitive function. FMPI was developed by the North Carolina University College of veterinary medicine and can be found at https://painfreecats.org/the-fmpi/. (Stadig, 2019)
7. Montreal Instrument for Cat Arthritis Testing (MI-CAT)—contains two tests to assess osteoarthritis pain in cats. One of the tests is for a veterinarian to take and one for the client to take (Klinck, 2017).
8. Feline Grimace Scale—this is a validated scale to gauge acute pain. The researchers are currently working on validation in chronic pain (Evangelista, 2021). More information can be found at https://www.felinegrimacescale.com/. They have an app for clients to download to score their pet.

Disease-specific scales

1. Cardiac—Fetch (Functional Evaluation of Cardiac Health) is a validated questionnaire for clients and veterinarians to assess the quality of life for patients with cardiac disease (Freeman, 2005). There are 18 questions, and the form is available from Tufts online.
2. Cancer in dogs—A validated Quality of Life (QOL) scale for animal cancer patients was published in 2005. There are 12 client observations. The scale is available from the authors by request (Yazbek, 2005).
3. Diabetes—A validated QOL scale for cats with diabetes (DIAQoL-pet) is client centered, measuring the impact of diabetes on the cat and the client (Niessen, 2010). Similarly, there is one for dogs (Niessen, 2012). They are available from the authors of the study.
4. Chronic kidney disease (CKD)—There is a validated quality of life scale for cats with chronic kidney disease called CatQoL (Bijsmans, 2016). It is a 16 question scale and can be found at https://www.surveymonkey.com/r/catquality (Fig. 6.4).

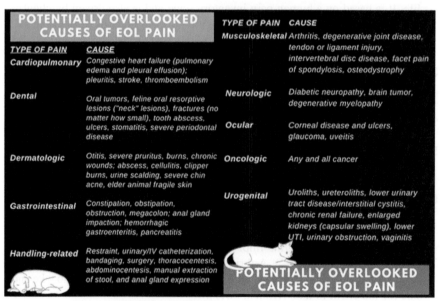

FIGURE 6.4

Potentially overlooked causes of EOL pain.

Used with permission and attribution from AAHA and Dr. Jessica Vogelsang 2021. Modified from original AAHA source and created on Canva by Lynn Hendrix © 2021.

Chronic pain in specific diseases
Cancer

Animals with cancer are the most commonly seen palliative veterinary patients. We can infer from human reporting that cancer causes pain, especially in the later stages. Cancer pain is multifactorial. The type and location of a tumor, comorbidities, paraneoplastic and metastatic involvement, chemotherapy, and radiation may all contribute to cancer pain. Tumors that may be destructive or invasive of the surrounding tissue may create ulcerations, inflammation, infarctions, or necrosis associated with substantial pain (Grant, 2019). For example, osteosarcoma causes local acidosis, which can cause pain in nearby tissues. When hemangiosarcoma tumors grow, the displacement of other abdominal contents can cause pain, and if they bleed into the surrounding abdominal space, the hemorrhage may produce inflammatory pain as well. Somatic pain develops when cancers affect muscle, skin, joint, or bone and is often described as a localized, constant throbbing or ache by humans experiencing this pain (Grant, 2019). Visceral pain can be due to stretching, distention, or obstruction of the viscera. Pain caused by cancer may be poorly localized and associated with deep, dull cramps or aches to unrelenting pain (Grant, 2019).

Cancer may initially grow without pain, but as the animal approaches the later stages of a neoplastic process, the pain level may increase and require pain management (Vendrell, 2015). Humans report cancer pain 33%−64% of the time; for those who report pain, 75%−90% will be moderate-to-severe pain (Vendrell, 2015). Cancer can have components of inflammatory, nociceptive (visceral or somatic), and neuropathic pain.

Measuring cytokines may help to predict the pain response in animals. The most common proinflammatory cytokines that cancer produces, which are known to cause pain, are IL-1β, IL-6, TNF-ɒ (Vendrell, 2015). A recent study looked at measuring cytokines and found that it may help to predict pain severity in human cancer patients. These cytokines had the highest predictability of being associated with pain, GM-CSF, IFN-γ, IL-1β, IL-2, IL-4, IL-5, IL-12(p70), IL-17A, and IL-23 (Fazzari, 2020). For example, osteosarcoma is known to cause pain, and increases in TNF-α and IL-1β have been observed to be associated with increased bone pain (Fazzari, 2020). The IL-1β binds to ion channels in local nociceptors; TNF-α stimulates the osteoclast, creating a local acidosis that stimulates the acid-sensing nociceptors (Fazzari, 2020).

Acute breakthrough pain can occur commonly in end-stage cancer. House call veterinarians should consider developing and providing a crisis kit for their cancer patients so that caregivers have pain medications readily available at home if the animals are experiencing breakthrough pain (McPherson, 2013).

Comorbidities that veterinarycancer patients may commonly experience include osteoarthritis, chronic renal or hepatic disease, dermatological or dental disease, chronic pancreatitis, and cystitis (Grant, 2019). Paraneoplastic syndrome can also generate cytokines, autoantibodies, hormones, and proteins that can be inflammatory, create comorbidities, and contribute to pain (Fig. 6.5) (Thapa, 2021).

Main category	Theme	Sub-themes	Descriptors
		Sensory aspects of pain	Intensity; frequency; nature
	Feeling cancer pain	Origin of the pain	Location; psychological contributors; physical
		Meaning of cancer pain	Suffering, disease progression fatalistic beliefs
Experiencing cancer pain		Behavioral reactions	Verbal and non-verbal behaviors
	Reacting to cancer pain	Emotional reactions	Anger; distress; anxiety; depression
		Cognitive reactions	Comparisons over time and with others; attitude
		Functioning with cancer pain	Losses; reduced functioning; reliance on others
	Living with cancer pain	Caring for a family member with cancer pain	Hyper vigilance; increased responsibility; new roles
		Cancer pain in the relationship	Changes in roles and relationship

FIGURE 6.5

Cancer-related pain in older adults receiving palliative care: patient and family caregiver perspectives on *the experience of pain.*

Used with permission from The Pulsus Group? McPherson, C. J. H. T. (2013). Cancer-related pain in older adults receiving palliative care: Patient and family caregiver perspectives on the experience of pain. Pain Research and Management, *293–300.*

Organ failure and other comorbidities

Late and end-stage CKD is often thought to be an easy way to die. However, in the literature on humans with end-stage renal failure, 60%—74% of patients reported that they had pain as they approached death. Of those, 70%—82% reported severe pain (Kafkia, 2011). In humans, uremia is known to cause nausea, pruritus, renal bone disease, osteoarthritis, peripheral neuropathy, and pain. In addition, comorbidities, such as heart disease, cancer, periodontal disease, or pancreatitis, may also cause pain, and uremia may exacerbate those conditions (Santoro, 2013). People with late-stage kidney disease may commonly have musculoskeletal pain, peripheral neuropathy, muscle weakness, and cramps, in addition to night waking, edema, and dyspnea in the late stages of renal disease (Caravaca, 2016). Abnormal metabolism of calcium and phosphorus may also contribute to pain.

Cats with late-stage chronic kidney disease or CKD may experience depression, dehydration, halitosis, diarrhea, vomiting, weight loss, decreased appetite, polyuria, polydipsia, and weakness (CVM Staff, 2019). Pain may be recognized in animals with acute renal failure; however, recognizing chronic pain in companion animals as a consequence of late-stage CKD can help us to palliate these animals better. Animals also have comorbidities with CKD that can cause pain including secondary hyperparathyroidism resulting in bone pain (O'Connor, 2012). Generalized musculoskeletal pain may be exacerbated by uremia. Cats and dogs that have osteoarthritis pain can be exacerbated by uremia (Marino, 2014). Weakness may be due to peripheral neuropathy, which is recognized as painful in humans. Weakness can also be exacerbated by cachexia or sarcopenia.

The use of NSAIDs has been considered contraindicated in CKD patients in the past. However, more current research has found that NSAIDs can and should be used with caution in animals with CKD. These studies also emphasize the importance of maintaining hydration during NSAID treatment of patients with CKD (Monteiro, 2019). Meloxicam was found to have no influence on creatinine at doses of 0.1 mg/kg SID between cats with CKD and the placebo subjects (Gunew, 2008). The International Society of Feline Medicine recommends that for patients with stable CKD and adequate hydration, a minimal effective dose may be used. Further changes to doses should be based on response to therapy, as well as the risks and benefits as discussed with clients, and should be followed with routine monitoring. More information on pain management for patients with CKD in the chapter on symptom management.

End-stage heart failure patients have common clinical signs, including dyspnea, and exercise fatigue. However, pain around end-stage heart failure does occur in people, and we should monitor for clinical signs of pain in animals. In a literature review in human medicine, people reported pain 23%−85% of the time, with around 50% of those reporting severe pain as they got closer to death. Chest pain was most reported with joint pain, peripheral edema, distended abdomen, shortness of breath, and osteoarthritis as additional areas of pain. Proinflammatory cytokines, IL-6, C-reactive protein TNF-α have been found to be increased in humans with congestive heart failure and may contribute to pain that may be associated with this condition (Alemzadeh-Ansari, 2017; Inamdar, 2016).

End-stage pulmonary disease may be due to chronic obstructive pulmonary disease (COPD), lung cancer or pneumonia, or pulmonary fibrosis. Pulmonary disease is reviewed in greater detail in the chapter on symptom management. In human patients with COPD, limb pain is common, with chest and back pain also frequently reported (Lee, 2016). In patients with pulmonary fibrosis chest pain is generally reported (Rajala, 2016). In human patients with lung cancer approximately 70% report pain in the late stages of the disease (Lim, 2016). There is little in the literature about veterinary patients with pulmonary disease experiencing pain, but given that we know humans with the pulmonary disease often experience pain we might surmise that our veterinary patients may as well.

End-stage liver failure in humans is reported to have pain associated with the cause of the liver failure (i.e., inflammation, infection, medications, neoplasia, Cushing's, hyperthyroidism, hypoperfusion, or cirrhosis) as well as the sequelae that can occur with those diseases, such as ascites and enlargement of the organ causing generalized abdominal pain (Potosek, 2014). Abdominal pain is recognized and reported in the ACVIM consensus statement with chronic hepatitis as well as hepatic neoplasia (Webster, 2019). Inflammation of the liver, musculoskeletal pain, joint pain, headaches, GI signs, such as diarrhea, are common symptoms of chronic hepatitis reported in humans (Lang, 2006). Hepatocellular carcinoma in humans may have abdominal pain, ascites, as well as metastatic bone pain (Christian-Miller, 2018). Other hepatic cancers may also have similar clinical signs. Pain may be due to inflammation of the peritoneum, mesentery, or omentum and can contribute to visceral hypersensitivity (Christian-Miller, 2018).

In animals with hepatic disease, the practitioner should be mindful of the potential need to modify pharmaceutical therapy in terms of pharmaceutical choices and doses. Integrative practitioners may also need to modify herbal treatments for patients with hepatic disease. There is additional information on the management of late-stage and end-stage hepatic failure in the chapter on symptom management.

In human patients with dementia, there may be unrecognized pain because the patient's ability to communicate is altered. In addition, they often have comorbidities that may contribute to pain, such as osteoarthritis. With our canine and feline patients with cognitive dysfunction, observing changes in behavior is our only way to assess for chronic pain. However, because their behavior is also altered, assessing pain in these pets may be more challenging.

There is a validated scale called Pain Assessment In Advanced Dementia (PAINAD) for humans with advanced dementia who may be nonverbal. This scale has five areas to assess, including breathing, vocalization, facial expression, body language, and consolability (Warden, 2003). Development of an associated veterinary pain assessment scale for animals with cognitive dysfunction would be valuable, and the author has proposed one based on the PAINAD scale, but modified for veterinary patients. The proposed scale has not been evaluated. The following figures include the PAINAD scale used in humans and the proposed scale for veterinary medicine (Figs. 6.6 and 6.7).

Items	0	1	2	SCORE
Breathing (Independent of vocalization)	Normal	Occasional labored breathing. Short period of hyperventilation.	Noisy labored breathing. Long period of hyperventilation. Cheyne-stokes respirations.	
Negative vocalization	None	Occasional moan or groan. Low level of speech with a negative or disapproving quality.	Repeated troubled calling out. Loud moaning or groaning. Crying.	
Facial expression	Smiling or inexpressive	Sad, frightened, frown.	Facial grimacing.	
Body language	Relaxed	Tense. Distressed pacing. Fidgeting.	Rigid. Fists clenched. Knees pulled up. Pulling or pushing away. Striking out.	
Consolability	No need to console	Distracted or reassured by voice or touch.	Unable to console, distract or reassure.	
TOTAL				

FIGURE 6.6

PAINAD scal.

Used with permission from Warden, V. H. A. (2003). Development and psychometric evaluation of the pain assessment in advanced dementia (PAINAD) scale. Journal of the American Medical Directors Association, *9–15.*

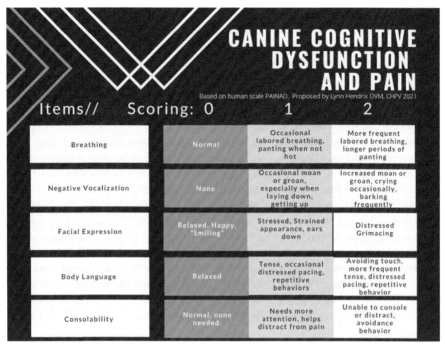

FIGURE 6.7

Canine cognitive dysfunction and pain proposed Pain/QoL Score.

Proposed by Lynn Hendrix DVM, CHPV 2021, Reproduced with permission.

Weakness or frailty is a condition that occurs in elderly humans and is often associated with pain (Chiou, 2018; Guerriero, 2020). Frailty does occur in companion animals and may also be associated with pain as it is in humans (Hua, 2016). Additional research needs to be done to assess pain in dogs with frailty, and symptom and pain management is further discussed in the chapter on symptom management.

Degenerative myelopathy in dogs is genetically related to amyotrophic lateral sclerosis (ALS) in humans with the same superoxide dismutase-1 gene or SOD-1 mutation. Pain is reported in 70% of people with ALS (Zarei, 2015). Pain with ALS patients tends to be mixed complex pain, neuropathy, nociceptive pain, muscle cramps, and spasms being the most common, which becomes more severe as the disease progresses (Delpont, 2019). Humans also report headaches, irritability, dyspnea, disturbed sleep, and fatigue (Delpont, 2019). Although it is commonly thought that degenerative myelopathy does not cause pain in animals, there may need to be a change in our understanding and treatment paradigms regarding this disease. There is a possibility that the weakness we observe in patients with degenerative myelopathy may be associated with some degree of pain as appears to be the case in humans with ALS. Dogs with degenerative myelopathy can also have known painful comorbidities, such as osteoarthritis, and it may be challenging for veterinarians to differentiate what disease process may be causing the pain.

A possible cause of pain in people with ALS may be a reduction in the number of astroglia glutamate transporters. Reductions of this transporter cause increases in extracellular glutamate, increased numbers of glutamate receptors, as well as neuronal degradation. This, in turn, causes increased blood calcium levels and increased firing of motor neurons (Zarei, 2015). As glutamate plays a significant role in pain transmission and central sensitization, it may be reasonable to hypothesize that if these changes exist in animals with degenerative myelopathy, they may have unrecognized pain (Pereira, 2019). There also appear to be changes in the mitochondria that may contribute to neuronal death and dysfunction (Pereira, 2019). As of this writing, no studies could be found that examined this aspect in dogs with degenerative myelopathy. Additional research could examine the biochemistry and genetic changes of degenerative myelopathy and pain. Treatment for pain management in patients with degenerative myelopathy patients is reviewed in the chapter on symptom management.

Osteoarthritis is the most common geriatric disease and late-stage comorbidity—causing pain that affects at least 20% of the dog population older than 1 year in the United States (Anderson, 2020). OA is a significant area of pain study in elder animals, and additional information on treatment can be found in the symptom management chapter.

Dental or periodontal disease is a common condition in geriatric pets. Many pets do not receive proper dental care in their later years, often due to client concerns regarding age and anesthesia as well as financial costs. Clients may not consider that their pet's severe dental disease may be painful because the animal continues to eat. When the animal stops eating, he or she may be prematurely euthanized (Gorrel, 2019). In addition to the accumulation of calculus and bacteria, older animals can have broken teeth that may not be recognized to be painful, worn teeth that are chronic sources of pain, neoplasia in the bone or soft tissue that can cause pain, as well as stomatitis (Gorrel, 2019). Periodontal cleaning should be considered as palliative care for older animals and should still be recommended to clients as animals age. In addition, it may be appropriate to place older animals on prophylactic antibiotics as well as pain medications to help temporarily relieve pain, until they can get their teeth cleaned. It may also be a last resort to make an animal comfortable with end-of-life patients.

Pain caused by procedures

House call veterinarians may find themselves also treating the pain associated with chemotherapy, radiation, catheter placement, surgery, biopsies, blood draws, epidurals, chest tubes, feeding tubes and care, abdominocentesis, thoracocentesis, or other invasive procedures that may have been performed in the clinical setting. Managing any pain associated with these procedures is of the utmost importance during end-of-life care.

Treatment: Pharmaceuticals for chronic pain in veterinary patients

NMDA receptor antagonists

NMDA antagonists—The activation of glutamate receptors plays a role in central sensitization. With prolonged or intense pain, there is an increase in glutamate release, which potentiates the NMDA receptor, enhancing the depolarization and increasing neuronal activation in the dorsal horn. This leads to depolarization of the postsynaptic nerve, enhancing the responsiveness of the nerve, which increases the modulation of pain. NMDA antagonists also help decrease glial activity and reduce neuropathic and "windup" pain (Childers, 2007). NMDA antagonists can also help decrease the required dosing of opioids and they can work as synergistic therapies (Fig. 6.8).

NMDA antagonists may have a neuroprotective property, particularly memantine, though more studies need to be done in companion animals to evaluate the efficacy (Mak, 2020). Human cognitive dysfunction seemed to be improved by

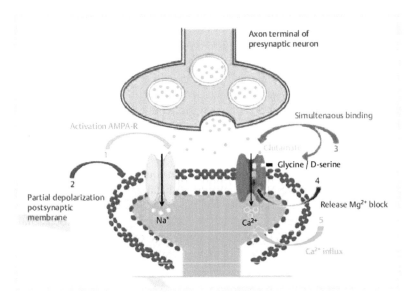

FIGURE 6.8

Activation of NMDA receptors. 1. NMDA receptors on the post synaptic memebrane are activated by glutamate. 2. Activation of NMDA receptor allows Na^+ into the cell causing depolarization of the post synaptic membrane. 3. This depolarization along with glutamate and glycine or D-serine bind to the NMDA receptor release a Mg^{++} block, allowing Ca^{++} to enter the cell.

Used with permission from Veerman, S. S. (2014). The glutamate hypothesis: A pathogenic pathway from which pharmacological interventions have emerged. Pharmacopsychiatry.

memantine in preclinical studies; however, other studies do not show a difference in efficacy (Folch, 2018). Patients with canine and feline cognitive dysfunction as well as degenerative myelopathy may benefit from early use of an NMDA antagonist, particularly ketamine or memantine. More research in companion animals may elucidate other ways to combat cognitive dysfunction in the future.

There are three commonly used NMDA antagonists in veterinary medicine: amantadine, ketamine, and methadone (an opioid with NMDA antagonist properties). Other NMDA antagonists less commonly used in veterinary medicine include memantine and dextromethorphan.

Amantadine is used in humans for Parkinson's disease and was used for influenza. It is no longer recommended for the flu because of viral resistance (Chang, 2020). It is also a first-line drug for multiple sclerosis and studied for use with restless leg syndrome and traumatic brain injuries. It has a weak affinity for the NMDA receptor (Pereira, 2019).

In dogs, the use of amantadine has risen recently (as of this writing) as a chronic pain management tool. However, few studies have evaluated the efficacy of amantadine in chronic pain in dogs or cats. One study looked at the using amantadine with an NSAID showed improvement with the combination (Lascelles, 2008). Amantadine may be difficult to dose for smaller animals and may need to be compounded to dose appropriately. Significant side effects can be behavioral changes, aggression, lethargy, and gastrointestinal. side effects such as anorexia, vomiting, and diarrhea. The recommended dose is 2−5 mg/kg PO SID to BID for dogs and cats (Moore, 2016).

Ketamine is more commonly used in human palliative medicine. Ketamine is an NMDA antagonist classified as a dissociative anesthetic used in many species. It may also have opioid receptor activity (Kronenberg, 2002). Ketamine can be used dosed with IV, SQ administration, and with continuous rate infusions (CRIs), at subanesthetic doses for palliative pain management. The research using ketamine in CRIs for acute pain in animals is more extensive. However, CRIs may not be practical in the home setting. Subanesthetic subcutaneous ketamine, an off-label use, may be more effective than oral amantadine as ketamine has a strong affinity for NMDA receptors, whereas amantadine has weak affinity. However, more research is needed to evaluate the use and efficacy in palliative veterinary patients. In addition, ketamine is a controlled drug in the United States, schedule III, and there is concern about diversion with use in the home.

The dosing for SQ subanesthetic dosing is 0.5 mg/kg SQ PRN (this is an anecdotal dose, there are no studies in dogs or cats as of this writing). A CRI can be given to dogs or cats at 0.5 mg/kg IV loading bolus followed by 2−10 μg/kg/min for 24 h (Shaffran, 2013). Another possible way of giving ketamine might be a subcutaneous CRI, with a new CRI pump from RxActuator but this modality needs to be researched to evaluate efficacy for chronic pain management. A 2018 study on intranasal use of ketamine in human patients with oral cancer found improved pain levels, heart rate, and blood pressure (Page, 2018). Another study in rats study found intranasal ketamine provided analgesia against inflammatory, neuropathic pain, and hyperalgesia (Claudino, 2018).

Memantine is an NMDA antagonist used in humans to treat dementia. It may be helpful for canine and feline cognitive dysfunction though more studies need to be done to assess efficacy in companion animals (Schneider, 2009). It may have a neuroprotective component as well (Mak, 2020). The dose is given orally at 0.3—0.5 mg/kg SID-BID (Wright, 2017).

Methadone—This is an opioid with some NMDA antagonist properties (see the opioid list for more information).

Dextromethorphan is a noncompetitive NMDA antagonist that is typically used as a cough suppressant (Kukanich, 2004). It is not commonly used in veterinary patients at the time of this writing.

Non-steroidal anti-inflammatory drugs (NSAIDs)

NSAIDs are generally used to treat inflammatory pain, most commonly in patients with osteoarthritis. There is also increasing evidence that NSAIDS which are cyclooxygenase-2 or Cox-2 selective inhibitors may have additional benefits when treating some forms of neoplasia. This table lists NSAIDs currently available for use with companion animals (Fig. 6.9).

Recommended NSAID dosages and indications

Washout periods for switching from NSAIDs to steroids or vice versa: There is no standard for washout periods. The standard of care in your area may apply to what is currently used in your area. In a study looking at concurrent administration to dogs of meloxicam at a dose of 0.1 mg/kg with prednisolone 0.5 mg/kg, these patients were found to have some gastric ulcerations and erosions, but not significantly more than in the control group. The study also looked at concurrent administration of a combination of ketoprofen 0.25 mg/kg and prednisolone 0.5 mg kg in dogs. In contrast, patients receiving this combination of NSAID and steroids were found to have severe gastric lesions (Ferguson, 2008; Narita, 2007). So it may depend on the NSAID and steroid. As of this writing, no study has examined specific washout periods directly to evaluate the most effective time period needed between the use of steroids and NSAIDS in companion animals.

Cox-1 inhibitors

Aspirin inhibits cyclooxygenase-1 (COX-1, prostaglandin synthetase), reducing prostaglandins and thromboxane synthesis (TXA2). These effects are thought to be how aspirin produces analgesia, antipyrexia, and reduces platelet aggregation and inflammation (VIN Staff, 2017). Aspirin is not currently recommended for pain use in animals; however, it may be recommended as antithrombotic therapy in low doses (Blais, 2019).

NSAIDs	Dosage/Route	Duration (PO)*	Indications	Comments: Common side effects, toxicities
Carprofen (tablet, chewable and injectable formulations)	Dog: 2-4 mg/kg divided into two equal doses P.O. or S.C. Injectable approved for S.C. administration.	12-24 hr	Mild to moderate pain; For perioperative soft tissue and orthopedic, acute pain and chronic osteoarthritic pain and inflammation in dogs.	Minimal toxicity in dogs with long-term use. For chronic use, titrate to the minimum effective dose. G.I. upset the most common side effect. Concern about use in hepatic and renal disease patients.
	Cat: 1.0-2.0 mg/kg; once only by the injectable route (not commonly used in palliative care for cats)			
	Cat: Not used			
Meloxicam (oral liquid suspension and injectable formulations)	Dog: 0.2 mg/kg initially; 0.1 mg/kg thereafter; IM, SC, PO	24 hr	Mild to moderate arthritis pain.	G.I. irritation; can be mixed with food; use in cats restricted to 2-3 days postoperatively. For chronic arthritic pain in cats, reduce the dose to 25% short-term dose. ***There is a black box warning about use in cats currently. (2021).
	Cat: 0.1 mg/kg initially; 0.025 mg/kg thereafter; IM, SC, PO	24 hr		

FIGURE 6.9

NSAID therapy. For animals in severe pain, combination therapy with opioids may be especially effective.

Used with permission from John Spahr at Teton New Media ©2021 Tranquilli, W. G. (2004). Pain management for the small animal practitioner: Teton New Media ©2004.

Ketoprofen (tablets and injectable)	Dog: 2.0 mg/kg SC, IM initially 1.0 mg/kg thereafter; PO, SC	24 hr	Mild to moderate pain.	Increase bleeding times, G.I. bleeding, ulcers, kidney damage reported; not recommended for more than five days. May increase bleeding times if given preoperatively. It can cause GI ulcers when given with tramadol. (Not commonly used in palliative care.)
	Cat: 1.0 mg/kg SC, IM initially, 0.5 mg/kg thereafter; PO, SC	24 hr		
Deracoxib Firocoxib	Dog: Deracoxib 3.0-4.0 mg/kg for seven days post-operatively and 1.0-2.0 mg/kg for chronic osteoarthritic pain. Firocoxib 5 mg/kg	24 hr	Mild to moderate pain. For acute perioperative orthopedic pain and chronic osteoarthritic pain and inflammation in dogs.	Deracoxib and Firocoxib are members of the coxib class of NSAIDs that seem to be a selective cyclooxygenase-2 enzyme. Coxibs may also have anti-neoplastic actions for canine mammary tumors and transitional cell carcinoma. (Saito, 2014) G.I. upset the most common side effect.
	Cat: Not used			
	Cat: Not used			
Tolfenamic acid (tablets and injectables)	Dog: 4.0 mg/kg S.C., I.M. initially, after that P.O.	24 hr	Mild to moderate pain.	May have antineoplastic properties for osteosarcoma, mammary carcinoma, and melanoma. (Wilson, 2012) Vomiting and diarrhea were reported; recommended for four days on and three days off in dogs and cats, which is not practical for chronic inflammatory pain.
	Cat: same as dog	24 hr		

FIGURE 6.9 cont'd.

Acetaminophen (tablets and oral liquid suspension)	Dog: 10-15 mg/kg; PO	8-12 hr	Mild to moderate pain; low anti-inflammatory action.	Toxic to cats; Do not use in cats. In dogs, it can be given in combination with codeine or hydrocodone. It can be used with NSAIDs or steroids
	Cat: Contraindicated			

FIGURE 6.9 cont'd.

Cox-2 selective inhibitors

Cyclooxygenase-2 (Cox- 2) inhibitors are commonly used in veterinary medicine for osteoarthritis and other inflammatory pain. The decrease of inflammation by inhibiting the COX-2 enzyme decreases the production of PGE2 (Prostaglandin E2). COX-2 inhibitors have also been shown to have some antineoplastic effects and may slow the progression of some cancers. Many cancers have overexpression of Cox-2, and the use of Cox-2 specific NSAIDs should be considered (Teske, 2010). The following cancer types have been found to have cyclooxygenase-2 expression: canine and feline transitional cell carcinoma, nasal carcinoma, canine and feline malignant mammary carcinoma, canine gastrointestinal cancers such as-colorectal stromal adenoma. Approximately ½ of the adenocarcinomas in one study had some expression, and although at lower levels, so did canine and feline squamous cell carcinomas, canine epithelial prostate tumors, osteosarcoma, anaplastic carcinoma, renal cell carcinoma, ovarian carcinoma, oral melanoma, and meningiomas (Dore, 2010).

Cox-3/Cox1-V1 inhibition

Acetaminophen/paracetamol is an antipyretic and pain reliever whose exact mechanism of action is not fully understood, but is thought to involve the inhibition of a third Cox isoenzyme called Cox-3 (also known as Cox1- V1) (Botting and Ayoub, 2005). Oral dosing for dogs is 10−15 mg/kg BID to TID. This medication may be contraindicated in animals with liver disease and for end-of-life patients the possible pros and cons may need to be discussed with the client before use. It can also cause methemoglobin in dogs, so it must be used caution. There are also reports of keratoconjunctivitis sicca or KCS developing in dogs after use (Fox, 2012). Acetominophen/paracetomol is toxic to cats and ferrets and should never be used with these patients.

Tylenol/codeine—Codeine has extremely low bioavailability in dogs, around 4% (from Plumb's) due to high first-pass metabolism (KuKanich, 2016). It does metabolize to codeine-6-glucuronide in dogs, which may contribute to pain relief, though more studies are needed to assess its efficacy (KuKanich, 2016). Dosing for dogs is based on the Tylenol dose.

Tylenol/hydrocodone—Hydrocodone is a better cough suppressant than codeine. The oral bioavailability of hydrocodone is between 40% and 80%, which is among the highest bioavailability reported for oral opioids (KuKanich, 2013). It can be given up to every 8 h with the dosing is based on the tylenol dose discussed earlier. Hydrocodone metabolizes to hydromorphone and because of diversion should be used with caution in the home (KuKanich, 2013).

PGE-4 receptor antagonist

Grapiprant (Galliprant®) is a newer medication of the piprant class. It is a non-COX inhibitor NSAID pain medication affecting prostaglandin E2 (PGE2), which binds to the EP4 receptor (Rausch-Derra, 2015). Galliprant® is more specific for the antiinflammatory process with fewer side effects from the COX inflammatory processes. Side effects can include vomiting and diarrhea, decreased appetite, and lethargy (Kirkby Shaw, 2016). There is one published study regarding safe use for cats (Rausch Derra, 2016). The small study with 24 cats found that a dose of <15 mg/kg given once daily was well tolerated, and no significant changes on necropsy were found.

Galliprant® is dosed for dogs as follows: to control pain and inflammation, 2 mg/kg PO q 24 h calculated to the lowest ½ tablet dose (VIN Staff, 2017). Dosing for less than a 3.6-kg animal cannot be done accurately (VIN Staff, 2017). It would be off-label use for cats and not recommended at the time of this writing although there is one study on safety there are no studies on the efficacy.

Steroids

There is a saying in veterinary medicine that, "No animal should die without the benefit of steroids." And while corticosteroids have been glorified in many ways, corticosteroids have been vilified as well. For patients in the late or end stages of their disease processes, steroids may be the correct choice. Animals with end-stage disease may need different options than what is the curative standard of care. However, examining all of the factors of the particular situation involved can help the veterinarian and the client decide whether it would be a beneficial choice to utilize steroids for your patient.

Possible clinical uses for steroids as a component of palliative care:

1. Inflammatory pain. While NSAIDs might be the best first-line inflammatory drug, having another comorbidity, such as OA and a brain tumor, steroids might be a better choice.

2. Hyporexia or anorexia. Again, steroids might be a better choice depending on the other disease process to help drive an appetite (where NSAIDs might depress it) (Miller, 2014).
3. Dyspnea. Steroids may help dyspneic patients with primary or metastatic lung cancer or patients with inflammatory respiratory disease, such as asthma or lung fibrosis.
4. Inflammatory diseases, such as neoplasia or FIP
5. Carcinomatosis
6. Hypercalcemia
7. Neoplasia/metastasis—Although many cancers may be responsive to an NSAID, consider steroids if they are not responding or have other comorbidities.
   a. Osteosarcoma
   b. Head and neck tumors
   c. Glucagonoma/insulinomas
   d. Brain neoplasia
   e. Mast cell tumors
   f. Mammary adenocarcinoma
   g. Lung neoplasia
8. Immune-mediated disease (although less likely to see in the home setting)
9. Addison's (Elkholly, 2020)

Clinical scenarios where steroids should be used with caution:

1. Congestive heart failure
2. Liver disease
3. GI bleeding
4. Other bleeding disorders
5. End-stage skin issues like decubitus ulcers.
6. Infectious disease (Elkholly, 2020)

Side effects of concern: gastrointestinal signs, such as vomiting, diarrhea, hematochezia, hematemesis, gastrointestinal ulceration, perforation, hepatopathy, body weight gain, or muscle loss, polyuria, and polydipsia. Adverse effects can also lead to immunosuppression, changes in behavior, panting heavily, delayed wound healing, urinary tract infections, or other infections (Elkholly, 2020). Polyphagia is listed as a potential side effect as well but this may also be considered a beneficial side effect for patients receiving palliative care.

Commonly used steroids in the home setting
Oral steroids

1. Oral prednisone, prednisolone—Dose 0.5–2 mg/kg PO q 12–48 h, starting with a higher dose and decreasing it until the side effects decrease or subside (VIN Staff, 2017)
2. Oral budesonide—Dose is 1–3 **mg** per **dog or cat** q 24 h (VIN Staff, 2017)

3. Oral dexamethasone—Antiinflammatory dose 0.25−1.25 mg per **dog** PO q 24 h for up to 7 days. For cats—0.25−0.5 mg per **cat** PO q 24 h for up to 7 days (VIN Staff, 2017)
4. Oral methylprednisolone (Depo Medrol)—2 mg for 5−15 lb dogs, 2−4 mg for dogs 15−40 lbs, and 4−8 mg per dog for 40−80 lb dogs, PO split into equal doses given q 6−10 h apart (VIN Staff, 2017).

Injectable steroids
Dogs and cats:

1. Dexamethasone sodium phosphate (Dex SP)—0.15 mg/kg IV q 24 h
2. Injectable methylprednisolone antiinflammatory dosing—0.9 mg/kg IV q 24 h (VIN Staff, 2017)

Gabapentinoids

Gabapentin is classified as an antiepileptic drug, but veterinarians most commonly use it to treat chronic neuropathic pain (VIN Staff, 2017). The mode of action occurs in the alpha-2-delta ($\alpha 2\delta$) subunits of the calcium channels in the spinal cord's dorsal horn and sites in the neocortex and hippocampus (VIN Staff, 2017). Gabapentin decreases calcium flow by binding to the $\alpha 2\delta$ subunit of voltage-gated calcium channels and inhibiting the release of excitatory neurotransmitters—such as substance P and glutamate (VIN Staff, 2017). It has a nonlinear absorption rate, which means practically, the drug can have varied effects on individuals, and the dose may need to be adjusted frequently throughout the disease (Quintero, 2017). In dogs, it has a bioavailability of 80% (VIN Staff, 2017). It is recommended for people with hepatic disease (Quintero, 2017). The bioavailability may decrease over time as well, also indicating a need for additional medication. The most common side effects reported are somnolence, dizziness (in humans), ataxia, and fatigue/weakness (Quintero, 2017). Gabapentin may also potentiate methadone (Quintero, 2017).

Dosing for gabapentin in dogs with neuropathic pain is 3−20 mg/kg PO q 8−12 h. The standard dosing for analgesia is 10−20 mg/kg PO q 8−12 h. The author recommends starting on the lower end of both the dose and the timing and increasing each over time with need. Taper off gabapentin if drug removal is needed, as there is a risk of rebound pain or seizures with abrupt discontinuation of this medication. For use as an anticonvulsant in dogs, the dose is 10−30 mg/kg PO q 8 h (VIN Staff, 2017). For cats, the analgesic dose starts at 5 mg/kg q 24 h and increases with need. The anticonvulsant dose for cats is 10−20 mg/kg PO q 6−12 h (Pakozdy, 2014).

Pregabalin is also classified as an antiepileptic drug. Pregabalin is a derivative of the inhibitory neurotransmitter gamma-aminobutyric acid (GABA). However, it does not bind directly to GABA receptors (VIN Staff, 2017). It does bind to the $\alpha 2\delta$ subunit of voltage-gated calcium channels in the dorsal horn and brain. It has a linear absorption rate, and therefore adjustment of dosing is typically not needed as compared to gabapentin. The oral bioavailability is 90% (VIN Staff, 2017). Pregabalin is more expensive than gabapentin as of this writing. And there are very few studies in companion animals on the efficacy of pregabalin when used to treat pain. However, prescribing pregabalin for patients that are not responsive to gabapentin, or where gabapentin makes them too sedate, may be another option to help treat neuropathic pain.

Pregabalin dosing for dogs as an anticonvulsant is 2—4 mg/kg PO q 12 h (VIN Staff, 2017). For cats, it is 1—2 mg/kg PO q 12 h (Pakozdy, 2014).

Antidepressants

Antidepressants have been used in human medicine for neuropathic pain. There are five main classes of antidepressants: selective serotonin reuptake inhibitors (SSRI), serotonin-norepinephrine reuptake inhibitors (SNRIs), tricyclic antidepressants (TCAs), monoamine oxidase inhibitors, and atypical agents.

Some commonly used antidepressants that are used as adjunctive therapies in the treatment of pain include amitriptyline (TCA), fluoxetine (Prozac) (SSRI), and clomipramine (Clomicalm) (TCA). Trazadone is not a tricyclic antidepressant, but an atypical antidepressant that has serotonin modulating effects. It is postulated that these antidepressants relieve pain via centrally mediated inhibition of presynaptic serotonin and norepinephrine reuptake. It is thought that tricyclic antidepressants tend to be more effective at addressing pain direction as compared to SSRI and SNRI antidepressants in people (Sindrup, 2005). Both trazadone and its active metabolite, *m*- chlorophenylpiperazine, are both serotonin receptor antagonists and serotonin reuptake inhibitors. They are weak analgesics but could be considered in addition to other pain management medications especially if anxiety is also an issue. These medications should be tapered when discontinuing an animal from the medication. Seizures have been reported if discontinued without tapering.

If compounding antidepressant medications for transdermal use, it has been recommended to use a sweetener in case of oral ingestion from grooming as these medications are often quite bitter or unpalatable (VIN Staff, 2017).

Dosing

1. Amitriptyline—Dogs: for chronic pain, 1—2 mg/kg PO q 12—24 h and neuropathic pain, 3—4 mg/kg PO q 12 h. Cats: 5 mg per cat PO q 24 h (VIN Staff, 2017)
2. Fluoxetine—Dogs: for anxiety 1 mg/kg PO q 24 h. Cats: management of psychogenic alopecia 2 mg per cat q 24—72 h. Management of behavior disorders 0.5—4 mg per cat (VIN Staff, 2017)
3. Clomipramine—Dogs: for behavior disorders 1—2 mg/kg PO q 12 h, Cats: For behavior disorders 0.25—0.5 mg/kg PO q 24 h.
4. Trazadone—Dogs: anxiety disorders 2—5 mg/kg PO q 8—24 h, Cats: 50 mg per **cat** for transport 1—1.5 h before transport

Cerenia® (maropitant)

Cerenia® is a neurokinin-1 receptor antagonist affecting the neurotransmitter, substance P. Cerenia® does prevent vomiting very well; however, it may not prevent nausea (Trepanier, 2017). Cerenia® also does appear to help reduce visceral pain (Trepanier, 2017). A study showed that Cerenia® decreases the need for inhalation anesthetic (Kinobe, 2020). In comparing morphine and maropitant when used as premedication's given before an ovariohysterectomy, there was little difference in the number of patients requiring rescue pain medication. The dogs who had received maropitant recovered faster and ate sooner (Marquez, 2015). NK-1 receptors are in the CNS, spinal cord, and peripheral nerves; they are also found in bronchial epithelium, bronchial vessels, and goblet cells in the lung and the bladder wall. However, to this date, no studies have seen significant effects with Cerenia® for nausea, asthma, bronchitis, or feline lower urinary tract disease (Trepanier, 2017). In humans, an NK-1 antagonist decreases visceral pain and lowered anxiety in women with irritable bowel syndrome (Tillisch, 2012). Compounding pharmacies can prepare a transdermal version of maropitant that may be helpful for animals who will not accept oral medications. However, at the time of this writing, there are no efficacy studies of Cerenia® when administered transdermally to animals.

Dosing: Dogs: 2 mg/kg PO q 24 h 1 mg/kg SQ q 24 h. Cats: 1 mg/kg PO, SQ q 24 h (VIN Staff, 2017).

Local anesthetics

1. Intravenous lidocaine has been used to treat humans with neuropathic pain (Corletto, 2019). Lidocaine has a reasonable margin of safety in dogs, and cats have a narrow margin of safety. Lidocaine is a sodium channel blocker that may decrease firing in damaged nerves (Corletto, 2019). Using intravenous lidocaine is not commonly done in the home setting. CRI dosing for dogs is 1−2 mg/kg IV followed by continuous infusion of 2−3 mg/kg/h. Side effects may be sedation, decreased appetite (Corletto, 2019).
2. Lidocaine patches are helpful in the home setting. They may work by inhibiting the small C and Aδ fibers (Corletto, 2019). They may be less effective in treating neuropathic pain than IV lidocaine (Corletto, 2019). Cardiovascular and neurologic toxicity are the major side effects. Seizures, arrhythmias such as ventricular tachycardia or ventricular fibrillation have been noted (Corletto, 2019). Toxicity occurs >2−3 mg/kg of bupivacaine IV or >10 mg/kg lidocaine IV (Corletto, 2019).
3. Viscous Lidocaine may also be used in "Magic Mouthwash".

Epidurals/joint infusions While these are commonly performed in specialty and general practice, these would be uncommon to use in the home setting for end-of-life care patients. Medications administered via the epidural route could include local anesthetics such as bupivacaine, or opioids. Joint infusions may employ local anesthetics, steroids, or opioids to decrease joint pain (Tranquilli, 2004).

Anti-NGF Antinerve growth factor is an up-and-coming monoclonal antibody medication (mAbs) that has shown promise in veterinary species with OA. Additionally, it may be useful in the pain management of osteosarcoma (see symptom management chapter for additional information). One anti-NGF mAbs has been approved in Europe for Zoetus under the name Librela (bedinvetmab). There is not and available product in the United States as of this writing (Melis, 2020).

α-2-Adrenergic Agonists are not typically considered for use with pain management though they have some analgesic properties. The mechanism of action for α-2-agonists is similar to opioids and can decrease the need for opioid use (Tranquilli, 2004). They activate membrane-associated G proteins that, in turn, open potassium channels, which hyperpolarize the nerve making it unresponsive to stimuli (Tranquilli, 2004). α-2 agonists may cause analgesia or sedation. The side effects include increasing vagal tone, decreased cardiac output, bradycardia, and vasoconstriction and may cause vomiting (especially in cats). Lower doses can help decrease the side effects (Tranquilli, 2004). Some α-2-agonists could be considered for inclusion as a sedative in a crisis kit. Dormosedan (detomidine) and Sileo (dexmedetomidine) are two oral preparations that can be used off-label for a crisis kit. The client would need education on how to use them for their crisis kit and would need to be informed that vomiting may occur.

Dosing—Dogs: Dormosedan gel (detomidine) 0.1 mL/kg transmucosally for sedation before euthanasia (anecdotal) (efficacy is variable.) $0.5-1$ mg/m^2 transmucosally (VIN Staff, 2017).

Dogs: Sileo gel 0.125 mg/m^2 transmucosal. It may take 30—60 min to take effect (VIN staff, 2017).

Medication to treat acute pain in the home setting
Opioids

Opioids have historically been a go to pain medication, especially for acute and surgical pain. However with the opioid crisis in humans, the use of opioids has changed. In house call practice, opioids can be utilized in crisis kits and for severe chronic pain or acute pain. Opioids, both endogenous and exogenous, mechanism of action is on the Mu or Kappa or Delta opioid receptor, which are G-protein coupled receptors that cause a release of potassium causing hyperpolerazation of the nerve. Most medically relevant opioids work on the Mu or Kappa receptors (Pathan and Williams, 2012). Opioids should be considered for palliative patients in the home setting for acute pain flare-ups, along with an NMDA antagonist or an alpha-2 agonist, which may help these animals be more comfortable. For animals with severe or unrelenting pain and who already have multiple pain medications in their treatment plan, opioids may be a final option to help manage their pain. A crisis kit should include medication for acute pain and other adjunctive therapies such as gabapentin and acepromazine that can help relieve pain and sedate.

Some drawbacks to opioid use: They must be used with discretion in the home setting due to the potential for diversion of narcotics. There should be an exceptional paper trail for any opioids left in the home, documentation with signatures acknowledging costs, side effects, and potential harm to humans. In human medicine, opioids for end-of-life patients are provided through a pharmacy only. Human hospice and palliative care doctors and nurses do not carry to the house, nor do they take them away, though removal from home had a recent change in the law. That law change does not affect veterinarians. Instead, veterinarians should consider leaving disposal information for animal caregivers. The other drawback to oral opioids is the degree of bioavailability in dogs (which varies by opioid) and cats due to the first-pass metabolism in the liver.

Mu-agonists opioids

1. Methadone (Schedule II)—Dogs: 0.25–0.5 mg/kg SQ q 3–4 h. Cats: 0.1–0.25 mg/kg SQ q 3–4 h. Methadone has some NMDA antagonist properties and could be useful with animals with central sensitization (VIN Staff, 2017). Oral bioavailability may be improved by giving a P450 inhibitor. A study looked at a novel formulation of methadone/fluconazole/naltrexone given orally the night before and the morning of surgery and post-op and found that none of the dogs getting this combination needed rescue medications (KuKanich, 2020).
2. Morphine (Schedule II)—Dogs: 0.25–1 mg SQ or 0.2–0.5 mg/kg q 6–8 h for liquid formulations. Cats: 0.1–0.25 mg/kg SQ q 2–4 h or 0.2–0.5 mg/kg q 6–8 h of oral liquid (can cause anaphylaxis, vomiting, dysphoria, constipation). Should have Naloxone (reversal agent) in case of side effects (VIN Staff, 2017).
3. Hydromorphone (Schedule II)—Dogs/Cats: 0.05–0.1 mg/kg SQ q 2–4 h (can cause hyperthermia in some patients). Use caution in MDR-1 mutation patients as they may be predisposed to toxicity (VIN Staff, 2017). It can cause vomiting, diarrhea, and panting. It can be partially reversed with butorphanol and naloxone.
4. Fentanyl patches may not be ideal due to variable uptake and the need for changing every 3 days, and the cost of the patch and the visit. However, they can help if that is the only option available to you.

Partial μ-agonists

1. Buprenorphine (Schedule III)—Dogs: 0.01–0.05 mg/kg SQ or TM q 8–12 h. Cats: 0.01–0.02 mg/kg SQ or TM q 4–12 h 0.12 mg/kg sustained-release formula is given SQ every 72 h, 0.24 mg/kg Simbadol only SQ q 24 h up to 3 days (this dose can cause profound sedation with other buprenorphine formulations). Use caution in MDR-1 mutation patients as they may be predisposed to toxicity from norbuprenorphine—the metabolite of buprenorphine (VIN Staff, 2017).

K-agonist/μ-antagonists

1. Butorphanol—Dogs: 0.1—0.5 mg/kg SQ q 1—4 h, 0.55 mg/kg PO q 6—12 h, though it may be more sedating than analgesic, not ideal for moderate or severe pain patients. First pass metabolism makes oral butorphanol ineffective for analgesia. Cats: 0.2—0.4 mg/kg q 1—4 h (VIN Staff, 2017). Butorphanol can be used in a crisis kit with other medications such as gabapentin and acepromazine or an α22-agonist.
2. Nalbuphine—This synthetic opioid analgesic is of particular interest, even though it is of limited efficacy for treating pain, because it is the only opioid marketed in the United States that is not controlled under the Controlled Substances Act, at this time. Dogs and cats: 0.2—0.5 mg/kg IV, IM, SQ. As a solo agent used extra-label for mild to moderate pain, it is considered of limited efficacy and of relatively short duration of action, similar to butrophanol (1+hours) (Plumb, 2021) (DEA). This is a synthetic opioid analgesic Nalbuphine causes fewer adverse effects than other opioid analgesics (Narver, 2015).

Recommended opioid dosages and indications
(Fig. 6.10).

Tramadol

Tramadol is classified as an opioid-like drug for humans. In humans, the first metabolite (M1) is O-desmethyltramadol. In dogs, it has been found that tramadol does not appreciably metabolize to the M1 metabolite (Schütter, 2017). Tramadol metabolizes to N-desmethyltramadol (M2) and behaves more like a tricyclic antidepressant in dogs. Research shows oral tramadol is an ineffective pain management medication for dogs in OA, spays, tumor removal, and other surgeries (Budsberg, 2018).

One study looking at the effectiveness of tramadol in canine patients with osteoarthritis found that there was no significant difference between the pain level in the animals treated with tramadol and the control group; however, the study found a big improvement in pain levels when carprofen was given (Budsberg, 2018). Potential adverse side effects in dogs may include serotonin syndrome, nausea, hypersalivation, and tremors (Itami, 2016).

Unlike in dogs, cats do metabolize tramadol into the M1 (O-desmethyltramadol) metabolite. The M1 metabolite has ½ life of approximately 5 h in cats (Pypendop, 2008). The M2 metabolite (n-desmethyltramadol) inhibits norepinephrine and serotonin reuptake, G-protein coupled receptors, α-2 adrenoreceptors, Neurokinin 1, muscarinic, and ion channels that include acetylcholine and NMDA receptors that may also be useful in pain management (Monteiro, 2017). Tramadol in cats may also help decrease central sensitization via both of these metabolites (Monteiro, 2017).

Opioid	Dose/Route	Duration (IM)*	Indications	Comments
Morphine (Schedule 2)	Dog: 0.2-2.0 mg/kg; IM, SC; 0.05-0.4 mg/kg; IV	3-5 hr	Moderate to severe pain; CRI at 0.05-0.3 mg/kg/h can be used for long term analgesia	Sedation, respiratory depression, bradycardia, nausea, hypothermia, dysphoria in non-painful cats, or large dosage. To avoid histamine release when given I.V., dilute or administer slowly.
	Cat: 0.05-0.2 mg/kg; IM, SC	3-4 hr		
Fentanyl (Schedule 2)	Dog:0.002-0.01 mg/kg; IM, IV, SC	0.5 hr	Moderate to severe pain; CRI at 0.002-0.01 mg/kg/h necessary for long term analgesia	Sedation, respiratory depression, bradycardia, nausea; inadequate duration of analgesia from single IV bolus or I.M. injection.
	Cat: 0.001-0.005 mg/kg; IM, IV, SC	0.5 hr		
Fentanyl Patch (Schedule 2)	Dog:0.005 mg/kg/h; Transdermal	3 days	Mild to moderate pain	The onset to effect ranges from 12-24 hours depending on location, skin adhesion, and transdermal absorption variability, resulting in inadequate analgesic effects.
	Cat: 0.005 mg/kg/h; Transdermal	3-5 days		

FIGURE 6.10

Table of opioids. *Duration varies with dosage and route of administration. Intravenous administration generally results in more rapid onset and shorter duration. In comparison, SC and PO administration usually results in a slower onset and longer duration than listed earlier for IM administration. Use the lower end of the dose range for initial IV administration (Tranquilli, 2004).

Reproduced with permission by John Spahr at Teton New Media ©2021.

Hydromorphone or Oxymorphone (Schedule 2)	Dog: 0.05-0.2 mg/kg; IM, IV, SC	2-4 hr	Moderate to severe pain	Similar side effects as those observed with morphine, but less vomiting and no histamine release.
	Cat: 0.05-0.2 mg/kg; IM, IV, SC	2-4 hr		Hydromorphone may provide a more extended period of analgesia in cats and has been associated with the occasional hyperthermia observed.
Methadone (Schedule 2)	Dog: 0.05-2.0 mg/kg; PO, IM, SC	4-6 hr	Mild to moderate pain	May also have NMDA antagonistic action.
	Cat: 0.05-1.0 mg/kg; PO	4-6 hr		
Butorphanol (Schedule 4)	Dog: 0.2-2.0 mg/kg; IM, IV, SC, PO	1-2 hr	Mild to moderate pain	Mild or no sedation, mild ventilatory depression. Butorphanol's analgesic effectiveness in dogs has been debated. Oral bioavailability is uncertain.
	Cat: 0.2-1.0 mg/kg; IM, IV, SC, PO	1-4 hr		

FIGURE 6.10 cont'd.

In cats, tramadol has been found to be beneficial for OA. Dosing in one study showed 2 mg/kg PO every 12 h was the most effective dose for cats, with more adverse events occurring at higher dosing (Guedes, 2018). Adverse events seen in cats may include dysphoria, sedation, decreased appetite, and diarrhea. They can also include mydriasis and euphoria (Monteiro, 2017). One challenge with using tramadol in cats is the taste and the size of the current tablet made for humans. It might be easier to give if compounded into smaller doses or liquid and is recommended to be compounded with a sweetener to help cut the bitter taste.

| Buprenorphine (Schedule 3) | Dog: 0.005-0.02 mg/kg; IM, IV, SC | 6-8 hr | Mild to moderate pain | The onset of analgesic action may require 15-30 min or longer. Prolonged sleep times may occur. They are administered orally for absorption through buccal mucosa in cats. It may be more challenging to antagonize than other opioid agonists. |
| | Cat: 0.005-0.02 mg/kg; IM, IV, SC, or transmucosal | 6-8 hr 6-8 hr | | |

FIGURE 6.10 cont'd.

While local blocks are used more often in the brick-and-mortar clinic for pre- or postprocedural patients, they may not be as practical for house call palliative medicine. However, they may find their place with patients undergoing surgeries, such as amputations, or surgical debulking, as well as palliative radiation.

Non-pharmaceutical pain management

A multimodal approach is conventional with end-of-life care and palliative medicine. Nonpharmaceutical approaches to pain management may be utilized and should be held to the same scientific standards of efficacy as any other therapy. That being said, regardless of the paradigm a veterinarian chooses to use to palliate and resolve pain in their patients, animal caregivers may ask questions regarding various therapies. Understanding a variety of therapies can help to support both the patient and the caregiver. Understanding a wide variety of therapeutic options will also help the clinician to feel more comfortable in terms of being informed about as many treatment options as possible. Utilizing nonpharmaceutical therapies as part of a multimodal approach may be additive or synergistic with pharmaceutical therapy. For integrative therapies, the evidence basis for use will be noted.

Palliative radiation

Palliative radiation is an excellent pain management option for animals with later-stage cancer, solid tumors, and osteosarcoma. Radiation can be used to palliate pain from melanoma, osteosarcoma, nasal carcinoma, mast cell tumors, ameloblastoma (Tollett, 2016), transitional cell carcinoma (Choy, 2016), and synovial cell carcinoma (Gibbons, 2011). A major drawback of palliative radiation, for some clients, may be the use of anesthesia to provide the radiation and the need and frequency of hospital visits needed for results. There is a solid evidence base for use of palliative radiation.

Weight loss therapy

Addressing obesity or nutritional overconditioning is not generally an area of focus with terminally ill dogs and cats. However, many elderly animals who suffer primarily from osteoarthritis pain or intervertebral disc disease may find relief when some degree of weight loss is achieved. Weight loss therapy can be complex beyond the scope of this chapter.

Physical therapy, rehabilitation

Physical therapy (the human term) and rehabilitation is covered in the physical support section. Rehabilitation type therapies are an essential part of veterinary palliative medicine and should be a comprehensive part of palliative care for animals. There is a substantial evidence base for use of rehabilitation with palliative patients.

Nutraceuticals

Nonpharmaceutical therapies have been utilized for pain management but are not regulated by the Food and Drug Administration (FDA). The scope of the information available is vast and beyond the scope of this text. The evidence is varied as to the efficacy of individual nutraceuticals.

Common nutraceuticals used to address pain from osteoarthritis include Glucosamine and Chondroitin, EPA (Omega-3) and DHA (Omega-6) found in the fish oils, as well as curcumin (turmeric).

There are additional references recommended at the end of the chapter for further information on nutraceuticals.

Herbal therapies

Western herbs, traditional Chinese herbal formulations, and ayurvedic herbal therapies may be recommended by an integrative practitioner to help with pain. Herbal formulas for animals come in different forms including liquids, tinctures, capsules, tea pills, and powders. There are numerous herbal therapies used to treat pain in humans as well as in animals. Some commonly used herbs used to treat pain include Boswellia serrata (Frankincense), Corydalis, Angelica and cannabis. There are additional references at the end of the chapter if you would like to read more about herbal therapies.

Cannabis

Cannabis has been used for medicinal purposes for thousands of years and, currently, is a common therapeutic treatment for humans in palliative care (Vučković, 2018). The prohibition of cannabis via the Controlled Substance Act put a halt to cannabis research in 1970 (Vučković, 2018; Hudak, 2018). But medicinal use and research have increased in recent years in both human and veterinary medicine, especially as cannabis has been legalized in many states in the United States.

Cannabis contains hundreds of substances, known as phytocannabinoids, that are currently being researched and have various pharmacological relevance (Richter, 2021). Phytocannabinoids and other components of cannabis such as terpenoids, have also been found in other plants such as carrots, black pepper,ginseng and echinacea (VanDolah et al., 2019). Cannabis is currently used to treat pain, nausea, inflammation, and anxiety, as well as seizures in humans. The primary phytocannabinoids of current therapeutic interest are cannabidiol (CBD) and tetrahydrocannabinol (THC). Cannabis plants containing more than 0.3% THC are considered marijuana. Plants containing less than 0.3% THC are considered hemp (Richter, 2021). Hemp was deregulated by the Farm Bill of 2018, which allowed for more research to be developed (Hudak, 2018.

THC is psychoactive, and has analgesic, antiinflammatory, antioxidant, antipruritic, bronchodilatory, and antispasmodic and muscle-relaxant properties in people (Rahn, 2009; Russo, 2011; Vučković S, 2018). CBD is considered to have analgesic, antiinflammatory, anticonvulsant, and anxiolytic activities, but without the psychoactive effects attributed to THC in people (Costa, 2013; Vučković, 2018). Research to evaluate these properties in companion animals are in progress as of this writing.

The endocannabinoid framework is a complex endogenous system designed to maintain homeostasis. The body has endogenous cannabinoids, in particular anandamide and 2-arachidonylglycerol (2-AG). The two identified receptors are CB1 and CB2. THC is an agonist and binds to the CB1 receptor, CBD is a partial agonist of the CB2 receptor. In the normal endogenous system the presynaptic neuron release gaba and glutamate, they in turn, stimulate the gaba receptors on the post synaptic nerve which release the neurotransmitters, anandamide and 2-AG, which in turn stimulates the CB1 and 2 receptors on the presynaptic nerve (VanDolah et al., 2019). Chronic pain is the most commonly cited reason for using medical cannabis in people. The proposed mechanisms of the analgesic effect of cannabinoids include inhibition of the release of neurotransmitters and neuropeptides from presynaptic nerve endings, modulation of postsynaptic neuron excitability, activation of descending inhibitory pain pathways, and reduction of neural inflammation (Vučković, 2018). CBD appears to have a more elaborate mechanism of action, affecting the reuptake of anandamide and 2-AG, and transient receptor potential vanilloid 1 and G-coupled protein receptor activation, and enhancing serotonin receptor activity (VanDolah et al., 2019).

Interestingly, cannabis and CBD can affect the metabolism of anesthetics and may cause an increase in the need for anesthetics, surgery, postoperative analgesia, or euthanasia (Richter, 2021). This may be due to the hepatic cytochrome P450 metabolism of cannabinoids. It has also been observed that medications that are metabolized by the P450s, phenobarbital, rifampicin, carbamazepine, and phenytoin may decrease the efficacy of CBD (Iffland, 2017). Medications that affect the inhibition of the CYP3A4 enzyme, such as ketoconazole, itraconazole, ritonavir, and clarithromycin, may increase CBD's effects (Iffland, 2017).

Research studies on efficacy for treating pain in humans and animals have, so far, yielded mixed results. Multiple studies have shown that cannabinoids are not effective in treating acute pain in humans (Beaulieu, 2006; Holdcroft, 2006; Kraft, 2008; Vučković, 2018). Clinical data also indicate that cannabinoids may only modestly reduce chronic pain (Romero-Sandoval, 2017).

In one human study, CBD inhalation increased THC plasma concentrations but decreased THC-induced analgesic effects, indicating that there may be antagonistic pharmacodynamic interactions between THC and CBD. This study illuminates the need for further research to determine THC—CBD interactions, and their role in pain relief (van de Donk, 2019).

A 2018 review looked at 47 studies (4743 participants) of cannabis or cannabinoids for various types of noncancer chronic pain in humans and found evidence of a small benefit, particularly with neuropathic pain (Stockings, 2018; Vučković, 2018). A study on dogs with osteoarthritis found that hemp-derived CBD decreased pain and increased mobility in a dose-dependent fashion (Verrico, 2020). Research in animal models (rodents) has shown that CB1, CB2, and G protein-coupled receptor agonists provided visceral analgesia (Larauche, 2012).

Despite the potential for cannabinoid-based pain medications to be helpful as adjunctive therapy for pain in our veterinary patients, there are several challenges that prevent the possibility to use them (at the time of writing this book). The primary challenge currently is that marijuana is still considered a schedule 1 controlled substance. Currently, federal law prohibits veterinarians from prescribing cannabis or any other schedule 1 substance. Laws and regulations, as well as research and evidence-based information, are changing quickly. Even though studies show promise, there are a relatively small number of these studies that show definitive significant evidence of efficacy in the treatment of pain. There are fewer human studies on understanding how to maximize the analgesic effects of cannabis-derived medications, and even fewer studies on this subject in companion animals. The therapeutic use of cannabis as an analgesic is an area that continues to be researched.

Acupuncture

Traditional Chinese veterinary medicine (TCVM) and acupuncture have been practiced for thousands of years (Alvarez, 2015). TCVM is based on two approaches: the Eight Principals (internal, external, hot, cold, excess, deficiency, yin, and yang) and the Five Elements (wood, fire, earth, metal, and water, which correspond to an organ system in the body). These are based on qi (life force) and meridians (or pathways) (Alvarez, 2015). Acupuncture is one of the four branches of TCVM. The other components are herbal medicine, food therapy, and Tui-na (a form of massage or medical manipulation). There are many identified acupuncture points in TCVM (Xie, 2006, 2012).

In the scientific understanding of acupuncture, one of many proposed mechanisms of action are that needle stimulation creates release of local inflammatory mediators such as prostaglandins, leukotrienes, bradykinin, and platelet-activating factor (Alvarez, 2015). These, in turn, create the release of histamine, heparin, and kinin protease leading to vasodilation. In addition, there may be direct stimulation of Aδ and C fibers, which send signals to the dorsal horn of the spinal cord, and travel to the brain via the spinothalamic tract and spinoreticular tract where they synapse in the thalamus (Alvarez, 2015). Endogenous opioids, serotonin, and monoamines are released. The release of neurotransmitters stimulates the substantia gelantinosa region of the dorsal horn to release enkephalin or dynorphin, inhibiting further transmission (Chiu, 2001). There may be additional stimulation of the sympathetic and parasympathetic nervous systems (Alvarez, 2015).

There are several different types of acupuncture. Dry needling is a technique in which a small sterile needle is inserted into the skin or deeper body tissues. Aquapuncture is a form of acupuncture, in which a small amount of a substance is injected directly into the acupuncture point, with the aim to prolong the effects of the acupuncture. Fluids that TCVM practitioners use in aquapuncture may include vitamin B12, Adequan, lidocaine, saline, or homeopathic solutions (There is a lack of conclusive evidence on the efficacy of homeopathy) (Alvarez, 2015; Jonas, 2003). Electroacupuncture is a type of acupuncture in which leads are attached to the needles that have been inserted into the body. The leads are connected toan electroacupuncture machine used to stimulate acupuncture points with electrical current. The current can be direct or alternating, and it can change frequency.

Acupuncture can be used alone or in combination with pharmaceuticals, nutraceuticals, and herbal formulations. Adverse effects following acupuncture are uncommon but may occur. These are reported to be sedation, "masking of symptoms," local pain, skin reactions, and bleeding. Acupuncture is contraindicated in animals with coagulopathies, thrombocytopathies, inflamed or infected skin, or placement of a needle directly through a tumor (Alvarez, 2015). Caution should be taken with animals who are weak, debilitated, or pregnant (Xie, 2006). Contraindications for use of electroacupuncture include animals with pacemakers, arrhythmias, or seizures (Alvarez, 2015).

Low-Level Therapeutic Laser

Therapeutic laser therapy is another often-utilized non-pharmaceutical therapy for musculoskeletal disease, joint, skin/wound healing, and rehabilitation. The evidence base is variable regarding efficacy, and the quality of the evidence also varies.

Laser units can be mobile and require training before having team members use them. The classification system developed by the FDA relates to the safety of the laser. The systems are classified I–IV, depending on the need for eyewear, with I and IIa not requiring eye protection and IIIa, IIIb, and IV requiring eye protection. The tissue penetration depends on wavelength and wattage (or the rate of electrical energy through the circuit). The wavelengths utilized are between 600 and 1000 nm and the wattage between 5 and 500 mW.

Further information on the efficacy of laser therapy is an area that continues to be researched .

Heat/Cold therapy

Warm compresses can help to soothe musculoskeletal and osteoarthritis pain in our veterinary patients. Cold compresses can provide relief for inflammatory pain and neoplasia. Further information can be found in the physical support chapter.

Music

Human hospices use music to aid in calming agitation in patients receiving palliative care. There is variable evidence that music may be therapeutic for easing pain in humans as well. For animals, it may be useful. A study looking at nine primates showed decreased heart rate and blood pressure when explosed to live harp music (Hinds, 2007). There is review of studies looking at classical music and decreasing stress in dogs, that may indicate it has a place in end-of-life care (Lindig et al., 2020).

Targeted pulsed electromagnetic field therapy

Pulsed electromagnetic field (PEMF) therapy is a treatment in which low levels of an electromagnetic field are pulsed through the tissue in order to promote healing and pain relief (Strauch, 2009). PEMF exposure leads to a release of intracellular Ca^{2+}, which in turn leads to increased binding of Ca^{2+} to calmodulin, which is thought to affect signaling pathways related to inflammation and vascular tone (Gaynor, 2018). Targeted PEMF treatment has also been shown to result in the production of low concentrations of calmodulin-dependent nitric oxide, which are associated with decreased inflammation and increased vasodilation (Bragin, 2014; Strauch, 2009).

PEMF has been used for postoperative pain, edema, and osteoarthritis in people. It has been approved by the US FDA for these conditions (Gaynor, 2018). There have been pain studies in animals that may support the use of PEMF. In one study, dogs receiving PEMF therapy following postoperative hemilaminectomy demonstrated improved wound scores at 6 weeks as well as a reduced mean number of owner-administered pain medications being required, as compared with the control group in the study (Alvarez, 2019). Additional information may be found in references at the end of the chapter.

Developing a crisis kit

What are crisis kits? Why do veterinarians need to utilize them? Crisis kits, also known as comfort kits or emergency kits, are medications and instructions for caregivers so that they can quickly provide emergency pain and symptom relief to their animals during an emergency or crisis. Defining what a crisis and distress is and might appear like in the caregiver's animal is also helpful. Crisis kits can give caregivers peace of mind to help their animals when they may be in distress. Crisis kits also empower caregivers to know there is something they can do, even if there is not a veterinarian available. The most common urgent issue for animals (and people) is a sudden and perhaps dramatic increase in pain levels. Pain medications are included in a crisis kit and can come in injectable, transdermal, and oral forms, and can include pain medications for different levels of pain. In addition to pain management, a crisis kit is also meant to help with a variety of other potential concerns in palliative patients such as acute hemorrhage, seizures, severe gastrointestinal flare-ups. Specific disease and symptom crisis information is in the medicine/symptom management chapter.

Veterinarians have been concerned about leaving controlled substances with clients in the home for crisis situations with their pets. However, they may have sent home many of the same medications for other reasons. One way to minimize diversion is to follow the example of human hospice. In human hospice programs, caregivers are provided with an emergency kit of specific instructions on how to and when to use medications in case of a sudden change in clinical signs (Yap, 2014). To minimize diversion, human hospice physicians' script out medications. Nurses do not carry controlled substances to the home, and the caregiver picks up medicines from the pharmacy. Veterinarians may consider scripting out medications as well, so there is a paper trail associated with a pharmacy. Removal of controlled substances after the passing of the pet is also a concern for diversion. The SUPPORT Act in the United States, passed October 24, 2018, allowed human hospices to remove controlled substances after a patient has passed and dispose of them (Gregory, 2018). This act does not include veterinarians at the time of this writing. The current recommendations for veterinarians are to have the client destroy medication in cat litter and place it in trash, or drop it off at a police station, or local medication waste drop-off day. The figure below sums up crisis kits and gives a few examples (Fig. 6.11).

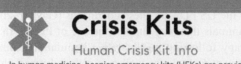

Crisis Kits

Human Crisis Kit Info

In human medicine, hospice emergency kits (HEKs) are provided to many patients near the end of life. Patients with HEKs can find relief from emergent symptoms like pain, agitation, dyspnea, secretions, and other problems. A pilot study created by Dr. Alexandra Leigh and colleagues (2011) wanted to determine the benefits of having a HEK at the home. The study interviewed hospice nurses and estimated that when a HEK was available, it was used in about 65% of patients. They found that it likely increased the comfort for patients dying at home. In addition, the study estimated that a vast majority of nurses (86%) believed that having a HEK to administer at home reduced both caregiver and patient anxiety

Utilizing Crisis Kits in Veterinary Medicine

Animals face similar emergent concerns at end of life, and thus can also use crisis kits. Below are examples of medications to utilize in a veterinary crisis kit. One column is designated for pain management, the other is for general symptom management

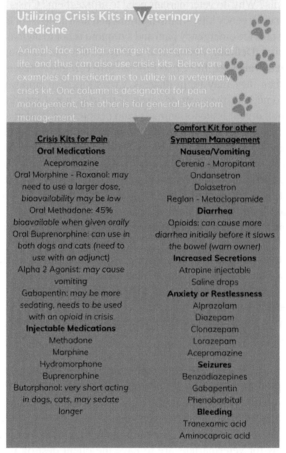

Crisis Kits for Pain
Oral Medications
Acepromazine
Oral Morphine - Roxanol: may need to use a larger dose, bioavailability may be low
Oral Methadone: 45% bioavailable when given orally
Oral Buprenorphine: can use in both dogs and cats (need to use with an adjunct)
Alpha 2 Agonist: may cause vomiting
Gabapentin: may be more sedating, needs to be used with an opioid in crisis
Injectable Medications
Methadone
Morphine
Hydromorphone
Buprenorphine
Butorphanol: very short acting in dogs, cats, may sedate longer

Comfort Kit for other Symptom Management
Nausea/Vomiting
Cerenia - Maropitant
Ondansetron
Dolasetron
Reglan - Metoclopramide
Diarrhea
Opioids: can cause more diarrhea initially before it slows the bowel (warn owner)
Increased Secretions
Atropine injectable
Saline drops
Anxiety or Restlessness
Alprazolam
Diazepam
Clonazepam
Lorazepam
Acepromazine
Seizures
Benzodiazepines
Gabapentin
Phenobarbital
Bleeding
Tranexamic acid
Aminocaproic acid

FIGURE 6.11

Crisis kit recommendations.

Created in Canva by Mina Weakley/Lynn Hendrix Used with permission and attribution from Elsevier ©2021 Bailey, F. A. W. B. (2014). Impact of a hospice emergency kit for veterans and the caregivers: A prospective cohort study. Journal of Palliative Medicine, 931–938.

References

Alemzadeh-Ansari, M. J.-R. (2017). Chronic pain in chronic heart failure: A review article. *The Journal of Tehran University Heart Center*, 49−56.

Alvarez, L. (2015). Acupuncture. In J. M. Gaynor (Ed.), *Handbook of veterinary pain managment* (pp. 365−379). St Louis: Elsevier.

Alvarez, L. M. (2019). Effect of targeted pulsed electromagnetic field therapy on canine post-operative hemilaminectomy: A double-blind, randomized, placebo-controlled clinical trial. *Journal of the American Animal Hospital Association*, 83−91.

Anderson, K. L. (2020). Risk factors for canine osteoarthritis and its predisposing arthropathies: A systematic review. *Frontiers in Veterinary Science*, 220.

Anekar, A. C. (2021). *WHO analgesic ladder*. StatPearls.

Arbuck, D. F. (2021). *Opioid prescribing and monitoring*. Retrieved from Practical Pain Management https://www.practicalpainmanagement.com/resource-centers/opioid-prescribing-monitoring/pain-assessment-review-current-tools.

Bailey, F. A.,W. B. (2014). Impact of a hospice emergency kit for veterans and the caregivers: A prospective cohort study. *Journal of Palliative Medicine*, 931−938.

Beaulieu, P. (2006). Effects of nabilone, a synthetic cannabinoid, on postoperative pain. *Canada Journal of Anesthesiology*, 769−775.

Bijsmans, E. S. (2016). Psychometric validation of a general health quality of life tool for cats used to compare healthy cats and cats with chronic kidney disease. *Journal of Veterinary Internal Medicine*, 183−191.

Blais, M. C. (2019). Consensus on the rational use of antithrombotics in veterinary critical care (CURATIVE): Domain 3-defining antithrombotic protocols. *Journal of Veterinary Emergency and Critical Care (San Antonio, Tex)*, 60−74.

Botting, R., & Ayoub, S. S. (2005). COX-3 and the mechanism of action of paracetamol/acetaminophen. *Prostaglandins Leukot. Essent. Fatty Acids, 72*(2), 85−87. https://doi.org/10.1016/j.plefa.2004.10.005

Bragin, D. S. (2014). Increases in microvascular perfusion and tissue oxygenation via pulsed electromagnetic fields in the healthy rat brain. *Journal of Neurosurgery*, 1−9.

Budsberg, S. C.,T. B. (2018). Lack of effectiveness of tramadol hydrochloride for the treatment of pain and joint dysfunction in dogs with chronic osteoarthritis. *Journal of the American Veterinary Medical Association*, 427−432.

Cachon, T. F. (2018). Face validity of a proposed tool for staging canine osteoarthritis: Canine OsteoArthritis Staging Tool (COAST). *The Veterinary Journal*, 1−8.

Caravaca, F. G. (2016). Musculoskeletal pain in patients with chronic kidney disease. *Nefrologia*, 433−440.

Chang, C.,R. K. (2020). *Amantadine*. StatPearls.

Childers, J. W. (2007). N-Methyl-D-Aspartate antagonists and neuropathic pain: The search for relief. *Journal of Medical Chemistry*, 2559−2562.

Chiou, J.-H. L.-K.-J.-N.-K. (2018). What factors mediate the inter-relationship between frailty and pain in cognitively and functionally sound older adults? A prospective longitudinal ageing cohort study in Taiwan. *Geriatric Medicine (BMJ Open)*, e018716.

Chiu, J. H.,C. H. (2001). Electroacupuncture-induced neural activation detected by use of manganese-enhanced functional magnetic resonance imaging in rabbits. *American Journal of Veterinary Research*, 178−182.

Choy, K. F. (2016). Tolerability and tumor response of a novel low-dose palliative radiation therapy protocol in dogs with transitional cell carcinoma of the bladder and urethra. *Veterinary Radiology & Ultrasound: The Official Journal of the American College of Veterinary Radiology and the International Veterinary Radiology Association*, 341–351.

Christian-Miller, N. F. (2018). Hepatocellular cancer pain: Impact and management challenges. *Journal of Hepatocellular Carcinoma*, 75–80.

Claudino, R. N. (2018). Analgesic effects of intranasal ketamine in rat models of facial pain. *Journal of Oral & Facial Pain and Headache*, 238–346.

Corletto, F. J. (2019). Pharmacological treatment of pain. In I. Self (Ed.), *BSAVA Guide to pain Management in small animal practice* (pp. 42–85). Quedgeley, Gloucester: BSAVA.

Costa, B.,T. A. (2013). The non-psychoactive cannabis constituent cannabidiol is an orally effective therapeutic agent in rat chronic inflammatory and neuropathic pain. *European Journal of Pharmacology*, 473–474.

CVM Staff. (March 2019). *Chronic kidney disease.* Retrieved from Cornell Feline Health Center https://www.vet.cornell.edu/departments-centers-and-institutes/cornell-feline-health-center/health-information/feline-health-topics/chronic-kidney-disease.

Delpont, B.,B. K.-P.-L.-B. (2019). Clinical features of pain in amyotrophic lateral sclerosis: A clinical challenge. *Revue Neurologuque(Paris)*, 11–15.

Dore, M. (2010). Cyclooxygenase-2 expression in animal cancers. *Veterinary Pathology*, 254–265.

Dueñas, M. O. (2016). A review of chronic pain impact on patients, their social environment and the health care system. *Journal of Pain Research*, 457–467.

Dureja, G. I. (2017). Evidence and consensus recommendations for the pharmacological management of pain in India. *Journal of Pain Research*, 709–736.

Edwards, H. L. (2019). Cancer-related neuropathic pain. *Cancers*, 373.

Elkholly, D. A. (2020). Side effects to systemic glucocorticoid therapy in dogs under primary veterinary care in the UK. *Frontiers in Veterinary Science*, 515.

Epstein, M. (October/November 2013). *Assessing chronic pain in dogs.* Today's Veterinary Practice.

Evangelista, M. S. (2021). Agreement and reliability of the Feline Grimace Scale among cat owners, veterinarians, veterinary students and nurses. *Scientific Reports, 11.*

Fazzari, J. S. (2020). Applying serum cytokine levels to predict pain severity in cancer patients. *Journal of Pain Research*, 313–321.

Ferguson, D. (2008). *Glucocorticoids+/- NSAIDs: why, why not, and washout.* DVM360 storage.

Folch, J. B.-L.-T.-Z. (2018). Memantine for the treatment of dementia: A review on its current and future applications. *Journal of Alzheimer's Disease*, 1223–1240.

Fox, S. (2012). *Chronic pain in small animal medicine.* London: Manson Publishing Ltd.

Freeman, L. R. (2005). Development and evaluation of a questionnaire for assessing health-related quality of life in dogs with cardiac disease. *Journal of the American Veterinary Medical Association*, 1864–1868.

Gaynor, J. H. (2018). Veterinary applications of pulsed electromagnetic field therapy. *Research in Veterinary Science*, 1–8.

Gaynor, J. M. (2015). *Handbook of veterinary pain management.* St. Louis, Missouri: Elsevier.

Gibbons, D. S. (2011). Palliative radiation therapy in the treatment of canine appendicular synovial sarcoma. *Journal of the American Animal Hospital Association*, 359–364.

Gorrel, C. (2019). Dental pain. In I. Self (Ed.), *BSAVA Guide to pain management in small animal practice* (pp. 137−141). Quedgeley, Glouchester: BSAVA.

Grant, I. H. (2019). Cancer pain. In I. Self (Ed.), *BSAVA Guide to pain Management in small animal practice* (pp. 153−168). Quedgeley, Gloucester: BSAVA.

Gregory, A. (November 1, 2018). *Hospice providers may dispose of controlled substances under new federal opioid law.* Retrieved from JDSupra https://www.jdsupra.com/legalnews/hospice-providers-may-dispose-of-19991/.

Guedes, A. M. (2018). Evaluation of tramadol for treatment of osteoarthritis in geriatric cats. *Journal of the American Veterinary Medical Association*, 565−571.

Guerriero, F. R. (2020). Linking persistent pain and frailty in older adults. *Pain Medicine*, 61−66.

Gunew, M. N. (2008). Long-term safety, efficacy and palatability of oral meloxicam at 0.01-0.03 mg/kg for treatment of osteoarthritic pain in cats. *Journal of Feline Medicine and Surgery*, 235−241.

He, Y.,K. P. (2020). *Allodynia.* StatPearls.

Hinds, S. B. (2007). The effect of harp music on heart rate, mean blood pressure, respiratory rate, and body temperature in the African green monkey. *Journal of Medical Primatology*, 95−100.

Holdcroft, A. M. (2006). A multicenter dose-escalation study of the analgesic and adverse effects of an oral cannabis extract (Cannador) for postoperative pain management. *Anesthesiology*, 1040−1046.

Hua, J. H. (2016). Assessment of fraility in aged dogs. *American Journal of Veterinary Research*, 1357−1365.

Hudak, J. (2018). The Farm Bill, hemp legalization and the status of CBD: An explainer. *The Brookings Institute.* https://www.brookings.edu/blog/fixgov/2018/12/14/the-farm-bill-hemp-and-cbd-explainer/.

Iffland, K. G. (2017). An update on safety and side effects of cannabidiol: A review of clinical data and relevant animal studies. *Cannabis and Cannaboid Research*, 139−154.

Inamdar, A. A. (2016). Heart failure: Diagnosis, management and utilization. *Journal of Clinical Medicine, 62.*

Itami, T. S. (2016). Comparison of pharmacokinetics of tramadol between young and middle-aged dogs. *Journal of Veterinary Medical Science*, 1031−1034.

Jonas, W. B.,K. T. (2003). A critical overview of homeopathy. *Annuals of Internal Medicine*, 393−399.

Kafkia, T. C. (2011). Pain in chronic kidney disease: Prevalence, cause and management. *Journal of Renal Care*, 114−122.

Katz, B. V. (2021). Neuroantomay and visceral pain. In D. Y. Pak (Ed.), *Interventional management of chronic visceral pain syndromes* (pp. 5−15). Elsevier.

Kaur, A. (2018). Phantom limb pain: A literature review. *Chinese journal of traumatology = Zhonghua chuang shang za zhi*, 366−368.

Kinobe, R. T. (2020). Evaluating the anti-inflammatory and analgesic properties of maropitant: A systematic review and meta-analysis. *The Veterinary Journal*, 259−260.

Kirkby Shaw, K. R.-D. (2016). Grapiprant: An EP4 prostaglandin receptor antagonist and novel therapy for pain and inflammation. *Veterinary Medicine and Science*, 3−9.

Klinck, M. G. (2017). Development and preliminary validity and reliability of the montreal instrument for cat arthritis testing, for use by caretaker/owner, MI-CAT(C), via a randomised clinical trial. *Applied Animal Behavior Science.*

Koga, K. L. (2016). Metabotropic glutamate receptor dependent cortical plasticity in chronic pain. *Current Neuropharmacology*, 427–434.

Kraft, B. F. (2008). Lack of analgesia by oral standardized cannabis extract on acute inflammatory pain and hyperalgesia in volunteers. *Anesthesiology*, 101–110.

Kronenberg, R. H. (2002). Ketamine as an analgesic: Parenteral, oral, rectal, subcutaneous, transdermal and intranasal administration. *Journal of Pain & Palliative Care Pharmacotherapy*, 27–35.

Kukanich, B.,P. M. (2004). Plasma profile and pharmacokinetics of dextromethorphan after intravenous and oral administration in healthy dogs. *Journal of Veterinary Pharmacology and Therapeutics*, 337–341.

KuKanich, B. (2016). Pharmacokinetics and pharmacodynamics of oral acetaminophen in combination with codeine in healthy Greyhound dogs. *Journal of Veterinary Pharmacology and Therapeutics*, 514–517.

KuKanich, B. K. (2020). Perioperative analgesia associated with oral administration of a novel methadone-fluconazole-naltrexone formulation in dogs undergoing routine ovariohysterectomy. *Journal of the American Veterinary Medical Association*, 699–707.

KuKanich, B. S. (2013). Pharmacokinetics of hydrocodone and hydromorphone after oral hydrocodone in healthy Greyhound dogs. *The Veterinary Journal*, 266–268.

Lang, C. A. (2006). Symptom prevalence and clustering of symptoms in people living with chronic hepatitis C infection. *Journal of Pain and Symptom Management*, 335–344.

Larauche, M. M. (2012). Stress and visceral pain: From animal models to clinical therapies. *Experimental Neurology*, 49–67.

Lascelles, B. D.-L. (2008). Amantadine in a multimodal analgesic regimen for alleviation of refractory osteoarthritis pain in dogs. *Journal of Veterinary Internal Medicine*, 53–59.

Latremoliere, A. W. (2009). Central sensitization: A generator of pain hypersensitivity by central neural plasticity. *The Journal of Pain*, 895–926.

Lee, A. L. (2016). Chronic pain in people with chronic obstructive pulmonary disease: Prevalence, clinical and psychological implications. *Journal of the COPD Foundation*, 194–203.

Lim, R. (2016). End-of-life care in patients with advanced lung cancer. *Therapeutic Advances in Respiratory Disease*, 455–467.

Lindig, A. M., McGreevy, P. D., & Crean, A. J. (2020). Musical dogs: A review of the influence of auditory enrichment on canine health and behavior. *Animals, 10*(1), 107. https://doi.org/10.3390/ani10010127

Mak, S. L. (2020). Pharmacological characterizations of anti-dementia memantine nitrate via neuroprotection and vasodilation in vitro and in vivo. *ACS Chemical Neuroscience*, 314–327.

Marino, C. L. (2014). Prevalence and classification of chronic kidney disease in cats randomly selected from four age groups and in cats recruited for degenerative joint disease studies. *Journal of Feline Medicine and Surgery*, 465–472.

Marquez, M. B. (2015). Comparison of NK-1 receptor antagonist (maropitant) to morphine as a pre-anaesthetic agent for canine ovariohysterectomy. *PLoS One*, e0140734.

McPherson, C. J.,H. T. (2013). Cancer-related pain in older adults receiving palliative care: Patient and family caregiver perspectives on the experience of pain. *Pain Research and Management*, 293–300.

Melis, S. (2020). What are the options for managing pain in a different way? *Veterinary Practice*.

Miller, S. M. (2014). Use of corticosteroids for anorexia in palliative medicine: A systematic review. *Journal of Palliative Medicine*, 482−485.

Mills, D. S.-B. (2020). Pain and problem behavior in cats and dogs. *Animals*, 318.

Monteiro, B. K.-P. (2017). Analgesic efficacy of tramadol in cats with naturally occurring osteoarthritis. *PLoS One*, e0175565.

Monteiro, B. S. (2019). Long-term use of non-steroidal anti-inflammatory drugs in cats with chronic kidney disease: From controversy to optimism. *Journal of Small Animal Practice*, 459−462.

Moore, S. (2016). Managing neuropathic pain in dogs. *Frontiers in Veterinary Science, 3.*

Muley, M. K. (2016). Preclinical assessment of inflammatory pain. *CNS Neuroscience & Therapeutics*, 88−101.

Narita, T. S. (2007). The interaction between orally administered non-steroidal anti-inflammatory drugs and prednisolone in healthy dogs. *Journal of Veterinary Medical Science*, 353−363.

Narver, H. (2015). Nalbuphine, a non-controlled opioid analgesic, and its potential use in research mice. *Lab Anim, 44*, 106−110. https://doi.org/10.1038/laban.701. In press.

Niessen, S. J. (2010). Evaluation of a quality-of-life tool for cats with diabetes mellitus. *Journal of Veterinary Internal Medicine*, 1098−1105.

Niessen, S. J. (2012). Evaluation of a quality-of-life tool for dogs with diabetes mellitus. *Journal of Veterinary Internal Medicine*, 953−961.

O'Connor, N. C. (2012). End-stage renal disease: Symptom management and advance care planning. *American Family Physician*, 707−710.

Ossipov, M. H. (2010). Central modulation of pain. *Journal of Clinical Investigation*, 3779−3787.

Page, N. N. (2018). Intranasal ketamine for the management of incidental pain during wound dressing in cancer patients: A pilot study. *Indian Journal of Palliative Care*, 58−60.

Pakozdy, A. H. (2014). Epilepsy in cats: Theory and practice. *Journal of Veterinary Internal Medicine*, 255−263.

Park, J. K. (2010). Current pharmacological management of chronic pain. *Journal of the Korean Medical Association*, 815−823.

Pathan, H., & Williams, J. (2012). Basic opioid pharmacology: an update. *Br J Pain, 6*(1), 11−16. https://doi.org/10.1177/2049463712438493

Pendergrass, J. (2018). New insights into the phantom complex for small animals. *DVM, 360.*

Pereira, V. G. (2019). Emerging trends in pain modulation by metobotropic glutamate receptors. *Frontiers in Molecular Neuroscience, 11.*

Plumb, D. C. (2021). Nalbuphine. *Plumb's Veterinary Drugs*. John Wiley & Sons. https://app.plumbs.com/drug-monograph/vTu5mODx1yPROD. In press.

Potosek, J. C. (2014). Integration of palliative care in end-stage liver disease and liver transplantation. *Journal of Palliative Medicine*, 1271−1277.

Pypendop, B. H. (2008). Pharmacokinetics of tramadol, and its metabolite O-desmethyl-tramadol, in cats. *Journal of Veterinary Pharmacology and Therapeutics*, 52−59.

Quintero, G. (2017). Review about gabapentin misuse, interactions, contraindications and side effects. *Journal of Experimental Pharmacology*, 13−21.

Rahn EJ, H. A. (2009). Cannabinoids as pharmacotherapies for neuropathic pain: From the bench to the bedside. *Neurotherapeutics*, 713−737.

Rajala, K. L. (2016). End-of-life care of patients with idiopathic pulmonary fibrosis. *BMC Palliative Care, 85.*

Rausch Derra, L. R. (2016). Safety and toxicokinetic profiles associated with daily oral administration of grapiprant, a selective antagonist of the prostaglandin E2 EP4 receptor, to cats. *American Journal of Veterinary Research*, 688–692.

Rausch-Derra, L. C. (2015). Evaluation of the safety of long-term, daily oral administration of grapiprant, a novel drug for treatment of osteoarthritic pain and inflammation, in healthy dogs. *American Journal of Veterinary Research*, 853–859.

Richter, G. (June 2021). The current state of cannabis research in veterinary medicine. *Today's Veterinary Practice*.

Romero-Sandoval, E. A.-V. (2017). Cannabis and cannabinoids for chronic pain. *Current Rheumatology, 67*.

Ross, R. (2003). Anandamide and vanilloid TRPV1 receptors. *British Journal of Pharmacology*, 790–801.

Russo, E. (2011). Taming THC: Potential cannabis synergy and phytocannabinoid-terpenoid entourage effects. *British Journal of Pharmacology*, 1344–1364.

Sandkühler, J. (2009). Models and mechanisms of hyperalgesia and allodynia. *Physiological Reviews*, 707–758.

Santoro, D. S. (2013). Pain in end-stage renal disease: A frequent and neglected clinical problem. *Clinical Nephrology*, s2–11.

Schmelz, M.,M. K. (2000). Which nerve fibers mediate the axon reflex flare in human skin? *NeuroReport*, 645–648.

Schneider, B. D. (2009). Use of memantine in treatment of canine compulsive disorders. *Journal of Veterinary Behavior*, 118–126.

Schütter, A. F.,T. J. (2017). Influence of tramadol on acute thermal and mechanical cutaneous nociception in dogs. *Veterinary Anaesthesia and Analgesia*, 309–316.

Self, I. G. (2019). Physiology of pain. In I. Self (Ed.), *BSAVA Guide to pain Management in small animal practice* (pp. 3–13). Quedgeley, Gloucester: BSAVA.

Shaffran, N. (2013). Constant-rate infusions for pain and anxiety in dogs and cats. In *World small animal veterinary association world congress proceedings, 2013*. Aukland, NZ: WSAVA/VIN.

Sikandar, S. (2012). Visceral pain: The ins and outs, the ups and downs. *Current Opinion in Supportive and Palliative Care*, 17–26.

Sindrup, S. O. (2005). Antidepressants in the treatment of neuropathic pain. *Basic and Clinical Pharmacology and Toxicology*, 399–409.

Stadig, S. L. (2019). Evaluation and comparison of pain questionnaires for clinical screening of osteoarthritis in cats. *The Veterinary Record*, 757.

Staff of IASP. (December 14, 2017). *IASP terminology*. Retrieved from IASP.org https://www.iasp-pain.org/Education/Content.aspx?ItemNumber=1698#Pain.

Stegall, P. (2020). *Feline grimace scale*. Retrieved from Feline Grimace Scale.com https://www.felinegrimacescale.com/.

Stockings, E.,C. G. (2018). Cannabis and cannabinoids for the treatment of people with chronic noncancer pain conditions: A systematic review and meta-analysis of controlled and observational studies. *Pain*, 1932–1954.

Strauch, B. H. (2009). Evidence-based use of pulsed electromagnetic field therapy in clinical plastic surgery. *Aesthetic Surgery Journal*, 135–143.

Teske, E. (2010). Cox-2 therapy and cancer. In *WSAVA 2010 proceedings*. Utrecht: WSAVA.

Thapa, B.,R. K. (2021). *Paraneoplastic syndrome*. StatPearls.

Tillisch, K. L. (2012). Neurokinin-1-receptor antagonism decreases anxiety and emotional arousal circuit response to noxious visceral distension in women with irritable bowel syndrome: A pilot study. *Alimentary Pharmacology and Therapeutics*, 360−367.

Tollett, M. A. (2016). Palliative radiation therapy for solid tumors in dogs. *Journal of the American Veterinary Medical Association*, 72−82.

Tranquilli, W. G. (2004). *Pain management for the small animal practitioner.* Teton New Media.

Trepanier, L. (2017). Maropitant Magic-Useful for more than just vomiting?. In *New York vet show conference proceedings 2017.* New York: NY Vet Show.

van de Donk, T.,N. M. (2019). An experimental randomized study on the analgesic effects of pharmaceutical-grade cannabis in chronic pain patients with fibromyalgia. *Pain*, 860−869.

VanDolah, H. J., Bauer, B. A., & Mauck, K. F. (2019). Clinicians' guide to cannabidiol and hemp oils. *Mayo Clin. Proc.* https://doi.org/10.1016/j.mayocp.2019.01.003

Varrassi, G. A.-R. (2019). Towards an effective and safe treatment of inflammatory pain: A delphi-guided expert consensus. *Advances in Therapy*, 2618−2637.

Veerman, S. S. (2014). The glutamate hypothesis: A pathogenic pathway from which pharmacological interventions have emerged. *Pharmacopsychiatry, 47*.

Vendrell, I. M. (2015). Treatment of cancer pain by targeting cytokines. *Mediators of Inflammation*, 984570.

Verrico, C. D.,W. S.-P. (2020). A randomized, double-blind, placebo-controlled study of daily cannabidiol for the treatment of canine osteoarthritis pain. *Pain*, 2191−2202.

VIN Staff. (2017). *VIN veterinary drug handbook.* Retrieved from VIN.com https//www.vin.com.

Vučković, S.,S. D. (2018). Cannabinoids and pain: New insights from old molecules. *Frontiers in Pharmacology*, 1259.

Warden, V.,H. A. (2003). Development and psychometric evaluation of the pain assessment in advanced dementia (PAINAD) scale. *Journal of the American Medical Directors Association*, 9−15.

Webster, C. C. (2019). ACVIM consensus statement on the diagnosis and treatment of chronic hepatitis in dogs. *Journal of Veterinary Internal Medicine*, 1173−1200.

Wessmann, A. (2019). Neuropathic pain. In I. Self (Ed.), *BSAVA Guide to pain Management in small animal practice* (pp. 131−136). Quedgeley, Gloucester: BSAVA.

Wright, B. (2017). Clinical advantages of ketamine and NMDA antagonist drugs. In *WSAVA congress proceedings 2017.* WSAVA/VIN.

Xie, H.,E.-R. C. (2012). Introduction to traditional Chinese veterinary medicine in pediatric exotic animal practice. *Veterinary Clinics of North America Exotic Animal Practice*, 311−329.

Xie, H.,O.-U. C. (2006). What acupuncture can and cannot treat. *Journal of the American Animal Hospital Association*, 244−248.

Yap, R., Akhileswaran, R., Heng, C. P., Tan, A., & Hui, D. (2014). Comfort care kit: use of nonoral and nonparenteral rescue medications at home for terminally ill patients with swallowing difficulty. *J. Palliat. Med, 17*(5), 575−578. https://doi.org/10.1089/jpm.2013.0364

Yazbek, K. F. (2005). Validity of a Health-Related Quality of LIfe Scale for dogs with signs of pain secondary to cancer. *Journal of the American Veterinary Medical Association*, 1354−1358.

Zarei, S. C. (2015). A comprehensive review of amyotrophic lateral sclerosis. *Surgical Neurology International, 171.*

https://www.deadiversion.usdoj.gov/drug_chem_info/nalbuphine.pdf, (2019—. (Accessed 24 November 2021).

Additional references for chronic pain

Canine brief pain inventory - https://www.vet.upenn.edu/research/clinical-trials-vcic/our-services/pennchart/cbpi-tool.

Feline grimace scale - https://www.felinegrimacescale.com/.

Feline musculoskeletal pain index - https://www.fourleg.com/media/Helsinki%20Chronic%20Pain%20Index.pdf.

Gaynor, J. S., & Muir, W. W., III (2014). *Handbook of veterinary pain management.*

Goldberg, M. E. (2014). *Pain management for veterinary technicians and nurses* (1st ed.).

Helsinki chronic pain index. Retrieved from https://www.fourleg.com/media/Helsinki%20Chronic%20Pain%20Index.pdf.

Ko, J. (2018). In *Small animal anesthesia and pain management: A color handbook (veterinary color handbook series)* (2nd ed.).

Self, I. (2019). *BSAVA guide to pain management in small animal practice* (A practical handbook you can carry with you).

Tranquilli, W. J., Grimm, K. A., & Lamont, L. A. (2004). *Pain management of the small animal practitioner* (This is a practical handbook you can carry with you).

Integrative text:

Additional information on Cannabis. Retrieved from https://www.nccih.nih.gov/health/cannabis-marijuana-and-cannabinoids-what-you-need-to-know.

American Holistic Veterinary Medical Association. Retrieved from www.ahvma.org.

International Veterinary Acupuncture Society. Retrieved from www.ivas.org.

Johns Hopkins medicine website. Retrieved from https://www.hopkinsmedicine.org/health/wellness-and-prevention/herbal-medicine.

Medical acupuncture for veterinarians offered by narda robinson at curacore vet.

Skidmore-Roth, L. (2009). *Mosby's handbook of herbs and natural supplements* (RN).

Veterinary Botanical Medicine Association. Retrieved from www.vbma.org.

Wynn, S. G. (2006). *Veterinary herbal medicine* (DVM).

Further reading

AAHA. (2007). AAHA/AAFP pain management guidelines for dogs and cats. *Journal of the American Animal Hospital Association*, 235—248.

Alexander, J. C. (2019). A review of the anesthetic implications of marijuana use. *Proceedings (Baylor University. Medical Center)*, 364—371.

Eskafian, H. S. (2017). Gastroscopic study of meloxicam, tramadol, and their combined administration on the development of gastric injuries in dogs. *Topics in Companion Animal Medicine*, 109—113.

Plumb, D. (2002). *Veterinary drug handbook* (4th ed.). Pharmavet Publishing.

Saito, T. T. (2014). Usefulness of selective COX-2 inhibitors as therapeutic agents against canine mammary tumors. *Oncology Reports*, 1637—1644.

Schneider, D. M. (2015). Application of therapeutic harp sounds for quality of life among hospitalized patients. *Journal of Pain and Symptom Management*, 836−845.

Shaiova, L. F. (2013). *Principals and practices of palliative care and supportive oncology.* Philadelphia, PA: Lippincott Williams and Wilkins.

Temel, J. e (2010). Early palliative care for patients with metastatic non-small cell lung cancer. *The New England Journal of Medicine*, 733−742.

Wilson, H. C. (2012). Effect of tolfenamic acid on canine cancer cell proliferation, specificity protein (sp) transcription factors, and sp-regulated proteins in canine osteosarcoma, mammary carcinoma, and melanoma cells. *Journal of Veterinary Internal Medicine*, 977−986.

Physical support

Lynn Hendrix, AA, BA, DVM, CHPV [1,2,3,4], **Carolyn Naun, DVM, CHPV** [5]

[1]*Owner, Veterinarian, Beloved Pet Mobile Vet, Davis, CA, United States;* [2]*Former Board of Directors, IAAHPC, Chicago, IL, United States;* [3]*Consultant, Hospice, Palliative Medicine, End of Life, VIN, Davis, CA, United States;* [4]*President, Founder, World Veterinary Palliative Medicine Organization, Davis, CA, United States;* [5]*Director, Medical Services, Arms of Aloha LLC, Kailua, HI, United States*

Supporting mobility and quality of life

Mobility problems are a significant subject with clients with elderly dogs and cats and account for many palliative appointments. Big or small, if an animal is having a tough time getting around, other matters start arising for the family. Urination and defecation in the house, on themselves, pressure sores, and watching their animal struggle can become life-limiting problems. The caregiver's ability to lift an animal, the animal's ability to stay on their feet, or even their ability to get up can decrease the physical quality of life and limit both the animal and the owner's autonomy. Dealing with pain management is a vital aspect of palliative care, and adding mobility aids may also improve the emotional and physical quality of life for both patient and caregiver. Many clients focus on the pain and suffering of end-of-life patients, but the loss of autonomy, loss of mobility, and having urine or feces in the house or outside the litter box can contribute to a euthanasia decision. An Oregon study on assisted death found that 40% of people choose assisted death due to loss of autonomy (Ganzini et al., 2009). Mobility plays a significant role in an animal's ability to live an autonomous life.

This chapter will discuss different physical aids for animals with mobility issues to improve their autonomy and physical and emotional quality of life. There are several suggested businesses to assist the reader in locating mobility assistance. The authors do not recommend an individual business or product.

Benefits of improving mobility

Mobility and quality-of-life (QOL) issues are closely related, and there exist substantial challenges to quantifying such a connection in veterinary medicine. Dogs in wheelchairs that have an improved emotional quality of life, and a will to live, may override the degree of loss of mobility and decline of physical quality. Many

Animal Hospice and Palliative Medicine for the House Call Veterinarian
https://doi.org/10.1016/B978-0-323-56798-5.00012-6

QOL assessments include mobility assessments. A pet's ability to engage with their environment, the caregiver's ability to manage their pet's unique needs, and the animal's preferences will influence their mobility needs.

Questions to ask and clients when assessing the effects of diminished mobility on QOL:

1. What is the animal's overall psychological or emotional well-being?
2. Are we able to improve or maintain decent emotional QOL? Physical QOL?
3. Do they still have a will to live?
4. Do they still show interest in their surroundings, family members, other people, and pets?
5. What are the animal's favorite activities, and can they still enjoy them?
6. Is it possible to modify activities so that the pet can still participate?
7. Is the patient isolated from the family and loved ones because of mobility issues?
8. Is this an issue that can be changed if given the right tools?
9. Is there more we could add to the pain management plan?
10. Are they in mild, moderate, or severe pain? Do they have acute pain signs?
11. How are the caregivers handling the increased burden (financial, emotional, and time) of care?
12. Are the caregivers prepared for the challenge of having the increased burden?
13. Are related needs such as hygiene and prevention of pressure sores adequately managed?
14. Is the animal able to be trained to a mobility aid? What kind of training will they need?
15. Are they able to be fitted with the proper equipment? Cost may also be a factor; consider renting equipment to clients for palliative patients.

Dealing with mobility complications in chronic and life-limiting disease

Pain and comorbidities

Pain is prevalent among animals with mobility problems. AAHA literature estimated 20% of adult canines suffer from osteoarthritis symptoms, with the likelihood increasing with age (Johnson, 1997). Felids have an even higher incidence; some estimates are 40%–92% (Cavenaugh, 2018). Arthritis, degenerative myelopathy, slack or ruptured ligaments, neuropathies, and other weak appearing animals may have unrecognized pain (by the owner). Chronic pain can be mild, moderate, or severe, and mild and moderate pain may be more challenging to assess in patients in the hospital setting and can also be tough to assess in stoic patients. Making house calls for these patients can increase pain assessment for these mild and moderately painful patients (see the Chapter on Pain Management for additional information).

For animals with mobility challenges, providing analgesia, often multimodal, can substantially change their quality of life. Patients who appear clinically weak may be reluctant to bear weight on one or more limbs due to pain. When adequate pain management occurs, owners note substantially improved mobility, even in patients where the pain is not apparent.

Worsening mobility complications may arise from systemic illness and may contribute to weakness, dehydration, and cognitive function, complicating comorbidities to worsening mobility problems. To identify new complications, offer a diagnostic workup. The workup may help identify additional effective interventions (Note: Clients may decline diagnostic workup with end-of-life patients).

Multimodal analgesia

Multimodal analgesia (or balanced analgesia) used in veterinary palliative medicine combines multiple medications and/or treatments and modalities to control pain. A combination of drug therapies, physical modalities, and mobility aids may help the down patient. The multimodal pain management protocol could incorporate one or more of the following interventions:

- One or more pharmaceutical agents (see chapter on pain management)
- Nutraceuticals (see chapter on integrative modalities)
- Weight management
- Physical medicine such as massage, physical therapy, acupuncture, and other modalities
- Modification of the environment to enhance mobility and reduce the burden of care
- Mobility aids

A personalized plan for mobility

Personalized plans should include mobility. Providing a personalized plan based on the medical management options available, considering the owner's goals and priorities can help owners provide management for the animal, and returning for additional checks can help give them time to digest the amount of information provided—this may need to happen over several visits. Checking in with caregivers to make sure they understand and provide the plan's care and getting feedback on what works (and what does not work) for clients will confirm you advance a personalized care plan together.

Consider:

- The needs of both the patient and caregiver. Meeting the animal's needs may depend on the caregiver being able to provide care. Caregivers are responsible for carrying out the plan—if they cannot provide care, the plan will go without being instituted. Caregiver burnout may occur, resulting in noncompliance from the medical perspective and the animal's needs will not being met. Caregiver needs will vary, but common themes seen with end-of-life plans are simplicity, frugality, or a sense that one has "left no stone unturned" in doing everything they can to help their beloved pet feel comfort at the end of their lives.

- What interventions will best address the identified needs of the animal?
- What obstacles to carrying out the plan can the veterinarian and the caregivers anticipate?
- What is the caregiver's perception of what the animal is going through, and how can this plan help them help their animal?
- A palliative plan for mobility should include the following:
  - Pain management
  - Environmental management
  - Mobility aids
  - Physical therapy

Managing the environment

Transforming the pet's home environment can augment their mobility and significantly change their quality of life.

Flooring—Slick surfaces such as hardwood, tile, and laminate can be problematic for animals with weakness and pain. Often seen and especially challenging may be rising from a sitting or lying position. Throw rugs, carpet runners with nonskid bottoms, yoga mats, and foam flooring may improve traction. Do-it-yourself home stores often carry large indoor/outdoor carpets and tape to cut and move to the area that needs coverage. Caregivers can come up with very creative solutions to this challenge! The pet's usual travel routes around the home should be covered with traction assisting flooring.

Resources—Consider the animal's ability to access food, water, potty, and resting areas with ease. Improving accessibility of food and water dishes can help by raising bowls and providing gripping surfaces around dishes. Dogs may be able to be taught to eliminate on a puppy pad indoors. If an animal spends long periods inside or cannot get outside, diapers or belly bands may help. For the nonmobile, diapers/belly bands may be invaluable. For dogs trained to eliminate on grass, remnants of artificial turf can often be purchased at little or no cost to provide a "bathroom" in an easier-to-access location. In the authors' experience, cats may need significantly lower litter boxes with the lip that they must walk over very low, often 1 in. or less. Making a litter box out of a plastic tote can be an innovative way to approach this problem. Many do-it-yourself types can find all sorts of ideas on the internet for creating their low litter box.

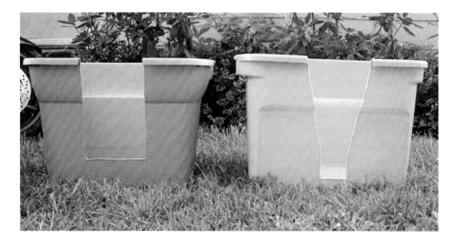

Bedding—The more time a disabled dog spends in its preferred resting area, the more influential the bedding quality becomes. The ideal dog bed has a padded layer 3 (for small and medium dogs) to 6 in. thick surrounded by a waterproof/washable layer and topped with absorbent material such as towels or puppy pads or a crib sheet. Getting to a sleeping area and ease of accessing a bed or a chair may also contribute to night waking. Steps or a ramp to a bed or a chair may help the disabled patient to obtain their previous sleep area. The ability to get on and off a bed may contribute to the animal sleeping on the floor, with minimal support for pressure points. For the floor sleepers, one-inch memory foam beds for dogs may help provide relief for pressure points while still maintaining the ability to get on and off a bed. Dogs that prefer to lie on hard surfaces such as tile might be convinced to use a bed topped with a passive cooling gel mat made for pets. A raised cot is an alternative that is easy to clean, provides some cooling and air circulation, and may be used outdoors; however, very weak or painful dogs may not be able to maneuver themselves on and off unless it is a shallow cot.

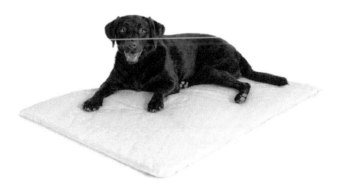

Other Hazards—Examining the house for tripping hazards, stairs, clutter, and obstacles can help the mobility impaired animal and should be barricaded or removed if possible. A thorough history may reveal less obvious problem areas—some dogs with cognitive issues routinely get stuck behind couches, in corners, or between kitchen table chairs, for example. Helping clients with ideas beyond the pet store for affordable barriers, rugs, yoga mats, and other household items discussed in this section can help owners with costs and may not have been previously considered by the caregiver. Baby gates, for example, can often be found at yard sales, garage sales, thrift, or second-hand stores or second-hand through online platforms such as Craigslist and local Facebook groups.

Shelter—Animals that spend time alone outdoors should be able to reach shelter from wind, rain, and sun without assistance. It may be necessary to partition part of the yard or provide shade in preferred resting locations. Screened tent structures can be set up for disabled patients and help protect them from insects and bugs and provide a shaded area. These may be found at the previously discussed second-hand places.

Ramps—Commercially available or homemade; these can help a dog navigate a few stairs or assist a larger dog into the car. Animals need the training to use ramps, and in the authors' experience, they should be at least 3 feet wide and have a railing. The angle of incline between the lower level and ramp should not exceed 20 degrees if possible. It should attach securely to the upper level without slippage. The walking surface should offer adequate traction. Especially for unstable dogs, the ramp should be next to a vertical surface or wall for safety and security. Many dogs will still need assistive devices (see next section) to use the ramp.

Assistive devices

Assistive devices are items around the home or specialized products that may be installed or utilized to help with mobility or improve the emotional quality of life for the disabled patient.

Wagons and strollers—Wheeling a pet around in a stroller, beach cart, or wagon can help them enjoy sights, sounds, smells, and opportunities for socialization. It's important to note that all pets will accept riding in a wagon or stroller, and the clinician should follow the client's lead on this.

Footwear for Pets—Adding traction to the feet may help the pet gain purchase on smoother surfaces and rise from resting. Depending on animal and owner preferences, options include booties, traction socks, or cuffs applied to the toenails.

Toe grips and pad treatments

Dr. Buzby developed rubber grips to place on the nails to help the dog grip the floor better. They are easy to apply and tend to work better with other gripping tools. However, they do seem to come off some dogs easily.

There are several pad treatments that a caregiver can paint or stick on the pads to help the dog better grip the floor. Some of the challenges with these aids are that some dogs do not like their feet touched and they may need to be reapplied frequently.

Where to find: Dr. Busby's Toe Grips https://toegrips.com/

Show Foot http://www.biogroom.com/dog/finishers/show-foot/

Paw Pads http://pupgearcorporation.com/products/Paw-Pads

Paw Friction https://pawfriction.com/

Wheelchairs/carts—an option for selected pets that may allow engagement in some normal activities. Before arranging for a cart, it is crucial to consider the following:

- What activities is the client hoping to use the cart for, and are their expectations realistic?
- How does the animal respond to being touched, moved, manipulated? Will they tolerate a stranger handling them to assist them into the cart during the training process?
- What motivators (e.g., treats) can be used to help acclimate the dog to the cart?
- Does the client have time to spend 5—10 min a few times a day for training?
- Are there any other helpers besides the primary caregiver? Ideally, every responsible person should be present for fitting and education.
- Is/are the primary caregiver(s) physically capable of assisting the animal into a cart?
- Will there be adequate supervision while the cart is in use?
- Are there narrow doorways, stairs, or other obstacles that could be a hazard or where the pet could get stuck? Can these be worked around, blocked, or secured?
- Is the yard fully fenced with secure gates? Is the ground even and level?
- Is there heavy street traffic outside the home?
- How has owner compliance been in the past?
- Are there other medical conditions (e.g., front limb disability or systemic illness leading to generalized weakness) that might preclude or complicate the use of a cart? Is the animal able enough to stand if the pelvic limbs are supported?

Business aspects of wheelchair/cart sales and rentals

- Ideally, one or two team members should be trained and familiarized with measuring, fitting, and assembling the cart. When setting prices, consider the cost of this training and the time needed for fitting and client education.
- Consider marketing carts as a professional service rather than a retail item. Clients can and will purchase devices over the internet at a lower cost than veterinarians may be able to offer—the value the veterinary professional brings

is the hands-on assistance with selecting, assembling, fitting, and client education.

- Before investing the veterinarian's time and the client's money on a fitting appointment, it is wise to ask screening questions such as those in the previous section.
- It is not required to have a valid Veterinary, Client, Patient Relationship to purchase carts over the internet. The veterinarian can help with case selection and treatment/prevention of complications.
- Follow-up will be needed, either with a doctor or a technician, to check for pressure sores and other complications with use, and to provide any additional client education and training.
- The client also needs to be educated about the initial time investment needed to acclimate the pet to the chair.
- Even after careful patient and client selection, carts often do not wind up working out. Return policies, fitting fees, and restocking fees should be established.
- There may be liability issues around renting carts, and the practice owner or management should discuss liability and waivers with an attorney.

In summary, there are more than a few options for improving mobility and function in dogs affected by neurological or orthopedic conditions. This presents a creative challenge, but it can be gratifying and satisfying when the veterinarian's efforts pay off!

Other mobility aids
Slings and harnesses

Slings—Slings are regularly used in the hospital or clinical setting to help animals get up and around after surgery and patients with back and hip problems. However, they can be more difficult for the owner to use in the chronic recumbent patient and often place stress on areas of the body where the animal has the most pain in their lower back and hip joints. A better way of helping these patients with lower back and hip problems may be to place them in a padded harness with a handle, or if all four legs need support, then a specialized harness may be offered to clients. These harnesses support the front weight-bearing limbs and give the animal better support with the sternum.

Gingerlead has a handle at the end of the sling, which can help minimize the strain on owners, and it can also attach to the collar to give a little extra assistance with stability and the ability to take for a walk.

Handicapped Pets have several different slings and carry a front and rear harness.

Labra Sling is a lightweight sling with adjustable straps to minimize strain on the owner.

Komfy Fleece Mobility sling has a fleece lining for comfort.

My Busy Dog carries numerous diverse slings and harnesses and can be found on multiple websites.

Harnesses—There are several products on the market designed to help lift and support larger dogs. There is usually a trade-off between simplicity of use (e.g., absence of many buckles and straps to be adjusted) and functionality (proper distribution of load-bearing and ergonomic for the owner) (Fig. 7.1).

There are many places to find harnesses. The veterinarian and team may find them on Amazon and Chewy.com, and 1000s other sites online.

Handicapped Pets, My Busy Dog, Labra Co. all carry harnesses as well.

Help 'Em Up Harness (Blue Dog Designs) is useful for the quadriparetic or quadriplegic patient. helpemup.com

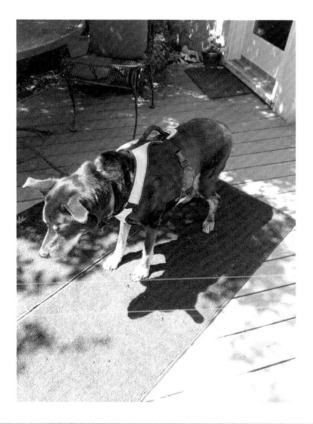

FIGURE 7.1

Photo of Buddy Deering with a harness.

Used with permission by Roberta Deering ©2018.

Orthotics and prosthetics

Orthotics for animals are dynamic braces that have a hinge at the joint, helping with support and immobilization of a joint and aligning a limb, and can support weak muscles and benefit the limb's function (Mich, 2011).

There are online orthotic businesses that provide premade and custom-made orthotics and prosthetics for animals. This list is not comprehensive. However, it will give the veterinarian a place to start.

Handicapped Pets have developed some premade orthotics and braces that the vet may purchase, and then the animal may be fitted with the help of the veterinarian.

OrthoVet Inc works with the veterinarian to develop custom-made orthotics and braces with hinges to stabilize joints.

Hero Braces will also work with the veterinarian to build a custom brace for dogs and cats.

Splints

Splints are rigid braces that can help keep the leg in a rigid and stable position and immobilize the joint movement. Veterinary distributors may carry splints.

Booties and socks

Booties are another way to help with gripping slippery floors. Pros—they are removable, can be used on any surface. Cons—leaving them on too long can cause pressure sores. Some dogs do not like them on their feet.

Where to find them:

Socks can also help with gaining purchase, and they may have different shape grips on the bottom ranging from a slight to a significant amount of rubber gripping. Baby socks (socks for infants) and socks specifically made for dogs (such a Power Paws, https://www.woodrowwear.com) work well.

Physical therapy

A veterinarian or team member may employ many different physical therapy techniques to help with hospice and palliative care patients. In a human study with advanced cancer patients, physical therapy helped with sleep, balance, pain, fatigue, and fewer falls (Kowalski, 2016). A study in 2013 showed that walking stairs and using a ramp can help improve mobility in the thoracic limbs (Carr et al., 2013). Another resource in the Veterinary Clinics of North America discusses various treatments for ambulatory and nonambulatory patients (Drum, 2010). There have been several physical therapy studies in animal patients, though they lack studies with end-of-life animal patients. The authors would encourage the veterinarian to refer to a veterinary professional trained in canine rehabilitation therapy or gain additional training in rehabilitation to help your patients. It should be noted that in some jurisdictons, the term "physical therapist" can only be used by individuals trained and licensed in human physical therapy. This section provides an introduction to physical therapy and consideration for use with the end-of-life patient. Physical therapy for end-of-life patients is a broad topic and beyond this book's scope and should be dedicated to a separate palliative medicine/physical therapy book.

Physical therapy and rehabilitation for animals are used for musculoskeletal diseases to build muscle and strength, stability, and balance (Levine et al., 2005). Finding a good housecall rehab veterinarian or learning more about rehab techniques will help veterinarians build a unique service and assist many palliative veterinary patients.

Tools utilized by veterinary physical therapists/ rehabilitators

Water therapy

Whirlpools or other water therapy can help those with joint problems, hip dysplasia, elbow dysplasia, or moderate to severe osteoarthritis. A useful tool is an underwater treadmill. In the home setting, aquatic therapy would entail a pool or a whirlpool to assist the dog (or cat if they will tolerate it). Cats are not likely to tolerate if the water is not heated.

Other therapies

Physical therapists utilize massage (commonly used in human hospice), balance skills, stretching exercises, muscle strengthening techniques, range of motion physical therapy, and aquatic therapy to help balance, strength, and pain.

Equipment that veterinary physical therapists may commonly use are the following:

- Physioball or Physio Roll
- A balance board
- Carts and slings to help support during therapy.
- Ice packs
- Cavaletti rails
- A-Frames
- Padded floor space
- Therapeutic ultrasound
- Outcome measurement devices: goniometer—measures joint flexibility and ooliometer—measures muscle diameter (Hudson, 2007)

Heat or cold therapy

Heat and cold therapy may be an adjunct that may add to the therapy of different diseases and be included in a multimodal approach to therapy in hospice and palliative patients. Heat (and Capsaicin) can increase TRPV1 receptor activity, facilitating calcium channel opening in the afferent synapse (Fox, 2012). Heat therapy may facilitate an increase or decrease in pain sensation and may be dependent on time used and temperature. It can also cause vasodilation, increasing blood flow that can help remove accrued metabolites. It can cause relaxation of muscle and may be helpful for osteoarthritis (Millis, 2015).

Cold therapy (and menthol and peppermint) can help many chronic, inflammatory diseases, especially cancer pain. It can cause numbness of the area with short-term use; constriction of blood vessels can reduce edema. It can also reduce cellular metabolism and oxygen use (Millis, 2015). Cold activates TRPM8 in A-δ fibers opening Na^+ and Ca^{++} channels and activating inhibiting fibers to decrease pain (Fox, 2012).

TENS unit

TENS stands for transcutaneous electrical nerve stimulation. In humans, it appears to stimulate both peripheral and central neurotransmitters. The TENS unit stimulates opioid, serotonin, and muscarinic receptors; peripherally, opioid and α-2 noradrenergic receptors are the receptors reported (DeSantana, 2008). The "dosage" seems to affect what receptors may be involved in the analgesic effects. It has also been proposed that it may help with the hyperalgesia of inflammation (DeSantana, 2008).

It can be an inexpensive way to help patients with musculoskeletal issues.

Assisi loop

Assisi loop uses electromagnetic current, and it is suspected to increase the calcium to Calmodulin that increases nitric oxide production, which in turn increases growth factor hormone to help with inflammation (Shearer, 2016; Pilla, 1996).

Chiropractic

The chiropractic theory uses high velocity, short lever device, or hands-on joints or cranial sutures to adjust vertebral subluxations (AVCA staff, 2000). Used in equine and canine species most, finding a veterinarian who does chiropractic may be difficult in many countries. A full physical exam is required (AVCA staff, 2000). There is a certification program in veterinary chiropractic by American Chiropractic Veterinary Association. Certification is not licensure (AVCA staff, 2000). In a Cochrane systematic review of the literature, there appears to have little to no evidence-based studies in veterinary chiropractic.

Conclusion

An animal's ability to ambulate will affect its quality of life, as well as the owner's quality of life, and may affect end-of-life decision-making. Owners have many physical medicine options to assist disabled and mobility-challenged pets, and utilizing them, may improve the quality of life of both the animal and the owner. Physical therapy for people with disabilities increases muscle tone balance and improves innervation and is being used more frequently with end-of-life patients to improve their capabilities. Further research in mobility aids, physical therapy, and other modalities could improve our understanding of assisting mobility for chronically debilitated animals.

References

AVCA staff. (2000). *AVCA doctors*. Retrieved from American Veterinary Chiropractic Association http://www.animalchiropractic.org/avca-doctor-find.htm.

Carr, J. G., Millis, D. L., & Weng, H. Y. (2013). Exercises in canine physical rehabilitation: Range of motion of the forelimb during stair and ramp ascent. *Journal of Small Animal Practice*, 409−413.

Cavenaugh, M. (2018). *Mobility matters*. Retrieved from AAHA.org https://www.aaha.org/graphics/original/professional/resources/other%20resources/mobilitymatters.pdf.

DeSantana, J. W. (2008). Effectiveness of transcutaneous electrical nerve stimulation for treatment of hyperalgesia and pain. *Current Rheumatology Reports*, 492−499.

Drum, M. (2010). Physical rehabilitation of the canine neurologic patient. In *Veterinary Clinics of North America small animal practice* (pp. 181−193). Elsevier.

Fox, S. (2012). *Chronic pain in small animal medicine*. London: Manson Publishing LTD.

Ganzini, L., Goy, E. R., Dobscha, S. K., & Prigerson, H. (2009). Mental health outcomes of family members of Oregonians who request physician aid in dying. *Journal of Pain and Symptom Management*, *38*(6), 807−815. https://doi.org/10.1016/j.jpainsymman.2009.04.026

Hudson, S. (March 8, 2007). *Top 10 rehabilitation tools*. Retrieved from VIN https://www.vin.com.

Johnson, S. (1997). Osteoarthritis. Joint anatomy, physiology, and pathobiology. In *Veterinary Clinics of North America: Small animal practice* (pp. 699−723). Philadelphia: WB Saunders Company.

Kowalski, S. (2016). Physical therapy and exercise for hospice patients. *Home Healthcare Nurse*, 563−568.

Levine, D., Millis, D. L., & Marcellin-Little, D. J. (2005). Introduction to veterinary physical rehabilitation. In *Veterinary Clinics of North America small animal practice* (pp. 1247−1254). Elsevier.

Mich, P. (July 01, 2011). *Orthotics and prosthetics in veterinary rehabilitation*. Retrieved from DVM 360.com http://veterinarynews.dvm360.c0m/orthotics-and-prosthetics-veterinary-rehabilitation.

Millis, D. (2015). Physical therapy and rehabilitation in dogs. In J. M. Gaynor (Ed.), *Handbook of veterinary pain management* (pp. 386–389). St Louis, MO, USA: Elsevier.

Pilla, A. E. (1996). *Journal of Athletic Training, 53*.

Shearer, T. (2016). *IAAHPC certification program*. IAAHPC.org.

Creating your interdisciplinary team

Lynn Hendrix, AA, BA, DVM, CHPV [1,2,3,4]

[1]*Owner, Veterinarian, Beloved Pet Mobile Vet, Davis, CA, United States;* [2]*Former Board of Directors, IAAHPC, Chicago, IL, United States;* [3]*Consultant, Hospice, Palliative Medicine, End of Life, VIN, Davis, CA, United States;* [4]*President, Founder, World Veterinary Palliative Medicine Organization, Davis, CA, United States*

Creating an interdisciplinary team will be important as you grow. What is an interdisciplinary team? The word interdisciplinary is defined as involving two or more academic, scientific, or artistic disciplines (Staff of M-W Dictionary.com, 2018). It may be more multidisciplinary, as defined by Merriam-Webster Dictionary.com as combining or involving more than one discipline or field of study: interdisciplinary (Staff of M-W Dictionary.com, 2018). Either way, there are multiple disciplines involved in the care of the end-of-life pet and the people who love them, and this chapter is about team building.

Human hospice uses the interdisciplinary team model to provide coverage of care 24 hours a day, 7 days a week and to provide the best care for the physical and social and psychological and spiritual needs of the patient and family. This human hospice model was utilized when creating the guidelines for the International Association of Animal Hospice and Palliative Care (IAAHPC) best practices in animal hospice and palliative care written in 2013. The core members of the team identified by the IAAHPC guidelines are the veterinarian as the medical director, the registered veterinary technician (or certified or Licensed), and a mental health professional (Shanan, 2017). These team members are ideal to have for a veterinary hospice team; however, they do not have to be employed directly by the veterinarian in a start up practice. It is a reasonable practice to refer to other businesses that provide the care that you are looking for, to add to your team, especially when you are first starting out. Other team members can include groomers, extended family members, pet sitters, their regular veterinarian and their team, respite workers, chaplains, churches, chaplains that are focused on animals and pet loss, compounding pharmacists, accredited pharmacists are preferred, volunteers, crematoriums, memorial homes, and pet cemeteries. This is not an exhaustive list. Anyone who can help in the care of the animal and their people can be helpful to your team.

The ideal team

Hospice and palliative trained veterinarians

Veterinarians is the core team medical provider, to provide the highest standard of medical care for the animal and to guide additional support for the family caring for their beloved animal. The veterinarian is involved in the decision-making regarding diagnosis, prognostication, medical planning, prescribing medications, other physical and emotional support of the animal as well as emotional support for the family. Veterinarians need further training in communication and palliative medicine to be considered palliative medicine veterinarians. Veterinarians can obtain certification in hospice and palliative care through the IAAHPC. The IVAPM has a pain management certification program. And eventually the goal may be to become a diplomate in a specialty of hospice and palliative medicine (however, at the time of this writing, that is years off).

Providing at-home palliative care can start with a sole practitioner. As you grow your practice, you may begin adding to your team of providers to assist clients in providing care day in and day out.

Veterinary hospice nursing

RNs or registered nurses, play a key role in the in-home care for human hospice. Ideally, veterinary hospice nursing care should be provided by registered veterinary nurses (called veterinary technicians in the United States) and veterinary assistants. Registered veterinary technicians can play a vital role in the care of dying patient. They can be more readily available for clients and can provide support for families by helping with medications, changes in the disease process, behavior, mobility, education, and respite for families. Every team member needs to have a clear goal of what the family's wishes, needs, and wants from the initial consultation and carry through to the end of the life of the patient, supporting the family postdeath, if needed by the family.

Registered veterinary technicians can become certified in Animal Hospice and Palliative Care through the IAAHPC's certification program. As a certified Hospice and Palliative Care Technician, veterinary nurses are an essential part of the animal hospice team, fulfilling the important function of managing the day-to-day health care of your end-of-life patients, and guiding and supporting their caregivers. The ideal goal of the animal hospice nursing staff should be the implementation of the plan created by a veterinarian.

Additional skills needed by veterinary technicians in veterinary hospice and palliative care

This section reviews the specifics for additional training for veterinary technicians in hospice and palliative care, and important topics for veterinary nurses to consider for a job in the field of hospice and palliative care.

Communication

The relationship between the veterinarian, the nurse, and the caregivers or family is the key to providing the best care to a dying patient. Communication between each of the parties is an essential component to providing an excellent relationship between the team and the caregivers. The team of providers, the veterinarian, and the nursing staff and any other members of your team should also have planned communication. Veterinary nurses skilled in effective communication can help educate and address all the concerns, worries, and fears of the family. Empathy is essential. Additional training can be provided through the IAAHPC certification course or through the Hospice and Palliative Nurses Association (this is for Registered Nurses—but they may provide training through Continuing Education(CE)). Communication classes may also be found at conferences and workshops at some conferences.

Analytical skills

Because veterinary technicians would be working in the field, they need to be able to analyze the current situation and advice the veterinarian of status changes. Competency in analytical skills and problem-solving adds to providing palliative care for patients and changing situations withcaregivers (Millburn, 2017).

Technical patient skills

Veterinary technicians or nurses providing care to hospice patients and their caregivers should have training and demonstrate skills in the following areas:

RVTs that have specific training in hospice and palliative care should be knowledgeable in the following:

1. Clinical sign recognition and patient triage—based on knowledge and training in animal physiology, behavior changes, and disease recognition.
2. Veterinary nurses need to be able to recognize physical and behavioral signs of acute, chronic, and terminal pain. They should be able to assess distinctive types

of distress, the clinical signs of imminent death, including terminal delirium, and the physical changes that take place during death and dying.

3. Basic knowledge of disease progression and disease trajectory progress to death, if euthanasia is not elected, is necessary.

Nursing skills that are helpful to have to provide palliative care:

1. Assessment of patient's status, recognizing changing clinical signs, some of which may change rapidly.
2. Ability to administer and teach the use of medications, including medications not typically given in the hospital setting. Many palliative or hospice patients are on transdermal, liquid oral, rectal, or injectable medications that the client or family may need training to use at home.
3. Application of palliative measures and pain management techniques. Certification in pain management through IVAPM or certification in hospice and palliative care would be a useful certification.
4. Charting progression through the disease process to provide consistant care for the patient and the family.
5. Understanding the difference between suffering and distress points to help the clients make decisions.
6. Be aware of language that may generate fear and avoid language that does not support the goals of the caregivers.
7. Ability to perform the following: IV catheter placement.
8. Urinary catheter placement.
9. Recognizing and monitoring bed sores and treating according to veterinarian's orders.
10. Feeding tube care.
11. Knowledge and use of IV pumps and syringe pumps.
12. Knowledge of medications given to an individual patient.
13. Assisting the veterinarian in examination and treatment procedures.
14. Maintaining timely and accurate medical records.
15. Feeding, watering and medicating of animals for respite care for the caregivers.
16. Monitoring safety issues for the pet and the caregivers within the home.
17. Daily, weekly progress reports to the team. Team meetings for rounds.
18. Providing enemas if needed for constipated animals.
19. Assisting the pet and family with mobility issues. Assisting families in finding ramps, braces, wheelchairs, and other mobility tools.
20. Managing medical waste.
21. Dealing with recumbent care, turning schedule (as provided by the veterinarian), lubrication of eyes, nose, mouth, and providing medications via a treatment plan to keep patient comfortable if they are recumbant.

Caregiver/client skills

1. Training caregivers to recognize patients' symptoms and needs, especially with behaviors that may indicate pain.
2. Training caregivers to administer treatments to their pet. These may include oral, injectable, and transdermal medications, and subcutaneous fluids administration by caregivers at home.
3. Training caregivers in provide comfort measures, including enviromental changes, and helping the animal with activities of daily living .
4. Empathy. Assessing caregivers' status/needs/feelings. Recognizing normal manifestations of grief, and recognizing those manifestations suggesting that complicated grief may be present.
5. Advanced communication skills. Providing support for common grief and bereavement situations. Actively listening with caregivers. Demonstrating empathy and having open-ended conversations with caregivers regarding palliation, grief, and death and dying. Validating spiritual and social concerns without judgment or interjection of own personal beliefs.
6. Provide information and guidance about the normal manifestation of grief and body care options.
7. Provide referrals to mental health professionals and for spiritual guidance as needed.

Body care of deceased animals

1. Assist the family with preparation of the body after a euthanasia or the animal has passed.
2. Supporting the client regarding decisions for cremation, burial, or other body services. Ideally, discussion of body care should happen before euthanasia or death; however, the author recognizes this does not always happen.
3. Providing information for the caregivers on disposal of medication and removal of any medical paraphernalia.
4. Treating the animal with respect and dignity is honoring the bond between the person and their beloved pet. Significant consideration of caring for the body. Swaddling an animal in a blanket and gently placing on a stretcher or gurney or in a basket to remove from the home for burial or cremation.
5. Honoring the caregiver's spiritual beliefs and providing a safe space for them to practice their personal rituals.

Hospice/Palliative additional team skills

1. Team communication—updating the hospice team regarding the patient's and the caregivers' status on a regular basis. Charting all communications with team members and outside service providers.
2. Coordinating care—ensuring all service providers are up to date on what others on the team and otherwise are doing. Ensuring plan of care is up to date and tasks performed as planned.

Knowledge of animal hospice ethics

Understanding ethics is a part of the medical profession. We do not have a code of ethics written for the Animal Hospice veterinary technician, so we will list the code written for the human hospice nurses. From the Hospice and Palliative Nurses Association, the code of ethics contains the following topics:

- Respect for persons: to honor the intrinsic worth and uniqueness of each person; to respect the basic human rights and the dignity of all patients, without consideration of social or economic status, race, religion, age, gender, sexual orientation, national origin, disability, personal attributes, nature of the health problem(s), or any other factors.
- Beneficence: to promote good and prevent or remove harm; to promote the welfare, health, and safety of society and individuals in accordance with their beliefs, values, and preferences.
- Justice: to be fair and promote equity, nondiscrimination, and the distribution of benefits and burdens based on needs and resources available; to advocate on another's behalf when necessary.
- Confidentiality: to safeguard patients' protected information, except when disclosure is required by law.
- Role fidelity: to respect one's own self-worth and professional integrity, and the integrity of the profession; to maintain the knowledge and skill necessary for competent practice within one's scope of practice (AEC staff, 2018).

To modify this code of ethics and update it for Animal Hospice Technicians:

1. Respect for both the animal patient and the humans that love them: to honor both parties intrinsic worth, and their basic rights without judgment or discrimination.
2. To promote quality of life, for the welfare and safety of the animal, and address the concerns, fears, and values of the caregivers and listen to their preferences.
3. To maintain confidentiality.
4. To maintain professional integrity, preserve self-worth, set and maintain boundaries and to upkeep the knowledge and skills necessary to provide the maximum quality of life for the end-of-life animal.

Other team members
Mental health professionals

Pet loss is discounted as a mode of grief in many circles in the United States, though the paradigm is changing. Mental Health Professionals can provide emotional and social support for caregivers of a dying pet. Mental health providers may be a resource, helping clients understand the dying process, supporting them through anticipatory grief, and postdeath grief, handling mental illness in the family, difficulties between family members. Grief support is deserved and since pet loss creates grief for those who love their pets, having additional support is significant. Postdeath counseling available for at least 6 months postdeath can make a significant impact for people. This can be in the form of a pet loss group facilitated by a mental health professional, an online chat room or pet loss hotline or individual counseling.

In addition to helping the client/caregiver, the mental health professional can also assist the other members of the team with the mental health stresses of caring for the dying animals. Grief can bring up mental illness issues and can become complicated grief. People can become angry or be in denial in grief, depression and anxiety issues may arise. Or they may become suicidal and may require additional psychological support.

There is a program for Veterinary Social Work through the University of Tennessee.

The chapter on grief support has more information, and numbers for crisis and pet loss support. The scope of all the mental health professionals can provide is beyond the scope of this text.

Spiritual support

Chaplains, ministers (Christian), Imam (Muslim), lama (Buddhist), Rabbi (Judism) are spiritual leaders that can provide spiritual support to clients, and be involved with grief support for your families. Finding a person who is interested in providing a wide range of spiritual support for families for their pets can be challenging. Spiritual leaders can also help provide rituals for grieving families. Consider approaching a community church or other nondenominational church or other spiritual house to provide services to support the spiritual needs of your clients, including memorial services, body care rituals, funerals, and spiritual counseling.

Groomers

Groomers can provide grooming care for the dying patient. They may need further training in the challenges of senior and life-limited care. Services that groomers could provide include, keeping nails short, pad care, placing nail grips, skin care, cleanliness, de-matting, and general grooming. Groomers should be able to provide physical support for the animal in the form of a sling that an animal can rest in if they are often unable to stand for extended periods of time. Groomers should recognize signs of chronic pain and be able to report if noted, to the team. They can also report indications of changing the physical needs of the animal. Veterinarians can employ mobile groomers or refer to them. Mobile groomers who have been trained to provide care for chronically ill and elderly pets are preferable.

Pet sitters

Pet sitters are another important provider of care for families caring for an end-of-life patient. They can give respite for the clients during a very physically and emotionally draining time in the family's lives. They also can be observers of changing physical signs in the animal, which could be communicated back to the veterinary team. They may be employed by the veterinarian or may be a trusted referral company. They ideally have previous experience or training working with elderly pets.

Respite care

Respite care is a needed service with animal hospice. As caregivers provide 24 hour care for their pets, they may need a break. Respite care for owners can be provided directly from a pet sitter, or a respite service, and there are programs to help with the elderly and can provide a break for caregivers.

Volunteers

Volunteers play a vital role with human hospice services. Volunteers (check with your state regulations—volunteers may not be able to assist for-profit businesses in certain states) may be very helpful in providing additional services. They can provide respite, emotional support for the family, physical support for the animals, and support for the team. Volunteers can gain experience and education through a human hospice volunteer training program. AHELP (Animal Hospice, End of Life Care Project) is located in Seattle, Washington and is a program to provide volunteers provide end-of-life care for veterinary providers, to give them better coverage for their end-of-life patients (Nichols, 2018).

Crematoriums, memorial homes, and pet cemeteries

Crematoriums, memorial homes, and pet cemeteries can also provide important services for the family. Body care can be quite meaningful to many families. Being comfortable with the crematorium fundamental. Visit to the crematorium and tour the space. Get to know the staff. They provide additional support to the veterinarian and staff and the caregivers. The veterinarian wants to be able to assure your families of where their beloved is going after euthanasia or hospice-supported death. Pick a crematorium that is going to perform the type of services you are require.

The interdisciplinary team is an essential part of end-of-life care for animals. Utilizing the team approach helps the house call veterinarian build their practice. This will add to your services and help you provide quality care for both the animal patient and the caregivers who love them.

References

AEC staff. (2018). *Code of ethical conduct.* Retrieved from Advancing Expert Care https://advancingexpertcare.org/ethical-conduct/.

Millburn, N. (July 5, 2017). *Skills & competencies OF a hospice nurse.* Retrieved from Career Trend.com https://careertrend.com/skills-competencies-hospice-nurse-38861.html.

Nichols, M. (2018). *AHELP project home.* Retrieved from Ahelpproject.org http://www.ahelpproject.org/.

Shanan, A. C. (2017). *Practice guidelines.* Retrieved from IAAHPC.org https://www.iaahpc.org/resources-and-support/practice-guidelines.html.

Staff of M-W Dictionary.com. (2018). *Interdisciplinary.* Retrieved from Merriam-Webster Dictionary.com https://www.merriam-webster.com/dictionary/interdisciplinary.

Supporting grief

Lynn Hendrix, AA, BA, DVM, CHPV [1,2,3,4,5]

[1]*Owner, Veterinarian, Beloved Pet Mobile Vet, Davis, CA, United States;* [2]*Former Board of Directors, IAAHPC, Chicago, IL, United States;* [3]*Consultant, Hospice, Palliative Medicine, End of Life, VIN, Davis, CA, United States;* [4]*President, Founder, World Veterinary Palliative Medicine Organization, Davis, CA, United States;* [5]*Founder, Consultant, The Palliative Vet, Davis, CA, United States*

Grief is a significant aspect of Veterinary Palliative Medicine and Animal Hospice. This chapter will review different grief types for adults and include a section discussing grief with children and grief in other household pets.

- In this chapter, we will be able to recognize different mental health professionals and know when to refer to them:
- Expected grief
  - Mourning versus grief
  - Stages of "Normal" grief
  - Trajectories of grief
  - Postdeath grief
- Atypical grief
  - Anticipatory grief
  - Complicated grief
  - Disenfranchised grief
  - Delayed grief
  - Traumatic grief
  - Suicidal ideation
  - Secondary traumatic stress disorder (aka. compassion fatigue)—while not grief specific, an animal's caregivers can experience secondary traumatic stress or compassion fatigue.
- Grief support for children
  - Talking with children about grief
  - Cognitive stages of development from ages 0 to 18 and how to approach death
- Support options
  - Memorial options
  - Adult support
  - Children (0−18) support
- Grief in other animal family members

Animal Hospice and Palliative Medicine for the House Call Veterinarian
https://doi.org/10.1016/B978-0-323-56798-5.00013-8

A brief overview of mental health professionals

Mental health professionals are essential to helping both clients and the veterinary team. This is a shortlist of mental health professionals, veterinarians might consider utilizing: Psychologists, Counselors, Clinicians and Therapists, Clinical Social Workers, Psychiatrists, Psychiatric Or Mental Health Nurse Practitioners.

Psychologists have obtained a doctorate in psychology, either Ph.D. or PsyD. The PhD degree holder is more research based, whereas the PsyD holder is more clinical trained (Choosing Between a PhD and PsyD: Some Factors to Consider). They can evaluate, diagnose, and provide individual or group therapy.

Counselors, Clinician, or Therapists have master's degree training and can evaluate and treat with their specific training (i.e., marriage and family counseling).

Clinical Social Workers have a master's in social work and can evaluate and treat with specific training. They also have training in case management and advocacy.

Psychiatrists are medical doctors who have psychology training. They can diagnose, prescribe, and provide individual or group therapy.

Psychiatric Or Mental Health Nurse Practitioners can assess, diagnose, and provide therapy for mental illness or substance abuse disorders. Some states allow them to prescribe, and other states require supervision by a licensed psychiatrist (NAMI, 2020).

Local resources: A local mental health professional may help clients with a variety of grief issues including, complicated grief, disenfranchised grief, and anticipatory grief. Support hotlines may aid clients who feel they are in crisis due to their grief. Options for support for clients may include pet loss support hotlines at universities or crisis hotlines for suicidal clients. Veterinarians may find additional support in private organizations such as the Association for Pet Loss and Bereavement. Veterinary practices can partner with a local mental health professional and create their own pet loss support group. There are many options to consider to help support clients experiencing grief.

Common understanding of grief

Mourning versus grief

Mourning is the behavioral structure of grief (Zisook, 2009). Mourning can involve rituals, traditions, and religious beliefs and can give personal and social, and cultural structure to death (Zisook, 2009).

Grief involves the internal feelings produced by loss. Grief can occur with any loss, the more significant loss occurs with an in-depth relationship, whereas death is the end of a physical connection. Prolonged grief occurs when integration of the death into the person's life and the reintegration of the person back into their routine lasts longer than a year (Medicinenet.com Staff, 2012).

Stages of expected grief

Grief has an expected role in a loss or death. The experience of grief is very personal; whatever the unique experience is "normal" for them. People may experience the "typical" stages of grief; however, they may not experience all of them, or they may be jumbled, experiencing different stage at distinct times.

The stages of "Normal" grief that are generally accepted by the psychological community for adults are as follows:

1. Shock and denial
2. *Pain and guilt*
3. *Anger and bargaining.*
4. *Depression, reflection, and loneliness*
5. *The upward turn*
6. *Reconstruction and working through.*
7. *Acceptance and hope.*
   Or the Kubler-Ross model:
1. *Denial*
2. *Anger*
3. *Bargaining*
4. *Depression*
5. *Acceptance.*

Trajectories of grief

There have been five trajectories of grief established: (1) common grief and recovery (returning to established norms) within 6 months to a year, (2) resilience and stable low distress, (3) depression that improved during bereavement, (4) chronic grief, and (5) chronic depression. The first three trajectories are likely to reintegrate to normalcy within a timely manner (up to 18 months). The last two are less likely to improve without assistance through their grief (Bonanno, 2008).

The author would include one additional caveat that veterinarians might see with animal loss. When there is a complicated and complex relationship with their animal, people may be more likely to have complicated grief. This complex relationship may be due to the intricacy of their human—animal bond. For example, the relationship may be a more substantial relationship, such as a therapy animal, a service dog, or the only significant relationship with another being. It could be that the owner is terminally ill, or they have obtained the animal because of a family member or friend who has passed, and this is the relationship that they have left with the person that has passed (which may involve delayed grief).

Postdeath expected grief

Postdeath grief is what is discussed with pet loss and grief. Elizabeth Kubler-Ross defined grief stages as denial, anger, bargaining, depression, and acceptance in the 1960s. These stages are still often discussed as normal grief. However, examining postdeath grief more comprehensively can help expand our understanding of people in grief. There may be physical changes, emotional experiences, and changes in behavior (Zisook, 2009). People grieve at their own pace. Grief may never leave the person though the emotion surrounding grief may lessen over time.

People respond emotionally, physically, socially, culturally to grief and responses may vary for individuals, and families. Grief emotions may show up intermittently or be overwhelming. The intensity and length of the feelings of grief are unique to each individual and may be affected by age, personal history, personality, personal health, attachment, and relationship to the lost pet, spiritual or cultural influences, support in the family and community, and type of loss (traumatic or sudden vs. planned, euthanasia vs. palliated death, number of previous losses (Bonanno, 2001). Psychologists have found people can go through denial or shock, anger, guilt, regret, intrusive thoughts, sadness, depression, feeling lost, alone, and overwhelmed (Zisook, 2009). People can also have moments of happier feelings, relief, peace, and joy at times with uncomplicated grief. However, these feelings can sometimes bring feelings of betrayal of the loved one and guilt.

Acute grief occurs immediately after the loved one's death, with overwhelming feelings of sadness, missing the pet, and thoughts dwelling on the lost loved one. People can have distressing feelings during this time. Acute grief can cause physical pain. The initial feelings receed over time paving the way to reintegration.

Grieving people eventually will reintegrate back into their life routines. Reintegration can include continuing the relationship with the deceased pet, with stories, memories, pictures, videos, or other social or cultural activities. Individuals may dream, "see or hear" their pet, or find other reminders of them in music and nature, especially in the acute phase of grief. Some may want to memorialize by donating to a charity, creating art, and writing stories to integrate the loss further.

"Atypical" grief
Anticipatory grief

Anticipatory grief can include emotional concerns and fears that may arise before the death of the pet. These emotions may consist of depression, anger, concern, worry, fear around the dying process, or the death. Culture, social groups, and other family members may also influence the preoccupation with death and the feelings that arise (Rogalla, 2020). Anticipatory grief may also occur when people struggle with the decision of euthanasia, especially when they do not feel supported.

Complicated grief

Complicated grief, also known as maladaptive grief, occurs when normal post death grief does not progress toward reintegration into routine. Complicated grief is a mental disorder in the DSM-5 (Diagnostic and Statistical Manual of Mental Disorders fifth edition). Acute grief is prolonged with complicated grief. Intense and overwhelming feelings of grief for extended periods of time may contribute to despair. Depression, drug abuse, alcoholism, and PTSD may exacerbate grief feelings. Warning signs of complicated grief may include an unusually close relationship with the animal, a traumatic death or euthanasia, or known mental illness (Shear, 2011). Clients with complicated grief should be referred to a counselor, psychologist or psychiatrist.

Clinical signs of complicated grief

Individuals with complicated grief may express difficulty accepting the death of their pet. They may disclose an intense longing for the deceased, a preoccupation with their pet's death, or thoughts of their pet, or anger, bitterness, especially if the death or euthanasia was perceived by the individual as traumatic. They may have looping thoughts, referring over and over to the death, a previous death or other aspects of the loss. The loss becomes a substantial focus in their lives, and they may not be able to perform regular life tasks. People with complicated grief may feel like they are betraying their pet if they start enjoying life. They may not continue with relationships they previously had with other people, and the loneliness can exacerbate their grief without support, by the extended length of time of the symptoms, the interference in normal function caused by the symptoms, or the intensity of the symptoms (such as intense suicidal thoughts or acts).

Complicated grief may also appear as a complete absence of grief and mourning, an ongoing inability to experience normal grief reactions, delayed grief, conflicted grief, or chronic grief. Substance abuse may occur to avoid painful feelings and other clinical signs such as sleeplessness (Medicinenet.com Staff, 2012).

How complicated grief differs from "Typical" grief

Failure of integration—The "typical" grieving person given time accommodates the permanence of death. In time, thoughts and feelings regarding the loss decrease as the person integrates the loss of the relationship into their lives. With complicated grief, there is a disconnect between death and integration. There is a difficulty with the perception of the permanence of death for the grieving person. There may be searching, seeking behavior (The author's observation and in conversations with clients within a month of the death of the pet that we also may see seeking, searching behavior with the animal companions, especially if they were not present during the dying process or euthanasia).

Negative beliefs and misinterpretations—The person experiencing complicated grief may hold negative beliefs or misinterpret the experience of the death. Examples of negative beliefs are self-worthlessness, hopelessness, the meaninglessness of life, and ideas that they cannot bear emotional pain and loss of control. These feelings may also contribute to or drive grief based depression and anxiety and enhance negative emotions, such as anger and fear.

Avoidance strategies—Avoiding feelings that arise with the grief process may be expected, but persistence to avoid feelings tends to contribute to loss of integration. Individuals may avoid painful emotions, withdraw, and become anxious and depressed. Coping strategies tend toward avoidance of support, inactivity, and detachment from society, and typical integration back into life.

In addition, understanding the qualities of the griever, whether they tend toward intuitive grieving or instrumental grieving or fall in between the continuum, may help the veterinarian support people on their journey of grief. Intuitive grieving includes heightened experience and expression of emotion, and instrumental grieving is more of a problem-solving approach. Instrumental grievers want to manage their feelings and focus on problem-solving rather than grief. Grief may also be influenced by the individual's culture, social groups, or religion (Doughty, 2009; Martin, 2000; Nader, 2011).

Disenfranchised grief

Disenfranchised grief is that grief that goes unrecognized or is not legitimized by social standards or by social groups (Raypole, 2020). Pet loss is considered a form of disenfranchised grief and may need additional grief support for the individual.

Delayed grief

Delayed Grief is postponed grief, sometimes recognized as complicated grief.

Traumatic death

Traumatic death can contribute to a complicated grief scenario. Animals that have been through a trauma, such as being hit by a car or a sudden terminal diagnosis may become traumatic. If the person is not prepared to make a euthanasia decision, it can increase the likelihood they develop complicated grief.

Difficult euthanasias from the perception of the client (even if you thought it went well) may also cause post traumatic stress syndrome. An animal that jumps, cries out, seizures, has agonal breathing (or, as the author refers to, brain stem breathing), and even calling it agonal breathing may cause stress and change their perception of how the euthanasia went. Consider what the client might perceive during euthanasia, including the words said, the expectations, the concerns they may not verbalize.

Traumatic grief

Traumatic grief is defined as grief from a sudden or abrupt loss. It may also occur with traumatic euthanasia. Posttraumatic stress disorder may occur, and complicated grief may occur (Boelan et al., 2003).

Suicidal ideation

"Atypical" types of grief may have the endpoint of suicide. However, suicide may occur with normal grief or other mental illness. Depression and anxiety may contribute to complicated grief and suicidal ideation. This section is for those veterinarians who want to be aware of the signs of suicide ideation that may occur around grieving. This section also includes help if any team member is concerned about a person who may be providing some clues, verbal or nonverbal. The following information is taken directly from the American Foundation of Suicide Prevention and may be potential warning signs of someone considering suicide.

If a person talks about:

- Being a burden to others
- Feeling trapped
- Experiencing unbearable pain
- Having no reason to live
- Killing themselves

Specific things to look out for include:

- Increased use of alcohol or drugs
- Looking for a way to kill themselves, such as searching online for materials or means
- Acting recklessly
- Withdrawing from activities
- Isolating from family and friends
- Sleeping too much or too little
- Visiting or calling people to say goodbye
- Giving away prized possessions
- Aggression

People who are considering suicide often display one or more of the following moods:

- Depression
- Loss of interest
- Rage
- Irritability
- Humiliation
- Anxiety

Suicide risk factors

Risk factors are characteristics or conditions that increase the chance that a person may try to take their life.

Health factors

- Mental health conditions
  - Depression
  - Bipolar (manic-depressive) disorder
  - Schizophrenia
  - Borderline or antisocial personality disorder
  - Conduct disorder
  - Psychotic disorders, or psychotic symptoms in the context of any disorder
  - Anxiety disorders
- Substance abuse disorders
- Serious or chronic health condition and/or pain

Environmental factors

- Stressful life events that may include a death, divorce, or job loss
- Prolonged stress factors that may include harassment, bullying, relationship problems, and unemployment
- Access to lethal means, including firearms and drugs
- Exposure to another person's suicide or graphic or sensationalized accounts of suicide

Historical factors

- Previous suicide attempts
- Family history of suicide attempts (AFSP Staff, 2021)

Talking to children about end-of-life issues

Many adults fear death and dying in the United States and often pass that fear along from generation to generation. Children may have their first dying and death experience with a pet. Their well-being and their concept of dying and death will be healthier if they can discuss all their feelings around the death and dying of their beloved animal. Death is commonly a complex topic for many parents, who also have their own attachments to the animal they are losing. It is also a trying topic for many veterinarians to feel comfortable talking about with parents.

The signs of grief that are generally accepted by the psychologic community for adults are:

1. Shock and denial
2. Pain and guilt
3. Anger and bargaining.
4. Depression, reflection, and loneliness
5. Vacillating between positive and negative emotions
6. Reconstruction.
7. Acceptance and hope.

Symptoms of grief in children:

1. Many of the same ways as adults but often shortened with some differences, denial, then crying, bewilderment, anger, guilt, depression, and attempts to rationalize loss.
2. More common with children, fear of abandonment, nightmares, insomnia, and anger toward siblings or playmates.
3. They can develop learning problems, anxiety, guilt from "Magical Thinking." Often, children do not tell the parents or other adults about their grief.

There is no order to grief—As in adults, grief can jump from stage to stage. Children may go through all or just a few, or seemingly none. Issues revolving around death may repeat as their brain ages. Younger children are much more reality-based, they are not cognitively advanced in their thinking as adults are, and their brains are still maturing, including memory and perception. Children to teens can also develop complicated grief (Nader, 2011).

Four cognitive stages for child development: infancy through adolescence

Cognitive age is a crucial factor in discussing death and dying of pets with children. As the child's brain matures and increases their perception of their world increases, we may change how we discuss death and dying topics with children. These are the primary cognitive stages as described by the psychologist Jean Piaget as they relate to death and grief (*disclaimer, not every child follows these general rules. Be sensitive to unusual circumstances regarding cognitive skills*).

Infants and toddlers (birth to 2 years)

Infants and toddlers are developing their understanding of their world with body movement and their senses, taste, touch, sight, smell, and hearing. Rational thinking is unlikely, and the concept of time is not likely in this age group. Infants are naturally egocentric and unable to see things from another person's viewpoint. Young children respond to their caregiver's emotions and physical changes in their environment. Children at this age do not understand the meaning of death. As they do not have an adequate death concept, they do not necessarily need to be present during either a conversation about palliative care or euthanasia unless the client wants them to be present. If they have a strong attachment to an animal, it is ok to have them there (Malik & Marwaha, 2021).

Preschoolers (2—5 years)

Magical thinking and fantasy predominate a child's thinking between the ages of 2—5, and they are also acquiring their fine motor skills. They tend to think about objects as if they were human, they are still egocentric, or have human traits. For instance, if a child's stuffed animal is left in the car overnight, he might worry that the stuffed animal is lonely or sad. Children of this age group feel and express their emotions deeply, and they may need additional support for their grief. Preschoolers often view death as temporary and reversible. Children in this age range may confuse death with sleeping or being away with the expectation that the animal will wake up at some later time or return. Preschoolers' thoughts are egocentric, and therefore they may equate or believe that death is a punishment for something they did or thought. Children these ages sometimes want to present during the conversation around death. Be very direct and straightforward in terminology and brief. For example, do not use put to sleep, as in, we are going to put your dog to sleep, instead use the term die or death, as in your dog is going to die, or has died. Answer questions directly, no euphemisms as they tend to confuse or scare children this age. Parents occasionally want the veterinarian to lie to a child to help "save their feelings". Lying to children is not recommended. Instead, discuss how important it is for children to feel included and that it can help them have a more healthy outlook on death and grief. Use recognizable life functions to help describe death, not breathing, etc. Children may ask the same question repeatedly. Children this age, because they are egocentric and still developing their experience with the physical world, will sometimes want to watch you give injections, or ask specific questions about the physical part of what you are doing (Malik & Marwaha, 2021).

School-age (6—11 years)

Children begin to comprehend logic between 7 and 12 and in a more concrete, less abstract way. They begin to lose their egocentricity and can start to see things from another person's perspective. School-aged children begin to understand the irreversibility of death and that they, or their parents, grandparents could also die. At this age, children may start to show interest in the biological aspects of death and the cultural events surrounding a death (i.e., funeral, wake, etc.). If the veterinarian is palliating the animal, giving school age children a task to participate in their animals final days can help them understand what the animal is going through, and may strengthen the bond between the pet, child and parent.

School-age children should be presented with a choice to be present or not during palliative discussions, or euthanasia. They may want to participate in the caregiving of a palliative patient or euthanasia. Veterinarians should encourage questions around the process of dying and death of their pet. Children may personalize death and may have nightmares about the death of the pet or family members. Children up to 8 years old may not need details of what you are doing. It may be better to say a little, then let them ask more. They may have concerns around the death of parents, themselves, and around their pet's death (Malik & Marwaha, 2021).

Tweens and teens (12—18 years)

The tween to teen develops abstract reasoning skills, and their logic skills improve as they age. At this stage, cognitive development continues through adulthood. At this developmental level, teens are beginning to think more like adults. Teens can comprehend not only the physical aspects of death but also the emotional impact of the loss. Teens should be part of the conversation regarding death and dying if they choose to. They understand the concept of death and often want to participate in the caregiving of a palliative pet. This age group should be encouraged to ask questions. Be wary of mental health issues, teens may be extremely attached to their pet, often having grown up with them, and euthanasia of a pet may be an inciting event around suicide. Suicide ideation is a concern in teens for other reasons as well. Teens need more information than the other age groups. Teens are also testing limits, boundaries and independence, and the questions they may ask will reflect that. Teens may also not express any emotions or have outbursts of emotions at appointments, this is part of boundary testing. Veterinarians can help support the parents of teens by having a mental health professional referral (Malik & Marwaha, 2021).

At-home discussions with children

Initial discussions for hospice or palliative care can be a time to emotionally support children. Discussing the pet's situation in age-appropriate ways for each child involved and giving each child the ability to express their feelings can help them feel included in the conversation about their pet.

Ask the parent's permission to talk with the child directly about end-of-life issues. If possible, get on the child's level. Talk openly with the child. Discuss planning or a euthanasia in age-appropriate terms. Discussions with the parents can happen while talking to the child regarding the process and planning. If discussing euthanasia, give the child permission to be present or leave as they feel they need to and provide them with support in making the comfortable choice for them.

The bond with a pet is forever. Part of a child's reintegration is continued connection with the pet and what it meant in their lives. Connection to the pet may occur in dreams. Adding rituals or other ways of memorializing the pet can help them continue their association. Children may re-grieve as they get older and their brain develops further.

"Prepare for death. If you can help the children deal with their feelings about it (the death), it becomes natural to them" (Atkins, 2015).

Memorializing

There are many ways to help a family memorialize their pet. Some suggestions that the author includes are journaling, photo albums, scrapbook, writing stories, candle lighting rituals, and setting up a special place in the home to memorialize. Burial, scattering of ashes, or memorial service for the pet can help support the grieving process for both parent and child. Giving flowers to clients, paw prints, or locks of hair that are lovely commemorative items may cherish them. Art therapy can also help children and adults with their emotions around grief.

Adult support: finding mental health professionals to help you help clients

Whether people have "typical" or complicated grief mental health professionals utilize tools to support people through their grieving process. Having a questionnaire with the initial consultation may help you identify who may need help (or have a mental health professional you work with and help them identify a more complicated situation). Veterinarians working with a mental health professional can create a questionnaire to help identify mental illnesses you may be dealing with and factors that may indicate they might develop complicated grief.

Having back up with pet loss support groups may not be enough support for some people. Check with your local resources. In addition, the US states, Canada, and Great Britain provided links to mental health information for further services.

Alabama- http://www.mh.alabama.gov/UT/FindServices.aspx.

Alaska—http://dhss.alaska.gov/dbh/Pages/default.aspx.

Arizona—https://dcs.az.gov/services/prevention-and-family-support/behavioral-health-services.

Arkansas—http://humanservices.arkansas.gov/dbhs/Pages/default.aspx.

California—http://www.dhcs.ca.gov/services/mh/Pages/default.aspx.

Colorado—https://www.colorado.gov/pacific/hcpf/behavioral-health-organizations.

Connecticut—http://www.ct.gov/dmhas/site/default.asp.

Delaware—http://www.dhss.delaware.gov/dhss/dsamh/mental_health_cmhc.html.

Florida—http://www.floridahealth.gov/programs-and-services/wic/health-providers/index.html.

Georgia—https://dbhdd.georgia.gov/providers.

Hawaii—http://health.hawaii.gov/amhd/.

Idaho—http://healthandwelfare.idaho.gov/Medical/MentalHealth/tabid/103/Default.aspx.

Illinois—https://www.illinois.gov/hfs/MedicalProviders/behavioral/Pages/default.aspx.

Indiana—http://in.gov/fssa/dmha/2578.htm.

Iowa—http://dhs.iowa.gov/ime/members/find-a-provider.

Kansas—https://kdads.ks.gov/commissions/behavioral-health.

Kentucky—https://dbhdid.ky.gov/ProviderDirectory/ProviderDirectory.aspx.

Louisiana—http://dhh.louisiana.gov/index.cfm/subhome/10/n/328.

Maine—http://www.maine.gov/dhhs/ocfs/cbhs/provider-list/home.html.

Maryland—https://health.maryland.gov/ohcq/mh/Pages/Home.aspx.

Massachusetts—https://www.mass.gov/orgs/massachusetts-department-of-mental-health.

Michigan—http://www.michigan.gov/mdhhs/0,5885,7-339-71550_2941_4868_4899-178824–,00.html.

Minnesota—https://mn.gov/dhs/people-we-serve/adults/health-care/mental-health/programs-services/.

Mississippi—http://www.dmh.ms.gov/providers/.

Missouri—https://dmh.mo.gov/docs/mentalillness/providerdirectory.pdf.

Montana—https://dphhs.mt.gov/amdd/Mentalhealthservices.aspx.

Nebraska—http://dhhs.ne.gov/behavioral_health/Pages/beh_mh_mh.aspx.

Nevada—http://dpbh.nv.gov/Programs/ClinicalBehavioralServ/Clinical_Behavioral_Services_-_Home/.

New Hampshire—https://www.dhhs.nh.gov/dcbcs/bbh/centers.htm.

New Jersey—http://nj.gov/humanservices/dmhas/home/hotlines/MH_Dir_COMPLETE.pdf.

New Mexico—http://www.hsd.state.nm.us/Behavioral_Health_Services_Division.aspx.

New York—https://www.omh.ny.gov/.

North Carolina—https://dma.ncdhhs.gov/providers/programs-services/mental-health/Behavioral-Health-Services.

North Dakota—https://www.nd.gov/dhs/services/mentalhealth/.

Ohio—http://mha.ohio.gov/Default.aspx?tabid=347.

Oklahoma—http://apps.okhca.org/providersearch/.

Oregon—https://www.mhaoforegon.org/resources/mental-health-providers/.

Pennsylvania—https://dbh.dc.gov/page/list-community-based-service-providers.

Rhode Island—http://www.bhddh.ri.gov/mh/index.php.

South Carolina—http://www.ddsn.sc.gov/consumers/findaprovider/Pages/QualifiedServiceProvidersList.aspx.

Tennessee—http://www.tennessee.gov/behavioral-health.

Texas—https://dshs.texas.gov/mentalhealth.shtm.

Utah—https://medicaid.utah.gov/mental-health-services.

Vermont—http://cvmhp.org/.

Virginia—http://www.dbhds.virginia.gov/individuals-and-families/licensed-providers.

Washington DC—https://dbh.dc.gov/page/providers.

Washington State—https://www.dshs.wa.gov/bha/division-behavioral-health-and-recovery/mental-health-services-and-information.

West Virginia—http://www.dhhr.wv.gov/bhhf/Pages/default.aspx.

Wisconsin—https://www.dhs.wisconsin.gov/regulations/mentalhealth/providerinfo.htm.

Wyoming—https://health.wyo.gov/behavioralhealth/mhsa/treatment/cmhc/.

Canada—https://www.canada.ca/en/health-canada/services/first-nations-inuit-health/non-insured-health-benefits/benefits-information/mental-health-counselling-benefits/guide-mental-health-counselling-services-first-nations-inuit-health.html.

Canada—http://www.ementalhealth.ca/Canada/Mental-Health-Providers/index.php?m=heading&ID=129.

Great Britain—http://directory.independent.co.uk/mental-health-services/in/great-britain.

Adult and youth support books

> ### Books you can offer to parents for ages 2—12
>
> Boo I'll Always Love You by Hans Wilhelm (Ages 2—6)
> For Every Dog An Angel by Christine Davis (all ages)
> Heal Your Grieving Heart for Kids by Alan D. Wolfelt, Ph.D. (adult)
> Annie Loses Her Leg but Finds Her Way by Sandra J. Philipson (Hospice)
> The Legend of the Rainbow Bridge by William N. Britton.
> The Rainbow Bridge by Niki Behrikis Shanahan
> Jasper's Day by Marjorie Blain Parker illustrated by Janet Wilson (6—10)
> Saying Goodbye to Lulu by Corinne Demas
> Annie and the Old One by Miska Miles (Ages 6—12)
> The Day Tiger Rose Said Goodbye by Jane Yolen, illustrated by Jim LaMarche (6—9)
> Dog Heaven by Cynthia Rylant (4—11)
>
> **Books for teens** My Grief Journal: for grieving teens (offers the opportunity to draw or write about memories and feelings after death) OUR HOUSE. Ages 11—18.
> Healing Your Grieving Heart for Teens: 100 Practical Ideas Alan D. Wolfelt, Ph.D. Ages 12—18
> Straight Talk about Death for Teenagers: How to Cope with Losing Someone You Love. E. Grollman, Boston: Beacon Press, 1993. (AD).
> The 10th Best Thing About Barney by Judith Viorst (4—9)
>
> **Books for adults** Goodbye, Friend: Healing Wisdom for Anyone Who Has Ever Lost a Pet by Gary Kowalski
> Losing My Best Friend: Thoughtful support for those affected by dog bereavement or pet loss by Jeannie Wycherley
> The Grief Recovery Handbook for Pet Loss by Russell Friedman.
> When Your Pet Dies: A Guide to Mourning, Remembering, and Healing. By Alan D Wolfelt Ph.D.
> When Children Grieve: For Adults to Help Children Deal with Death, Divorce, Pet Loss, Moving, and Other Losses by John W. James.

Grief in animals

It is worth mentioning in the section about grief, that grief does seem to occur in animals. And there is a growing body of literature that shows various species do grieve for one another. It is the observation of the author that other animals in the household will also grieve for housemates. A recent example was a kitty named Cookie. Cookie was not doing well, quite dehydrated, and no longer moving, and when the author got there, the other kitties in the household seemed to be holding vigil all around Cookie. There were 6 other kitties in the room, however only Blob (Cookie's son) and Cookie's niece were on the bed with him. The other kitties were in various spots in the periphery of the room. At the time, Blob would not look at Cookie, instead laying at the end of the bed facing away from him, whereas his niece laid down on top of Cookie as he slept with medication and as Cookie died. Animals, like children, should be given the space they need to participate. It may help them with their grief (Figs. 9.1 and 9.2).

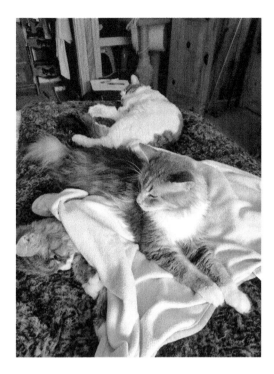

FIGURE 9.1

Cookie, Cookie's niece (on top of Cookie) and Blob (Cookie's son on the end of the bed)
Tromborg cats

Photo by Dr. Lynn Hendrix Copyright 2021. Used with permission from Chris Tromborg. 2021.

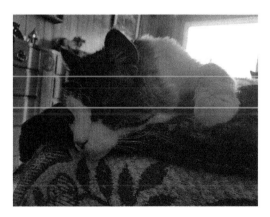

FIGURE 9.2

Blob did not want to look at Cookie or us.

Photo by Dr. Lynn Hendrix copyright 2021. Used with permission from Chris Tromborg. 2021.

References

AFSP Staff. (2021). Risk Factors and Warning Signs. *American Foundation for Suicide Prevention*. https://afsp.org/riskfactors-and-warning-signs. (Accessed 15 November 2021).

Atkins, M. J. (2015). *Martha Beck radio show. (M. Beck, interviewer).*

Boelan, P. A., van den Bout, J., & de Keijser, J. (2003). Traumatic grief as a disorder distinct from bereavement-related depression and anxiety: a replication study with bereaved mental health care patients. *American Journal of Psychiatry, 160*(7), 1339–1341.

Bonanno, G. A. (2001). The varieties of the grief experience. *Clinical Psychology Review*, 705–734.

Bonanno, G. A. (2008). Trajectories of grieving. In *Handbook of bereavement research and practice: Advances in theory and intervention*. Washington DC: American Psychological Association.

Doughty, E. A. (2009). Investigating adaptive grieving styles: A Delphi study. *Journal of Death Studies*, 462–480.

https://www.psychologytoday.com/us/blog/careers-in-psych/201603/choosing-between-phd-and-psyd-some-factors-consider, (2016–. (Accessed 11 November 2021).

Malik, F., & Marwaha, R. (2021). Cognitive Development, *E. StatPearls*. Treasure Island,Fl: StatPearls Publishing. https://www.ncbi.nlm.nih.gov/books/NBK537095/.

Martin, T. L. (2000). *Men don't cry…women do: Transcending gender stereotypes of grief.* Philadelphia: Brunner/Mazel.

Medicinenet.com Staff. (June 14, 2012). *Medical definition of complicated grief.* Retrieved from Medicinenet.com https://www.medicinenet.com/loss_grief_and_bereavement/article.htm.

Nader, K. a (2011). Complicated grief reactions in children and adolescents. *Journal of Child & Adolescent Trauma*, 233–257.

NAMI. (April 2020). *Types of mental health professionals.* Retrieved from National Alliance on Mental Illness https://www.nami.org/About-Mental-Illness/Treatments/Types-of-Mental-Health-Professionals.

Raypole, C. (2020). Disenfranchised Grief: When No One Seems to Understand Your Loss. *Healthline.* https://www.healthline.com/health/mental-health/disenfranchised-grief#finding-support, 2020. (Accessed 15 November 2021).

Rogalla, K. B. (2020). Anticipatory grief, proactive coping, social support, and growth: Exploring positive experiences of preparing for loss. *Omega, 81*(1), 107–129. https://doi.org/10.1177/0030222818761461

Shear, K. M., et al. (2011). Complicated grief and related bereavement issues for DSM-5. *Depression and Anxiety, 28*(2), 103–117. https://doi.org/10.1002/da.20780

Zisook, S. S. (2009). Grief and bereavement: What psychiatrists need to know. *World Psychiatry*, 67–74.

Further reading

Berman, R. (June 15, 2018). *The chance to text with the dead via AI is creepy or wonderful.* From bigthink.com https://bigthink.com/robby-berman/the-chance-to-text-with-the-dead-via-ai-is-creepy-or-wonderful.

Supporting a palliated death★

10

Lynn Hendrix, AA, BA, DVM, CHPV [1,2,3,4]

[1]*Owner, Veterinarian, Beloved Pet Mobile Vet, Davis, CA, United States;* [2]*Former Board of Directors, IAAHPC, Chicago, IL, United States;* [3]*Consultant, Hospice, Palliative Medicine, End of Life, VIN, Davis, CA, United States;* [4]*President, Founder, World Veterinary Palliative Medicine Organization, Davis, CA, United States*

Changing our definitions

The term natural death is in much of the current end-of-life animal literature. The author believes "natural" death is a controversial and inadequate term, much like the terms "organic" or "toxin". These perception of this term is vague and confusing to the public and veterinarians alike. To improve upon this term, the authors of the 2013 IAAHPC guidelines used "Hospice-Supported Natural Death". "Hospice-supported natural death" has become interchangeable with "Natural Death" by early adoptors in the palliative care and hospice field (Shanan, 2013). What does "Hospice-Supported Natural Death" mean? To begin unraveling the confusion, let's examine each term. To some veterinarians natural death is the same as an un-supported or unassisted death, while others interpret it to avoid emphasizing eutha-nasia as a means to death. Natural death is a term used in human law as a cause of death, a legal term defined as a death that occurs because of age or disease, not an accident or trauma (Staff of Merriam-Webster, 2020). It may be thought of as the non-hastened, non-prolonged, non-induced death, but what does that mean? (Selter,

---

★ "Natural death" is a controversial topic to discuss, so some clarifications before we continue. This chapter may evoke feelings of discomfort. Remember, the change in thinking about end-of-life care takes time and thoughtful study and early adopters. Not everyone will be immediately comfortable with this concept. That is ok. You may have to read this chapter more than once, and you may never feel comfortable with the idea of a palliated death that ends with the disease. And that is ok too. How-ever, you may run into a client who is not comfortable with euthanasia and to keep that animal from suffering through their dying process, you need to have additional support on how to accomplish a palliated death or have a conversation about it. Education on how to proceed and support the patient and the client in their decision-making can assist you in preventing unnecessary suffering of a dying patient. This chapter is meant to give you a broader perspective on helping an animal through their disease until death occurs or the client's choose euthanasia. All that said, there are undoubtedly acute diseases, such as gastric dilatation and volvulus, where bearing in mind, waiting would be inhumane, and euthanasia would be the only best option if surgery or medical intervention was not elected. The veterinary field considers euthanasia as the standard of care for end-of-life diseases. This chapter has been written with those parameters in mind.

Animal Hospice and Palliative Medicine for the House Call Veterinarian
https://doi.org/10.1016/B978-0-323-56798-5.00014-X

Persson, Risse, Kunzmann, & Neitzke, 2021). If palliative sedation is an inducement of pain management, and perhaps hastens death does "natural death" still apply? So is "natural death" or even "hospice-supported natural death", an ideal term?

"Hospice-supported natural death" was meant to convey a palliated "natural" death, one that was supported by a medical team to the conclusion of the disease as opposed to an unpalliated or unassisted passing or euthanasia provided at the end. "Palliative supported death" or "Palliated death" is more specific and may include animals who have euthanasia offered as an option to them. The medical team can then support the animal until death occurs, either because of the terminal end of the disease or with euthanasia. The palliative team must include a veterinarian as the medical director and may also includetechnicians and mental health professionals, preferably trained in animal hospice or veterinary palliative medicine. Henceforth, the term Palliated Death will be used in the following discussion.

Death is the natural conclusion of life

Death can occur from disease, age-related changes, malnutrition, hypo or hyperthermia, or trauma and may not be what veterinarians or clients consider an ideal or pain-free death (Ward, 2016). The dying process may be associated with pain, and other unpleasant symptoms, such as nausea, vomiting, diarrhea. Continuing with the disease unassisted may be challenging for a client to treat or emotionally deal with, especially without further education in end-of-life care.

Veterinarians may recommend euthanasia to a client, and there may be situations where the client does not want to proceed with euthanasia. The client may not believe in euthanasia due to religious or spiritual beliefs or may not perceive, understand, or mentally process what the veterinarian has evaluated and discussed with them. Veterinarians may wonder, "If the animal leaves against medical advice, will there be additional care for the animal, or will it suffer?" These are sources of concern for many veterinarians.

In addition, traumatic deaths are distressing for a client (or veterinarian) to watch and can cause complicated grief. Traumatic euthanasia may also cause emotional suffering and mental trauma for a client. The client who has witnessed a past traumatic euthanasia may choose a different path for their next pet. Terminal delirium is arduous to watch in humans and can be equally difficult to watch with beloved pets. By having an animal go home against medical advice and not palliating or having minimal palliation for these animals may create physical suffering for the pet and emotional suffering for the persons observing.

Death is the natural conclusion of life. It occurs with all life. Discussing death and dying with clients needs more clarification for clients. Educating clients on specific disease trajectories, disease progression, what to expect, what they can do for an emergency are topics that may help them make better and more informed choices. No client wants their animal to have an unpalliated death, although they do not always understand that likely means their animal will suffer. Clients more frequently state, "I don't want my animal to suffer", but do not understand what suffering really means, what it may look like for their individual pet. If theyare educated on what a palliated dying process can look like and that it will help them achieve that goal, then they are more likely to want additional support. They may ultimately help the animal have a peaceful death.

Utilizing veterinary palliative medicine at the end of life

Ethicists, moralists, and medical practitioners may argue the question of how death comes to us for years to come. Science and medicine have made enormous strides in understanding what happens to a body with disease and trauma and how we can intervene. The practice of medicine is about intervention. Medicine intervenes from birth to death and has the goal of averting death, and providing health and comfort. Palliative medicine continues intervention with advanced, progressive, chronic disease and terminal illness; however, the intent shifts. The goal shifts from health to comfort and support until euthanasia is provided for animals or the disease reaches its natural conclusion.

"Death is the endpoint of terminal illness, defined as a disease that will likely cause death" (Staff of MarieCurie.org.uk, 2020). Utilizing palliative medicine early in the diagnosis can help increase the quality of life and potentially extend life with better quality (Temel, 2010). The result of a palliated death, regardless of how the death occurs, is a better life for the time that they have left.

The physiology of death

To help support client's in making the best decision for their pet, understanding the dying process up to the occurrence of death can help veterinarians educate clients on their pet's needs and what is involved in nursing care as they proceed through the dying process. We do not know some of the mechanisms of death and are still studying the dying process. For example, the precise cascade in molecular biology that stops the body from functioning is still unknown. Cellular metabolism continues in many cells after death. There is more literature in human medicine on the physiology of death, and we will utilize the human experience and literature. We will begin with clinical signs of imminent death and then continue with the known physiology of dying.

Clinical signs of impending death

With people, there are two recognized phases of the dying process. The first phase may be called the pre-active period and may last from a few hours to a few weeks in humans. The observed (anecdotal) timelines in animals may be shortened compared to those in humans. We need more research to get better timelines for animals and whether palliation makes a difference in the timeline. Animals may have one or more of these clinical signs. Clients may consider euthanasia during the pre-active stage, as some animals can linger with these signs. These may also be changes that the client may want to call their veterinarian to discuss (in parenthesis are suggested writing for modified client communication for handout purposes).

Signs of the preactive phase of dying seen in animals may be:

1. *Withdrawal from the family, hiding more, leaving the room, not wanting as much attention (client communication tip: this seems to be a key sign for considering euthanasia for many families).*
2. *Increased sleeping patterns (they are staying asleep for extended periods).(Or decreased awake times.)*
3. *Increased lethargy (they are not as active when they are awake).*
4. *Breathing changes, some apnea can occur (see the chart in the active phase of dying for different breathing patterns.) (Client communication tip: show them what the breathing pattern might look like).*
5. *Decreased appetite, withdrawal of food intake (appetite decreases first, before decreased fluid intake, may not eat for days to weeks before death so it may be a poor qualifier to make a decision about letting them die a death from their disease).*
6. *Diminished fluid intake, withdrawal from drinking (second to* occur post appetite loss, *usually occurs within a day to a few days preceding to passing, though there is no predictability of death occurring-can be a short time, maybe longer).*
7. *Decreased to absent ability to heal from wounds, or infections (bedsores can become a problem during this time, tumors may start oozing or* rupture).
8. *Edema of extremities or the entire body (peripheral edema can occur as the kidney function declines, protein levels decrease, and lymphatic or circulation changes occur. Client communication tip: this may be a time to consider euthanasia).*
9. *Humans will start reporting glimpses of heaven and seeing people that are not there (often deceased family members). While animals cannot say what they are witnessing to us, there is often a vacant look, staring into space for more extended periods as they get closer to death (client communication tip: if they are noticing this, it may be time to consider euthanasia, and they can also know that the animal is getting closer, within days to a couple of weeks).*
10. *Weight loss is common as animals approach death (usually due to decreasing intake of nutrients, loss of muscle mass, fat, and increasing cytokines from tumors).* (Staff of HPA, 2018).

Active signs of death occur a few hours to a few minutes before death occurs in animals. Things can also change rapidly. They may have one or more clinical signs.

The clinical signs active dying is happening are:

1. Comatose or stuporous state. The animal is only responsive to noxious stimuli (painful) or not responsive at all. They will quickly return to the semicoma state from the noxious stimuli (painful stimuli such as a toe pinch, a powerful smell). They may become agitated and vocalize with no stimulation.
2. *Severe agitation (can be terminal delirium).*
3. *Brain stem breathing patterns—more extended periods of apnea, Apneustic, Cheyne–Stokes, agonal breathing (client communication tip: Call all abnormal breathing patterns, brain stem breathing. Using the term agonal breathing often makes people believe their animal is painful or in agony).*

—cont'd

---

4. *Open-mouth breathing can occur (most common in cats at the end of life, but can also be seen with dogs in severe respiratory failure).*
5. *Pulmonary edema (client communication tip: also called death rales, owners may have heard this term).*
6. *Increased viscosity of saliva, causing increased upper airway stridor (client communication tip: called the death rattle in people).*
7. *Inability to swallow fluids (generally not taking food or water at this point, which is expected in the progression of dying).*
8. *Urinary or bowel (or both) incontinence.*
9. *A marked decrease in urine output and often darkening of urine, brown or red.*
10. *Blood pressure drops (though we may not take it in animals, this occurs in humans and is likely to occur in animals).*
11. *Extremities cool, feet, limbs, and ears may be very cool to the touch and may become mottled, dusky, or bluish. The color change may be difficult to see unless the skin is usually pink (e.g., cat nose, cat pads, pinna, even gums sometimes, can also occur in dogs with pink skin).*
12. *Their body may stiffen, their head may contract towards their spine in the final moments of death if they are not euthanized. There may also be gasping-like breaths, these are brain stem reflexes.*

They can get "jaw drop," though it is more common to see in humans than animals (in the author's clinical experience) (Staff of HPA, 2018).

Animals may show some or all these signs before dying. Educating clients on these clinical signs, instructing them to contact the veterinary office, and using their crisis medications can help them get through these phases.

Pathophysiology of death

Depending on the type of disease the animal is dying from, the early cellular changes may differ from patient to patient. However, in the active phase of dying, a series of biochemical and physiologic changes occur.

Cardiopulmonary

A cascade of cardiopulmonary and cerebral events happens as an animal goes into the active phase of dying. Each of the cascades will be discussed in separate sections, however, they can occur at the same time or because of each of the changes that occur. Acidosis, shock, altered oxygen and carbon dioxide with alterations in circulation, and cerebral changes may drive death. The dying animal may already be in a systemic metabolic acidosis due to their current disease, such as renal failure, diabetes ketoacidosis, severe diarrhea, or shock. They may have developed a respiratory acidosis if the animal has pneumonia, COPD, ARDS, pulmonary thromboembolism, or increased intracranial pressure. As the respiration rate starts decreasing in the dying animal, the increased CO_2 will begin to amplify respiratory acidosis. As both the metabolic and respiratory acidosis increases, the brain begins to lose consciousness and the brain stem will initiate Cheyne–Stokes breathing. O_2 levels continue to decrease with the decreasing respiratory rate.

As acidosis affects the cardiovascular system, peripheral blood vessels constrict, causing limbs and other peripheral areas to begin to cool. Humans get mottling of the skin, which may be noted on animals with little hair or pink skin but may not be noticed by clients (veterinarians may note muddy gum color). Tachycardia may occur as they become more hypotensive. Animals develop coolness of limbs due to peripheral vasoconstriction.

Third space fluid build up may have occurred with their disease, distending the abdomen, or may increase pleural effusion or peripheral edema. This may contribute to shock.

Animals may die from shock. There are four types of possible shock: hypovolemic shock, septic shock, obstructive shock, and distributive shock. These algorithms are for humans provided by medical doctors on The Calgary Guide found on their web page, https://calgaryguide.ucalgary.ca/, can help us review the kinds of shock we may encounter when dealing with an end-of-life patient. Hypovolemic shock is the most common type of shock seen with end-of-life patients (Fig. 10.1).

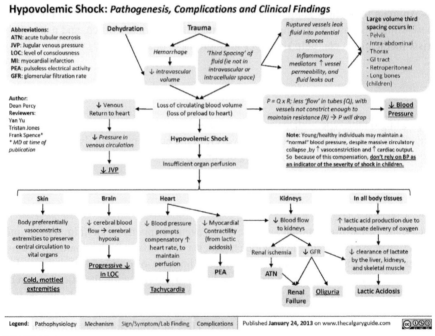

FIGURE 10.1

Hypovolemic shock.

An algorithm from The Calgary Guide, Authored by Dean Percy, reviewed by Yan Yu, Tristan Jones, and Frank Spence MD, and used with permission from The Calgary Guide. ©2021.

Hypovolemic shock may be the most common form of shock seen in many cancer, organ failure and dementia patients. As third spacing occurs, eating and drinking decrease with the disease, and fluids may be lost via vomiting, diarrhea, renal failure, and as dehydration take over; they may go down the pathway of hypovolemia. Animals who develop sepsis develop septic shock (Fig. 10.2).

Sepsis and septic shock may also contribute to the changes seen as animals go through the dying process. Bacterial translocation may happen as the animal's circulation decreases, cytokines are released, microclot formations may occur, the bowel slows, and the endothelium becomes permeable. Obstructive shock may occur with cardiac tamponade, pulmonary embolism, or a tension pneumothorax (clinical signs house call veterinarians are less likely to see but will include the algorithm for completeness) (Fig. 10.3). Distributive shock may occur with liver failure, pancreatitis, Addison's, and neurologic injuries (Fig. 10.4).

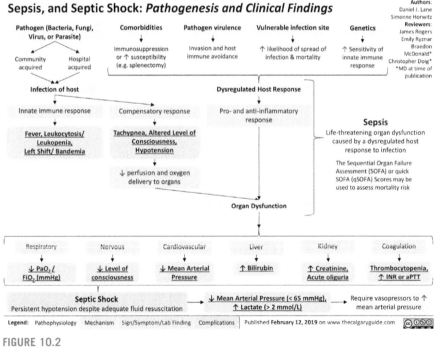

FIGURE 10.2

Sepsis, and septic shock.

Authored by Daniel J. Lane, Simmone Horwitz and reviewed by James Rogers, Emily Ryznar, Braedon McDonald MD, and Christopher Doig MD. Used with Permission from The Calgary Guide ©2021.

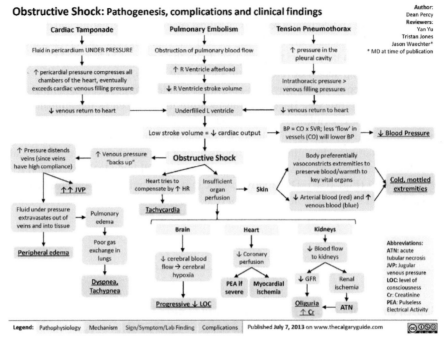

FIGURE 10.3

Obstructive shock.

Authored by Dean Percy and reviewed by Yan Yu, Tristan Jones, and Jason Waechter MD. Used with permission from The Calgary Guide© 2021.

Neurologic changes

As the circulatory system is declining, the brain becomes affected by the decreaing levels of oxygen and the increasing levels of carbon dioxide. Brain cells require a high level of oxygen to continue to function. With decreasing oxygen levels, there is a resulting increase in brain edema and intracranial pressure. The decreasing perfusion to the brain may result in either eventual herniation or further reduced blood flow and aseptic necrosis of the brain (Starr et al., 2021).

Altered oxygen and carbon dioxide levels

The brain cells become damaged as oxygen levels decline from hypoventilation (Starr et al., 2021). The carbon dioxide levels increase, and the level of consciousness will decrease as a result. As the level of consciousness decreases, clients may note with their animal either stupor or coma, or delirium (Starr et al., 2021). Humans can go down two different clinical neurologic paths as they approach death.

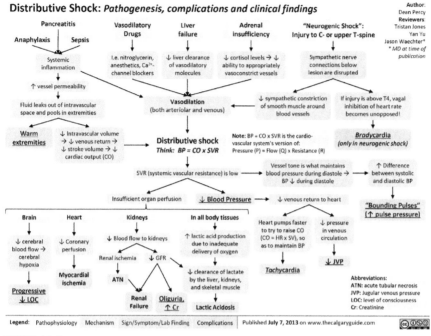

FIGURE 10.4

Distributive shock.

Authored by Dean Percy and reviewed by Tristan Jones, Yan Yu, and Jason Waechter MD. Used with permission from The Calgary Guide ©2021.

Increased sleep time may be one pathway for the brain to take as they progress toward death (Fig. 10.5).

Animals may get more lethargic, then obtunded, stuporous, and then unconscious, and then die. The other type of neurologic changes people experience follows a course of restlessness, confusion, tremors, hallucinations (we do not know if animals have this issue), myoclonic jerking, +/− seizures, semicomatose and comatose, and death (Starr et al., 2021). Hearing and touch are the last senses preserved documented with humans (Blundon et al., 2020).

Altered blood flow

Hypoxemia can lead to ischemia. Ischemia leads to anoxic brain injury and death (Starr et al., 2021). These two algorithms show the pathway to cellular death. A decrease in cardiac output, blood flow obstruction, or oxygen-carrying capacity reduction will result in ischemia, resulting in hypoxia or anoxia (Figs. 10.6 and 10.7).

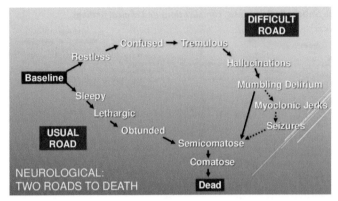

FIGURE 10.5

Neurological Two Roads to Death, one appearing peaceful , the other road appearing dramatic.

Slide created by Kyle P. Edmonds, MD, Palliative Physician Reproduced with Permission of Dr. Kyle Edmonds ©2021.

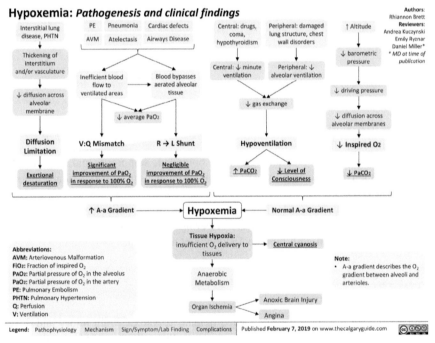

FIGURE 10.6

Hypoxemia.

Authored by Rhiannon Brett, reviewed by Andrea Kuczynski, Emily Ryznar, and Daniel Miller MD. ©2019 Used with permission from The Calgary Guide 2021.

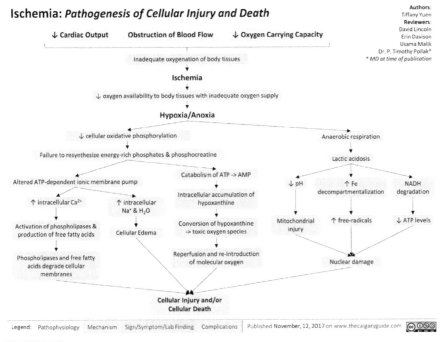

Ischemia: *Pathogenesis of Cellular Injury and Death*

Authors:
Tiffany Yuen
Reviewers:
David Lincoln
Erin Davison
Usama Malik
Dr. P. Timothy Pollak*
* MD at time of publication

↓ Cardiac Output   Obstruction of Blood Flow   ↓ Oxygen Carrying Capacity

Inadequate oxygenation of body tissues

Ischemia

↓ oxygen availability to body tissues with inadequate oxygen supply

Hypoxia/Anoxia

↓ cellular oxidative phosphorylation   Anaerobic respiration

Failure to resynthesize energy-rich phosphates & phosphocreatine   Lactic acidosis

Catabolism of ATP -> AMP

Altered ATP-dependent ionic membrane pump   ↓ pH   ↑ Fe   NADH
                                                              decompartmentalization   degradation

Intracellular accumulation of hypoxanthine

↑ intracellular Ca^{2+} ↑ intracellular Na^+ & H_2O

Activation of phospholipases & production of free fatty acids   Cellular Edema   Conversion of hypoxanthine -> toxic oxygen species   Mitochondrial injury   ↑ free-radicals   ↓ ATP levels

Phospholipases and free fatty acids degrade cellular membranes   Reperfusion and re-introduction of molecular oxygen   Nuclear damage

Cellular Injury and/or Cellular Death

Legend: Pathophysiology   Mechanism   Sign/Symptom/Lab Finding   Complications | Published November, 12, 2017 on www.thecalgaryguide.com

FIGURE 10.7

Ischemia.

Authored by Tiffany Yuen, reviewed by David Lincoln, Erin Davison, Usama Malik, and P. Timothy Pollak MD.
©2017 Used with permission from The Calgary Guide 2021.

Increased intracranial pressure

There can be multiple etiologies of increased intracranial pressure with the end-of-life patient. Primary or metastasis tumors may have increased intracranial pressure from the expansion of the mass, cerebral edema, increased cerebrospinal fluid, hypertension, increased intracranial blood flow, or clot formation (Pinto, 2021).

In addition, an animal can have a stroke, ischemic or hemorrhagic, that may also contribute to increased intracranial pressure (Pinto, 2021). Regardless of the etiology, increased intracranial pressure contributes to brain death (Starr et al., 2021).

Delirium

Terminal delirium in humans is associated with a declining consciousness, a change in cognitive ability, disturbance over time (minutes to hours), and a disease or medication that may alter brain function (Harris, 2007). In animals, these signs may manifest in vocalization, disorientation, consciousness changes. Terminal delirium can be exhausting or distressing for the caregiver family, and they may choose to help the animal with euthanasia at this stage. Decreasing acetylcholine and increasing dopamine may be the cause of terminal delirium (Moyer, 2010). The common differentials for humans are hypercalcemia, medications, hypoxia, prerenal azotemia, disseminated intravascular coagulopathy, hyperosmolarity, hepatic failure, infection, and damage to the CNS (Morita, 2001).

Summation of causes of terminal agitation in humans

Opioid toxicity: High or prolonged opioid administration can lead to sedation, neuroexcitation, and potentially agitated delirium.

Pain: Uncontrolled and severe pain can cause agitation; this should be ruled out. Note that communicating pain is difficult for cognitively impaired patients.

Drug interactions: Many drugs used in palliative care, such as hypnotics, antimuscarinics, and anticonvulsants, can cause agitation.

Fever or sepsis: The onset of delirium can occur with fever (reducing cerebral oxidative metabolism).

Hypercalcemia: Hypercalcemia is the most common life-threatening metabolic disorder in cancer patients. It can lead to a confused and agitated state, so calcium levels should be monitored.

Raised intracranial pressure: Brain tumors or cerebral metastasis can increase intracranial pressure, leading to an agitated state (Chand, 2013).

Haloperidol is commonly used in humans for terminal delirium. It is primarily a dopamine antagonist and has α1-adrenergic, histaminergic, and cholinergic antagonist properties. As Haloperidol is similar to phenothiazines in the mechanism of action, acepromazine, a veterinary approved medication, may also help with terminal delirium though it is not labeled for terminal delirium. If unable to resolve signs of terminal delirium, then euthanasia or palliative sedation should be utilized. Caregivers of terminal patients may become distressed when caring for a terminal delirium patient (Morita, 2007).

Owners need a crisis kit (discussed later in this chapter) to minimize the amount of time that the animal might be experiencing these issues. The crisis kit should include detailed instructions on how, when, and the technique to give each medicine. It is harder to say that the animal is experiencing discomfort or pain during delirium, but it is undoubtedly difficult for the caregivers to witness.

Palliated death

Supporting your client as well as the patient in a palliated death is of the utmost concern and in supporting the client, you will help them support the patient. Checking in with clients at frequent intervals, ensuring the animal is receiving medication, having the pet's medical needs met, and supporting and educating the client on the clinical signs as they approach death. If they are chosing to have the animal die of their disease, the animal may need increasing nursing support, especially if it needs palliative sedation. Palliative sedation may require 24 hour care, which is most commonly done in a 24 hour practice. If you are advanced enough in your end-of-life care practice to have 24 hour care, it may be done in the home. Veterinary nurses can provide additional support for treatments and be another person helping to support the patient. Before palliative sedation is instituted, clients may consider euthanasia.

It may be difficult for some veterinarians to understand why an client would want to provide a palliated death to the end of the disease. Palliated death occurs with humans, and some people may feel they have had loved ones suffer. Significant concerns about animals are that they will also suffer. Understanding why people choose assisted death (euthanasia) for themselves and how often they choose assisted death might help a client or a veterinarian understand the difference between a euthanasia decision versus a supported palliated death decision. The author finds for her clients and patients that euthanasia tends to fall along the same percentages. Very few people choose a palliated death from the disease, and almost all choose euthanasia once they understand the difference between dying and death, palliative sedation vs euthanasia drugs. Assisted death in humans (or euthanasia) occurs in less than 1% of people who die, in Oregon, 0.21% from a statistic in 2013, and in Washington State, 0.23% in 2012 (Figs. 10.8 and 10.9) (Staff for ANAS, 2018).

For those who choose assisted death in humans, about 32%−38% of the individuals that chose to seek medication had inadequate pain control or other disease-related symptoms, according to the 2020 Oregon Death with Dignity Act Annual report. More people choose assisted death due to loss of autonomy issues at 93%, which may also be consistant the choice of euthanasia for similar situations, like mobility issues, incontinence (Public Health Division, Center for Health Statistics, 2021). According to one study, 1 in 70 patients leave acute care against medical advice(AMA).(Ibraham et al., 2007). There are no studies found to look at how many animals leave AMA. In the author's experience, is was a higher percentage for animals in the emergency room. For animals who go home against medical advice or never seek medical advice, the number of animals who haveinadequate pain control is likely much higher than the number in the Oregon statistics for people.

The author postulates a smaller percentage of pets will suffer at the end of their life if we advance the pet-owning public's interactions with palliative medicine-trained veterinarians. Whether the clients decide on euthanasia or a palliated death, refining veterinarian's palliative medicine skills can make a difference and should be a part of the veterinary curriculum.

The education of caregivers on their journey with their animal's disease and the journey with which the animal will progress through their disease is paramount. It is also vital for caregivers to understand how much time will be needed in nursing care to help the animal be comfortable. Caregivers need to be educated how the disease will progress through the body and the disease trajectory that the animal may be on and what they can do to keep the animal comfortable during the progress. The disease itself and the animal's journey may be complicated, fraught with pain, distress, discomfort, and increased nursing care. If veterinarians follow what palliative

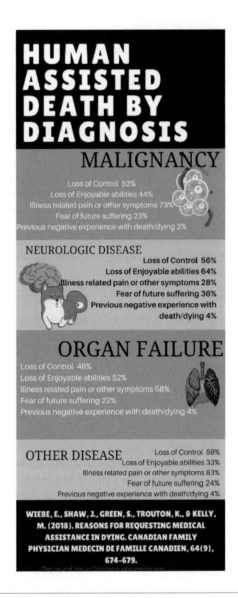

FIGURE 10.8

Human-assisted death by diagnosis.

Created on Canva by Author: Lynn Hendrix ©2021, Information from Canadian Family Physician, Authors E. Wiebe, J. Shaw, S. Green, K. Trouton, M.Kelly, ©2018.

medical doctors do to treat humans, pets may end up being hospitalized for palliative sedation to provide comfort and caregivers would need to be prepared for that eventuality.

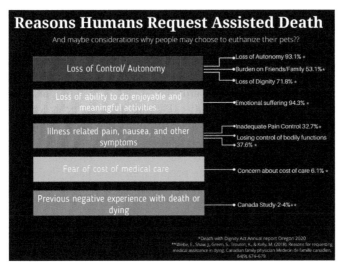

FIGURE 10.9

Reasons humans request assisted death.

Created on Canva by Author Lynn Hendrix ©2021, Statistics from the 2020 Oregon Death with Dignity Annual Report and, Information from Canadian Family Physician, Authors E. Wiebe, J. Shaw, S. Green, K. Trouton, M.Kelly ©2018.

Palliative sedation

A controversial topic among veterinarians, palliative sedation, is the active sedation of an animal to minimize pain and maintain minimal consciousness. Palliative sedation needs 24-h care and may not be adequately performed in a home setting without additional equipment, staff, and cost to the client. Caregivers need to be prepared and educated on giving extensive nursing care, cost, and length of time it may take to provide adequate palliative sedation. The author's experience is that once clients are educated on all the nursing challenges, medications, potential side effects to medications and what they may witness, they are less likely to proceed with palliative sedation, chosing euthanasia instead. However, there may be some religious beliefs that may make it challenging for them to consider euthanasia. There may also be locales in the world where the general population does not consider euthanasia as appropriate for their pets and supporting their veterinarians with palliative sedation techniques may minimize end of life suffering for those pets.

Holding vigil

Another concept in human medicine that may occur with a veterinary palliated death is the concept of holding vigil. The tradition of "keeping a vigil" or "holding vigil" when someone is dying occurs because we do not have an exact timeline and want to be present for the dying person or animal. Humans' timeframe can be days to weeks for the preactive phase of dying, and the active phase may be hours to days. The statistics are hard to find for timelines in animals. Anecdotally, the author observes they are shorter for animals. Caregivers may notice the other animals in the house, keeping vigil or behaving differently towards the animal as they progress through their dying process. As other animals start exhibiting different behaviors toward their housemates, caregivers may note that things are changing with the ill animal. If the caregiver wishes to "be there" with their loved one when death occurs, keeping a vigil at their beloved's bedside can be part of their emotional and grieving process. This can also be a difficult time for people with anticipatory grief and feelings around euthanasia. Caregivers may elect euthanasia if the process is prolonged or there is a need for palliative sedation.

In a semicomatose state, the dying animal may be able to hear, even if they do not respond (this seems to be true for humans with near-death experiences as well) (Staff of IANDS.org, 2017; Blundon, Gallagher, & Ward, 2020).

Planning for imminent death

If the client wants to continue palliative treatment to the conclusion of the disease, education of the client on what to do for their pet showing clinical signs of dying is an integral part of a palliated death. The housecall veterinarian may be intimately involved in the education and planning of their imminent death. A veterinary nurse or other caregivers can keep the veterinarian updated on the progression of the disease so that adjustments can be made to medications and other treatements. Giving the caregivers tools to help them assess the progression of their animal's disease is practical and empowering.

To provide a palliative death, planning for emergencies are essential. Creating a crisis kit, planning for palliative sedation if needed, and providing a plan for additional symptom management as they progress. There are some medications that should be used with caution that may cause distress in the patient's final days. For example, it may not be necessary to continue an appetite stimulant, or fluid therapy if the animal has stopped eating, or is retaining fluids and is near death. Giving medicines to the patient can also be challenging, especially if they are not eating. Consider switching to oral medications mixed with honey or Karo syrup to ease the act of giving the medication. Nasal drop preparations, transdermal pharmaceuticals, and injectables that can be given subcutaneously (SQ) to be provided by the caregiver to help alleviate clinical signs. IV drips with pain medications may be needed for severe and unrelenting pain and may need 24 hour monitoring.

As the animal enters the active phase of dying, relieving the distressing signs is significant for both patient and client. Pain, dyspnea, and congestion can be among the active phase signs to treat. The modified WHO cancer pain ladder may help determine the need for certain medications (Fig. 10.10).

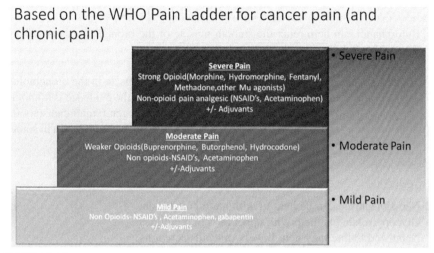

FIGURE 10.10

Modified WHO Pain Ladder slide created by Dr. Lynn Hendrix .

Adapted from the WHO Cancer Pain relief ladder from World Health Organization. (1986). Cancer pain relief. World Health Organization. https://apps.who.int/iris/handle/10665/43944 publication on page 19. Used with permission from the World Health Organization, 2021. Please note that WHO cannot verify the accuracy, cannot approve the content, and takes no responsibility for the adaptation.

Medications to have on hand for imminent death

Have a list of 24-h pharmacies to prescribe to or leave a crisis kit.

For pain:

1. Methadone injectable (best used for severe pain), or,
2. Morphine/hydromorphone injectable (best used for severe pain) (these can cause vomiting) or,
3. Fentanyl patches (not optimal, as it takes 12—24 h for full effect and the circulation is peripherally vasoconstricting in the dying patient, and therefore, it may be variable in efficacy).
4. Butorphanol injectable (but must give frequently, and often not adequate for anything but mild pain but is useful for sedation. Should be used in conjunction with other medications).
5. Buprenorphine (transmucosal or transdermal or injectable) is often used with cats and pocket pets. Best used for mild or moderate pain.
6. Gabapentin is used in conjunction with other medications for neuropathic pain. Best for mild to moderate pain.

Dyspnea

1. Butorphanol can help relax the smooth muscle of the bronchi for dyspneic patients. May help with air hunger.
2. Other opioids (see earlier discussion).
3. Magnesium sulfate nebulized may help relax smooth muscle in the bronchioles.
4. Nebulized furosemide may help decrease edema though the evidence is minimal.
5. Oxygen, either an oxygen concentrator or Pawprint oxygen (small canisters for short-term use) or compressed oxygen, which may be difficult to obtain in some states.

Congestion

1. Neo-synephrine can be helpful with nasal congestion.
2. Glycopyrrolate can help with upper airway secretions.
3. Nebulized Saline may help liquefy mucoid secretions.
4. Suctioning the nasal passage or back of the throat with a red rubber tube and syringe or a bulb syringe (may not be long enough for longer-nosed dogs).

Dry eyes and mouth

1. Artificial tears for eyes either drops q 1–2 h or ointment q 4–6 h to keep eyes from drying out.
2. Glycerin is helpful to keep the mouth moist q 1–2 h.

Restlessness/terminal delirium

1. Acepromazine
2. Benzodiazepines
3. Trazadone (may not be fast enough acting)
4. Haloperidol—not typically used with animals. Used in humans but may or may not be helpful for companion animals.

Antiemetics

1. Cerenia®
2. Ondansetron®
3. Both Cerenia® and Ondansetron®
4. Reglan®—Metoclopramide—can be a prokinetic as well.

IV or SQ fluids are contraindicated in the active phase of dying. They generally are not absorbed well in the final days due to a decrease in renal function and changes in circulation. They can create third space discomfort in the subcutaneous tissues, or intrathoracic or intraabdominally.

Post-palliated death
Client communications

The palliative support team may not be present at the time of death. Giving the client a list of postmortem changes they may witness can help them understand their beloved pet's transition after death has occured. Prior discussion about the body's care, the rituals they may wish to have performed, or what they may want to complete before body transport can help this transition progress smoothly. The clients may want to spend time with the body or want to have the crematorium come quickly. It is beneficial for the team to know the client's wishes before the death has occured, if they will assist in transporting to a crematorium or if the client wishes to bury the pet. Providing a list of crematoriums can also help caregivers make informed decisions on body care before the death of the pet.

Postmortem changes (0 min—2 h)

Discuss or give a whitesheet on postmortem changes with clients before the death occurs. Some clinical signs that may be noted before the death of the pet; eyes may stay wide open (for cats and brachycephalic dogs) or relax at "½ mast"-partially open (for longer snout dogs). The jaw may be slack; the tongue can fall out of the mouth. If the animal passes away, or with euthanasia, when moving a deceased patient, the veterinarian or the client should be cautious about cradling the head and neck. The client may note muscle fasciculations post-death. Occasionally, the animal will have a diaphragmatic twitch shortly after the heart has stopped, which will look like an "agonal" breath, the author uses the term gasp-like breath, or reflexive breath. This is similar to any other muscle twitch the caregiver may see. The animal will leak urine and sometimes will have a bowel movement as the gut muscles contract and the sphincters relax. It helps to have an absorbent item, such as a towel, diaper, or pee pad, to help catch urine and feces. Warn the caregiver that the animal's body might make a groaning sound if they move the animal postdeath, especially if the animal has been hyperventilating pre-death and developed aerophagia.

Postmortem changes (30 min—36 h)

Knowledge of post mortem changes may be important for clients who might want to keep the body for some time or have an animal die before euthanasia is performed.

Algor mortis—The body's cooling varies with the animal's size, obesity, covering (i.e., blankets), and ambient temperatures (Almuhim & Menezes, 2020). This timeline may be difficult to predict, but on average, the body cools about 1.5°F per hour until the body is at ambient temperature (Brooks, 2016). However, the author notes anecdotally that clients may notice body temperature changes fairly shortly after death, depending on the ambient temperature.

Livor mortis—Blood accumulation in parts of the body dependent on gravity and decomposing tissue/blood vessels (Brooks, 2016). It will cause a "bruising" appearance in the skin (Almuhim & Menezes, 2020). Livor mortis does occur in other parts of the body, notably the gums, lungs, heart, and abdominal viscera, though may not be noted by the caregiver (Brooks, 2016).

Rigor mortis—Stiffening of the body's muscles due to the depletion of ATP in muscle and build-up of lactate prevents the actin-myosin bond's release (Almuhim & Menezes, 2020). In smaller animals, thin animals, this can occur more rapidly than in larger, obese animals. Average times are 30 min to 24 h. Ambient temperature, obesity, electrolyte composition at the time of death can also affect rigor. Rigor mortis ends on average 24–36 h later due to the enzymatic breakdown of the bond (Almuhim & Menezes, 2020).

Unusual postmortem phenomena

Cadaveric Spasm is the phenomenon where rigor mortis occurs very quickly after death (within a few minutes). It is also sometimes called instant rigor mortis. Cadaveric spasm is very rare and is associated with a traumatic death in people (Brooks, 2016). Cadaveric spasm has been reported anecdotally with euthanasia in animals but is also exceedingly rare.

The Lazerus sign—The Lazarus sign has been observed with people who have been declared brain dead. They have been noted to raise and lower and cross their arms, have toe twitching, have facial twitches, and entire leg twitches. In euthanized animals, a similar phenomenon has been anecdotally reported. The author theorizes that euthanized animals are brain dead for all intents and purposes due to the medications used, yet they may still have circulation for a time after brain death. The Lazarus sign is also very rare in euthanized patients.

Postmortem (within a few minutes to days, months)

Desiccation—The drying out of tissues post-death. Most commonly noted by clients is the eye changes, immediately after death ("their eyes look different" is a typical comment). Skin will also undergo immediate changes but may not be as noticeable because of the fur (Brooks, 2016). Desiccation may continue depending on the environment the body is located.

Decomposition—Decomposition begins in some cells shortly after death. As cellular changes occur, the collapse of ion gradients and cell membrane cohesiveness drive early decomposition. As cells degrade, enzymes are released to nearby cells, causing a cascade of local decompensation. Bacteria then can proliferate and continue to degrade tissues, a phenomenon known as putrification (Brooks, 2016).

Bloating of the abdomen is noted approximately 4 days postdeath. There can be significant gas pressure build up in the abdomen, and rupture of the abdomen may occur. Hair loss can start to appear during this time period. These changes may be noted 1–21 days postdeath (Brooks, 2016).

Advanced decomposition occurs sometime between 3 and 18 days. The skin and muscle and other soft tissues begin disintegrating off of the skeleton, with less than ½ the skeleton showing. The abdomen that was previously bloated will collapse. Heat and insect activity will assist in the breakdown of the tissues. Sepsis, diabetes mellitus, and obesity are diseases that decrease the time of decomposition (Brooks, 2016).

Skeletonization occurs between 2 and 9 months, defined as more than ½ the skeleton showing through the soft tissues (Brooks, 2016). Skeletonization that has bleaching or exposure of cancellous bone occurs somewhere between 6 months and 3 years (Brooks, 2016).

Mummification can occur in locales with low humidity. Mummification does not go through the typical decomposition. Instead, the skin and tissues become dehydrated quickly, and autolysis and putrification may be delayed or absent (Brooks, 2016).

One final aspect to consider: What to do with the medical supplies and other equipment: Providing instructions on proper disposal of medications and needles may also help the transition time of grieving and is a form of grief support. Clients may also want a list of disposal options for regular prescriptions, and controlled substances, which may differ. Check with your regulatory body for further legal instructions on disposal of medication. Also, knowing where clients can donate blankets, pillows, beds, food and other animal-related materials can also be immensely helpful. Provide grief support information and suicide or crisis hotline information, and pet loss support before the client has lost their pet.

Conclusion

Palliated death due to the disease for animals is not a common occurrence in veterinary palliative care. Providing support for the clients and the animal can be time consuming and challenging for the house call veterinarian and the team. Still, it may provide comfort and support for some people due to religious, spiritual, personal beliefs, or regional customs. Some diseases are not suited for assisting the animal to the natural conclusion of their condition due to the increased risk of suffering. While other diseases that may die fairly rapidly and be well supported with little suffering may be able to be helped. Euthanasia is a difficult choice, but frank, open, educational discussions, including (1) what the people involved are going to have to handle emotionally and physically, (2) what the animal may experience as they go through their disease, and (3) what the owners may witness with the dying process and imminent death, are necessary to prepare for the supported end. The caregivers must be willing to intervene medically to make sure the animal is comfortable throughout their dying process. They need to be prepared to potentially have major changes in their lifestyle to achieve those goals set out by both the client and the veterinarian working together as a team. Finally, if they choose to proceed, palliative sedation should be considered with 24 hour supervision, most frequently done in the 24 hour hospital setting.

Checklist for the veterinarian caring for a palliative-supported patient (regardless of the death)

Basic needs of the client/caregiver

Establish the goals of the owner/caregiver

- What are their concerns, worries, and fears?
- What do they understand about their animal's disease?
  - Give education materials regarding the end of life of their animal's disease
- Death due to illness—palliated
- Death due to euthanasia
- Establish DNR status
  - Do they want rescue status?
  - Do they want a do not resuscitate status if the animal ends up in an emergency room?
- Establish where they would like the death to happen—usually at home
- Create a timetable for their disease
  - Stable disease—likely has at least a year to live
  - Unstable disease—likely has 6 months or less to live
  - Deteriorating disease—likely has 2 months or less to live
  - Final days—likely have 2 weeks or less to live
- Check in's (times can vary depending on the situation)
  - For stable patients, at least every 6 months
  - For unstable patients, at least once a month
  - For deteriorating patients, at least weekly
  - For final days patients—daily
- Educate and create a plan for the client on common clinical signs to monitor for the disease.
  - Signs with stable disease
  - Signs with unstable disease
  - Signs with deteriorating disease
  - Signs of final days
  - Imminent death signs
- Create an advanced directive for both the patient and the client
- Give written educational information

- Quality of life
- Chronic pain information
- Other symptom management
- Crisis information
  - Where to call if there is a crisis—ER, your practice, the regular doctor of veterinary medicine (RDVM).
- Assess the need for other support
  - Nursing support
- Mental health support
  - Assess coping skills of family
  - Address for possible unfinished issues with family
  - Assess need for increase social worker intervention through visits, telephone calls
  - Bereavement risk
- Grooming support
  - Local groomers who are knowledgeable in caring for elderly patients
    - Animals can lay down while being bathed
    - They recognize the signs of pain
- Respite support
  - Pet sitting support
    - Local petsitters who understand the needs of an elderly, frail patient
  - Family respite support
  - Housesitting/pet sitting
- Spiritual support
  - Assess for cultural beliefs and values, and beliefs about death and dying
  - Establish resource list
  - Education for staff to improve sensitivity for the spiritual needs of all clients
- Aftercare support
  - Review cremation services
  - Review other bodycare options
  - Review memorial items
  - Review grief services
    - Pet loss support hotlines
    - Online support
    - In-person local support

Patient needs

- Create a personalized plan for the patient
  - Consider pain management
    - Mild, moderate, or severe chronic pain, or unrelenting pain
      - Use validated pain scales to assess pain with clients
    - Acute pain

- Acute pain flare-up on top of chronic pain
- Review pain management at each point of contact
  - Review current dosing—what is the owner giving, how often, and at what dose?
  - Review need for additional medication
  - Review need for refills
- Consider other symptom management
- Bleeding
  - Where are they bleeding from?
  - Skin
  - Spleen
  - Liver
  - Kidney/urinary tract
  - GI
  - Pulmonary
  - Head/neck
  - Third space—abdomen, pericardium, pleural space
- Breathlessness/dyspnea
- Constipation
  - Straining
  - Frank blood in stool
  - Dark stool
- Carcinomatosis/metastasis
- Chronic renal disease
- Delirium
- Dementia
- Diarrhea
- Dysphagia
- Dysrexia
  - Anorexic
  - Hyporexic
- Fever/chill
- Frailty
- Hydration
- Hypercalcemia
- Lethargy
- Liver disease, end-stage
- Lymphatic disease
- Neuromuscular disease
  - Degenerative myelopathy
  - GOLPP
- Nutrition
- Osteoarthritis
- Pancreatic disease

- Seizures
  - How long are the seizures lasting?
  - How often do they have them?
  - When did they have the last seizure?
  - Medications prescribed
- Sleep/wake disturbances
- Urination
  - Are they incontinent?
  - Are they urinating frequently?
  - Are they not urinating? Or oliguric?
  - Straining to urinate
  - Blood in urine
- Vomiting/nausea
- Skin health
  - Monitor for redness, irritation, licking at pressure points
  - Monitor for ulcerations, "bedsores"
  - Monitor for insects, fleas, flies, maggots
  - Monitor for petechiae, ecchymosis
- Eyes, nose, throat, oral hygiene
  - Keeping the ENT moist
  - Checking for ulcers on eyes, oral mucosa
- Anxiety/terminal delirium
- Interventional therapies/client declines/approves
  - Feeding tubes
  - Epidural pain management
  - IV infusions
  - Joint infusions
  - SQ port placement
  - TENS unit
  - Urinary catheters
- Review symptom management at each point of contact
- Establish a crisis kit
  - Address the concerns of the client—what are they worried about, concerned about, what are they most scared about happening
  - Address what you are, the veterinarian, concerned about happening with this particular disease as it progresses toward death
  - Establish medications that will address those concerns if you are not available
  - Have specific instructions for each medication
    - when to use
    - what it is used for
    - how to give
    - how long it will last before they may have to redose
    - possible side effects of each medication

- Decide what you are comfortable giving and what your client is comfortable giving, oral, transmucosal, transdermal, and injections (recognize that not all clients will be able to give injections or want to).
- Equipment needs
  - Animal wheelchair (does the client need education?)
  - Splint
  - Orthotic device
  - Harness/sling
  - Stroller/wagon
  - Raised dishes
  - Rugs
  - Foot covers/toe grips
  - Diapers/pee pads
  - Syringes for feeding, water
- As they approach imminent death
  - Educate owners on the imminent death
  - Monitor for preactive dying signs (possibly hours to a week or two before death-often the time when nursing care increases, owners may elect euthanasia at this time)
    - Weakness and fatigue
    - Disorientation
    - Withdrawal from family
    - Dyspnea, especially with heart failure patients
    - Increased respiratory rate due to pain
    - Increased risk of decubitus ulcers
    - Decreasing urine output
    - Decreasing food and water intake (can go weeks without eating, can go many days without water)
    - May have difficulties swallowing
  - Monitor for active dying signs (sometimes minutes to a day or so before death)
    - Decreasing mentation
    - "Death Rattle"—thickening of secretions in the pharynx
    - Dyspnea in heart failure patients
    - Brain stem breathing to include Cheyne—Stokes breathing,
    - Pads, ears, and nose (if pink) may become dusky, mottled, or blue
    - Limbs and ears are cold to touch
    - Decreased to absent urine output
    - Terminal delirium—vocalizations
    - Tachycardia, hypotension

Team support

- Create team plan of care for patient and caregiver(s)

- Review the best plan of support for the client
- Review updated plans/timetable
- Triage
- Check-in with team daily
  - How did the caseload go?
  - Medication check
    - Follow up drug logs
    - Are files complete?
  - Any challenges? What could we do to improve?
  - Any wins? How did we support a family well?
- Check-in with team weekly
  - Assess client interactions
  - Difficulties that have come up with clients/patients
  - Challenges with team efforts
    - What could we do better?
    - How could we support each other in this situation?
  - Wins-what went right?
  - Shout-outs
    - Who felt good about a case? Tell us about it!
    - Recognition of fellow team member
  - Working together shout-outs—who felt great about the team effort?
- Check-in with team monthly
  - How has the month has gone for each individual?
  - Challenges we have not addressed?
  - What could we do better?
  - Ideas to improve?
  - Best experience this month?
- Referral letters—summary of palliative visits—should minimally include current physical problem list, assessment, plan.
- Follow up with the client—sympathy card, ashes, memorial items, 1-year follow-up
  - Follow up postdeath with RDVM with a record of death and any palliative information not already sent.

References

Almuhim, A. M., & Menezes, R. G. (2020). Evaluation of Postmortem Changes. *StatPearls*. Treasure Island, Fl: StatPearls Publishing. https://pubmed.ncbi.nlm.nih.gov/32119351/.

Blundon, E. G., Gallagher, R. E., & Ward, L. M. (2020). Electrophysiological evidence of preserved hearing at the end of life. *Scientific Reports, 10*(1), 10336. https://doi.org/10.1038/s41598-020-67234-9

Brooks, J. W. (2016). Postmortem changes in animal carcasses and estimation of the postmortem interval. *Veterinary Pathology, 53*(5), 929–940. https://doi.org/10.1177/03009858166 29720

Chand, S. (April 1, 2013). *Dealing with the dying patient - treatment of terminal restlessness.* Retrieved from The Pharmaceutical Journal https://www.pharmaceutical-journal.com/learning/learning-article/dealing-with-the-dying-patient-treatment-of-terminal-restlessness-and-agitation/11119466.article?firstPass=false.

Harris, D. (2007). Delirium in advanced disease. *Postgraduate Medical Journal,* 525–528.

Morita, T. T. (2001). Underlying pathologies and their associations with clinical features in terminal delirium of cancer patients. *Journal of Pain and Symptom Management,* 997–1006.

Ibraham, S. A., Kwoh, C. K., & Krishnan, E. (2007). Factors associated with patients who leave acute-care hospitals against medical advice. *American Journal of Public Health, 97*(12), 2204–2208. https://doi.org/10.2105/AJPH.2006.100164

Morita, T. A. (2007). Terminal delirium: Recommendations from bereaved families' experiences. *Journal of Pain and Symptom Management,* 579–589.

Moyer, D. (2010). Review article: Terminal delirium in geriatric patients with cancer at end of life. *American Journal of Hospice and Palliative Medicine,* 44–51.

Pinto, V. L. (2021). *Increased intracranial pressure.* Retrieved from StatPearls https://www.ncbi.nlm.nih.gov/books/NBK482119/.

Public Health Division, Center for Health Statistics. (2021). Oregon Death with Dignity Act 2020 Data Summary. *Oregon Health Authority Public Health Division, 23,* 1–17. https://www.oregon.gov/oha/PH/PROVIDERPARTNERRESOURCES/EVALUATIONRESEARCH/DEATHWITHDIGNITYACT/Documents/year23.pdf.

Shanan, A. C. (2013). *Practice guidelines.* Retrieved from IAAHPC.org: https://www.iaahpc.org/resources-and-support/practice-guidelines.html.

Staff for ANAS. (2018). *Statistics and figures.* Retrieved from Advocates for National Assisted Suicide https://advocacyfornas.weebly.com/statistics-and-figures.html.

Staff of HPA. (2018). *Signs and symptoms of approaching death.* Retrieved from Hospice Patients Alliance http://www.hospicepatients.org/hospic60.html.

Staff of IANDS.org. (December 14, 2017). *Characteristics of the near death experience.* Retrieved from IANDS.org https://iands.org/ndes/about-ndes/characteristics.html.

Staff of MarieCurie.org.uk. (2020). *What does terminal illness mean?.* Retrieved from mariecurie.org.uk https://www.mariecurie.org.uk/who/terminal-illness-definition.

Staff of Merriam-Webster. (2020). *Definition of natural death.* Retrieved from Merriam-Webster Dictionary https://www.merriam-webster.com/dictionary/natural%20death.

Starr, R., Tadi, P., & Pfleghaar, N. (2021). Brain Death. *StatPearls.* Treasure Island, FL: StatPearls Publishing. https://www.ncbi.nlm.nih.gov/books/NBK538159/.

Temel, J. E. (2010). Early palliative care for patients with metastatic non-small cell lung cancer. *The New England Journal of Medicine,* 733–742.

Ward, J. Y. (2016). Why animals die: An introduction to the pathology of aging. *Veterinary Pathology,* 229–232.

Further reading

Event Medicine. (2020). *Respiratory patterns and causes*. Retrieved from Event Medicine https://www.eventmedicinegroup.org/patientassessment.

Ferreira, P. (2018). The effects of death and post-mortem cold ischemia on human tissue transcriptomes. *Nature Communications, 9.* https://www.nature.com/articles/s41467-017-02772-x.

Marchetelli, B. (2020). The pathophysiology of dying. In *Veterinary clinics of North America: Small animal practice* (pp. 513–524). Elsiever.

Selter, F, Persson, K, Risse, J, Kunzmann, P, & Neitzke, G (2021). Dying like a dog: the convergence of concepts of a good death in human and veterinary medicine. *Medicine, Health care and Philosophy.* https://doi.org/10.1007/s11019-021-10050-3

Staff for Lexico. (2020). *Clinical death*. Retrieved from Lexico https://www.lexico.com/en/definition/clinical_death.

Staff of MarieCurie.org.uk. (January 3, 2017). *Recognising the deterioration/dying phase*. Retrieved from MarieCurie.org.uk https://www.mariecurie.org.uk/professionals/palliative-care-knowledge-zone/symptom-control/recognising-deterioration-dying-phase.

Staff for Virbac. (2020). *Euthasol euthanasia solution*. Retrieved from Drugs.com https://www.drugs.com/vet/euthasol-euthanasia-solution.html.

Verheijde, J. L. (2018). Neuroscience and brain death controversies: The elephant in the room. *Journal of Religion and Health*, 1745–1763.

Providing a gentle death- Euthanasia

11

Lynn Hendrix, AA, BA, DVM, CHPV [1,2,3,4],
Anthony J. Smith, BS, DVM, MBA, CHPV [2,5]

[1]*Owner, Veterinarian, Beloved Pet Mobile Vet, Davis, CA, United States;* [2]*Former Founding Board of Directors, President, IAAHPC, Chicago, IL, United States;* [3]*Consultant, Hospice, Palliative Medicine, End of Life, VIN, Davis, CA, United States;* [4]*President, Founder, World Veterinary Palliative Medicine Organization, Davis, CA, United States;* [5]*Owner/Veterinarian, Rainbow Bridge Veterinary Services, Hercules, CA, United States*

"Dying is a process, and the individual has a right to pass in an individual way. Our goal is peace and comfort, which you provided, not speed." Katherine Carlson DVM The decision to euthanize another being is one of the most complex decisions a person might make in their lifetime. Guiding a person through that decision may be equally difficult for both the caregiver and the veterinarian. A companion animal may be having a down day but may be better the next day. The clients may be struggling with a decision or have the decision compounded with guilt. They may be in denial or frozen in emotional indecision. There is usually so much more going on behind the decision than may be assessed in a short appointment. In addition, the animal's physical quality of life may not match the emotional quality of life or their will to live and the client or family perspective may be based on the emotional quality of life, whereas the veterinarian focuses on the physical. The psychology of end-of-life decision-making for animals could probably fill another book.

So many factors are involved in the decision to euthanize an animal, that this time is challenging for both pet, client and veterinarian. In addition to guiding a client's plan for euthanasia, veterinarians may have moral and ethical dilemmas, and this could be compounded with compassion fatigue, or career burnout. In the clinical setting, a euthanasia decision may feel rushed for the client. The client may drop off and not stay with their animal, or be a decision based on finances, which may be stressful on the veterinarian and the team. Veterinary education may not focus on euthanasia or any of the challenges it may present. Death is a challenging subject for people to discuss in many countries, and a euthanasia decision, may come with complex feelings like the feeling of playing God or that they are killing their animal if they choose euthanasia. For some veterinarians, it may feel like the antithesis of medical training, where we learn to save a life and vow to "do no harm."

When veterinarians have patients who have entered the end-of-life stage of care, the focus shifts; death is the eventual outcome, and providing palliation is only part

309

of our job. Providing a gentle death, relieving suffering, and preventing distress are other goals for veterinarians, especially those who are focusing on end-of-life care and euthanasia.

In-home euthanasia can provide an end-of-life service more intimate than the clinical setting. Sitting with people and their pet in a living room or a bedroom where stress levels are decreased can be a profoundly emotional and trusted time for both the veterinarian and the pet owner and even the pet themselves. Providing care in the home embodies the human—animal bond as it can allow for more time. Making euthanasia personalized nourishes a vital relationship between pet, family and veterinarian, which is just as important as the setting, or the medications involved.

The goal of euthanasia is to provide a gentle death. Euthanasia comes from two Greek words, "Eu"—which means good or easy and "Thanatos"—death (Merriam-Webster Dictionary, 2018). To make a good and easy death is not always easy. Adverse reactions such as, agonal or brainstem breathing, muscle twitching, excitatory phases with medication, seizures, can occur during euthanasia. A veterinarian wants to be able to facilitate and curate an gentle death for an animal, whether it is in the clinic or the home. There are two significant factors to consider: (1) what the owner experiences and (2) what the animal experiences.

The client's experience

In the author's experience, the decision to have an euthanasia performed for a beloved animal is not one that people come to lightly. In doing house calls, veterinarians will likely get into more depth about why a client has decided on euthanasia as compared to the clinical setting. Meeting people where they are, in their home, where they are emotionally, and being able to spend time with people where they are comfortable, allows them to share more, and allows the veterinarian to ask more questions. Issues that may come up around a euthanasia decision may relate to a lack of understanding of the disease, having waited for an extended time because of fear, loss of quality of life for the pet or the client, or both, concerns about waiting too long, doing it at the wrong time, the role of suffering, ability to observe and understand chronic pain, and their personal history with other animals, and other family members around death. Consulting with the family on these issues will help veterinarians guide them with a euthanasia decision.

The discussion about euthanasia may start in the first phone call or the first palliative consultation with the house call vet. The client's questions may revolve around the quality of life and how their experience is going to be, and the veterinarian's questions may revolve around the logistics of the situation into which you will be walking. Common questions the veterinarian might ask: Do they want to be present (most do), or are they considering leaving the room, the house? Are there going to be other family members present? Do they have people who need to get home before you schedule an appointment? Do they want music, candles, a paw print, help with something else? Do they need help with cremation services? Can someone help carry their beloved pet to the car? Do they want you to take the animal to the car before they have passed?

The questions clients might ask are: Ist it time, or how will I know it is time? Discussions around quality of life may take place before a euthanasia. They have questions regarding the medications, how you will use them, and how long it will take for each medication? Are you going to give the medication subcutaneously (SQ), intramuscularly (IM), or intravenously (IV)? Does it make a difference in time or efficacy if you give SQ versus IM or IV? Are you going to place an intravenous catheter? Will you be giving one injection or several? Do you give oral medications before you give any injections?

Included in the discussion will also be body care (in Chapter 12 Aftercare). You may have clients who have researched or discussed with other veterinarians in your area, so it is best to be prepared for questions of this nature and if you are just starting out, the questions tend to be the same questions for most people who call. If you have a team to answer questions, having common questions in your team handbook can help with training.

Discussing all the steps you are going to take can help alleviate concerns and start to set expectations. It is best to discuss the medications you will use, the route you will use, any concerns they have. The clinical signs that may arise from the medications is best discussed if an adverse reaction arises. Giving people a litany of possible adverse reactions, adds to their stress level. Giving some people multiple choices can be overwhelming. Other caregivers appreciate being able to choose what their animal experiences. The author usually gives two choices, for example, oral or injectable, fast or slow experience. The client also knows their pet better and may know how they may react to oral medications versus injections. As a result, they may be able to help you make a better experience for both the animal and the client. The client's perception of SQ versus IM versus IV injections or intraorgan injections could also be discussed. In general, the author finds the family typically wants to cause the least amount of distress possible for the animal. The client's knowledge of how their animals have reacted in the past with veterinary visits and anesthesia can also help the veterinarian make the pet's euthanasia a much calmer experience.

The animal's experience

Veterinarians also need to consider the experience of the animal. In the clinical setting, the animal's experience leading up to any medication given can be a stressor. Stressors may include, the drive there, the waiting room with other animals, being taken from the client for catheter placement, and the act of placing a catheter are all stressors that may occur before medication is ever given. To minimize stressors in the home setting, the author uses the mantra "sedate, anesthetize, then euthanize."

With this mantra, we can achieve a smooth transition from an alert animal to quiet and sedate, then asleep, and finally, death. It is a slower process than the clinical approach. However, unless caregivers specifically request one-step euthanasia, it is a gentler transition for the animal than just giving pentobarbital.

A word on sedation vs anesthesia. Sedation can start the process for the animal. The veterinarian can begin the process by giving oral medications in food, which is often a good experience for both the pet and the client or start with injectable sedatives, premedicating the animal and achieving a sleepy disposition. The choice of what to start with may depend on what experience the family wants and can also depend on the disposition of the animal. Sedation is classified as having some level of consciousness. By definition, even with heavy sedation, the animal has a nociception response. Minimally, sedation should be considered prior to any hospital or home setting induced stressor, such as a catheter to provide a better experience for the pet.

Anesthesia is classified as loss of consciousness without nociception (Wilson, 2017). Considering the patient's experience, it is crucial to sedate, anesthetize, and then euthanize. Heavy sedation is acceptable according to the terms of the AVMA for IV and intraorgan injections (Leary, 2018). However, let us consider that heavy sedation means they still respond to pain. Placing a catheter, a butterfly catheter, and injection into a vein or organ means that the animal will feel the effect and therefore feel discomfort or pain and may react negatively. In considering the animal's experience, the author believes anesthesia, creating unconsciousness and relieving the animal of pain perception, improves their overall experience. This concept is different than the guidelines written for the AVMA.

This is the link to the AVMA guidelines for euthanasia: https://www.avma.org/ KB/Policies/Documents/euthanasia.pdf.

Routes for medication

Consider the route by which you are going to give medication. Which is the easiest route for the animal? How is it going to feel to them? Is it better to give oral medications first? SQ versus IM versus IV for premedication, sedation, and anesthesia? Do you do euthanasia IV, intraperitoneal (IP), intrarenal (IR), intracardiac (IC), and intrahepatic (IH)? How do you choose?

For most patients, SQ injections are more comfortable than IM or IV injections for both the sedation and the anesthetic. For an animal who has allodynia, any of these injection sites will be painful. Consider oral sedation for animals who have allodynia. After experiencing animals scream, cry, leap, and run away, with telazol or vomit with alpha 2's, the author has adjusted their protocol. Instead, when going very slow with the first and second SQ injection, animals tend not to object, do not act painful or are minimally uncomfortable or stressed, and can be eating as they start to fall asleep. Giving an IM injection, while effective, is painful, and from the client's perspective, pain is the last thing they want to have happen. The author has not given an IM injection in many years.

For aggressive animals, the author advises using a different protocol to achieve a gentle and minimally stressful death. For dogs, the author finds it is best to start with oral meds first, in some food. Pill pockets work well for many and you may try a variety of foods, such as raw hamburger, butter (soft or melted), ice cream, cat food, peanut butter, or canned food. Discussion with the client of favored treats can occur on the phone or at the appointment. There are also variations of oral medications you may choose, listed later in the chapter. For cats, oral medications are limited by what the cat might ingest. If the cat is feral or aggressive, having the animal in a cage or soft sided kennel and getting an anesthetic (and the author recommends either tiletamine/zolazapam or ketamine/midazolam) into the cat as quickly as possible with an injection in cat approach and then allowing them to be covered and minimally handled until they are asleep. Veterinarians should consider increasing doses of medications for the following animals; younger, alert, aggressive, good or obese body condition.

The author uses the IV route for most patients. However, if the vein is difficult to visualize, then it may be in order to change to IR, IH, and IC. The author does not use the IC route with owners present. Other veterinarians that do house calls may use the IC route routinely, and that is a matter of preference. For intraorgan injections, animals should be anesthetized.

Drugs currently available for premedication

There are many premedication options available to veterinarians. This section will discuss what is available and what is commonly used by house call vets as of this writing.

Oral medications

(Oral and injectable dosing recommendations are based on anecdotal discussion provided by house call veterinarian colleagues. They may vary from currently published dosing. These dosing suggestions are **for euthanasia only.**)

Phenothiazine derivatives

Acepromazine is one a commonly used drug for tranquilization and sedation. It comes in tablet and injectable forms. Sedation occurs via a dopamine blockade (Plumb, 2015a). The time of onset of tranquilization/sedation can be decreased by crushing the tablets and feeding via meatballs and pill pockets or another yummy treat. Sedation is enhanced with administration with an opioid or gabapentin (Plumb, 2015a). Injectable acepromazine can be given orally as well.

Dosing—dosing can vary based on weight, fat content, alertness, and tendencies toward aggression. Commonly used dosing is far higher than drug dosing in the literature (100 mg and up tablets can be used for small dogs, 150 mg and up tablets can be used in medium to large dogs). Anecdotally, it appears safe to use at much higher doses for euthanasia than doses used in the clinical setting for tranquilization. The author has not had an animal die from these high doses used in euthanasia only patients.

> Pros—can crush and place in meatballs or pill pockets. Injectable acepromazine can also be used in meatballs, though the author finds it less consistent with the onset of clinical tranquilization as compared to crushed tablets. Will increase dilation of blood vessels and decrease the need for a tourniquet or catheter. Has antiemetic and antihistaminic properties (Plumb, 2015a). It only takes 5 −10 min to take effect and works better with gabapentin or other sedating drugs than alone.
>
> Cons—not reversible. No analgesic properties. Effects can be variable and aggressive animals may be rousable (Plumb, 2015a). May lower the seizure threshold, though the studies vary in the conclusion of this (McConnell, 2007; Tobias, 2006).
>
> The author does not use it orally in cats as it tastes terrible and can cause heavy drooling.

Anticonvulsant/neuropathic pain medication

Gabapentin—can be used orally in very high doses for sedation. Can take medication out of capsules and mix in food for both cats and dogs.

Dosing—100−300+ mg for cats, 100 mg/kg for dogs (anecdotal). For Euthanasia patients only.

> Pros—can help with neuropathic pain and sedation (for euthanasia, using the sedating properties, especially at higher doses and along with acepromazine).
>
> Cons—animals do not always eat food with gabapentin mixed in, will spit capsules out, and −variable sedation effects. Should be used in conjunction with other medication.

Pentobarbital—comes in injectable and powder forms. Fatal Plus and Pentasol are the powder forms, Fatal Plus, Sleepaway, Socumb-6gr, Somlethol, and SP6 are the Schedule 2 Pentobarbital without the salt added (phenytoin sodium). Euthanasia III, Beuthanasia-D-Special, Euthasol, and Somnasol, are considered Schedule 3 controlled substances and include Phenytoin sodium as an additive (Plumb, 2015g).

Oral dosing—(written and used with permission from Dr. Anthony Smith, Rainbow Bridge Pet Services).

Oral Pentobarbital Sedation for Euthanasia.

Note: This information is based strictly on Dr. Smith's personal experiences and anecdotal infomation from other veterinarians who have tried oral pentobarbital. To date, there have been no published studies evaluating the safety or efficacy of orally administered Pentobarbital for sedation or euthanasia. Reactions to medication may vary. Please contact Dr. Smith with questions or to report your results.

There are some situations where it is advantageous to provide complete deep sedation/anesthesia for a pet via the oral route. Most commonly, this is useful for an aggressive dog that cannot be easily handled yet still has a good appetite. Other sedatives (e.g., acepromazine, benzodiazepines, trazodone, etc.) may work but have a variable effect, which may be undesirable when working with a potentially dangerous animal. In Dr. Smith's experience, when a sufficient amount of pentobarbital is consumed by the pet, the resulting sedation is relatively smooth and profoundly deep (even to the point of achieving euthanasia on occasion), allowing for a follow-up injection to achieve final euthanasia safely for everyone involved.

1. Before administration, the veterinarian must ensure that there is a valid veterinarian—client—patient relationship (however defined by your state's veterinary medical board) for both your protection as well as an excellent veterinary practice.
2. Ensure that the pet still has a good enough appetite that s/he will consume the medication in a favorite treat, ideally without stopping to taste the food. Discuss options with the client to find appropriate food.
   a. For liquid pentobarbital (Fatal Plus or Beuthanasia-type solution), the author find that soft foods typically work best. Flavored yogurt or melted ice cream have worked well for me. Firmer foods can be used, but the liquid often leaks out before the pet consumes the treat.
   b. For solid form pentobarbital (Fatal Plus powder or placed into gel caps), there are more options, the author has used Pill Pockets, cut up hot dogs, meatballs, and cheese with great success (see below for preparation).
3. 45—90 min before the desired time for euthanasia, have the caregiver administer the Pentobarbital hidden in the appropriate treat. There is no established dose, but the author has had consistently good results when we have administered a minimum of $1.5\times$ the standard IV euthanasia dose (e.g., 1.5 mL per 10 lbs of body weight). More is better, but the author has had satisfactory results even with less than 1 mL/10 lbs.
4. During the induction time, make sure that the pet is contained someplace quiet and relatively safe from falling hazards, as induction may not be rapid. As with any induction of anesthesia, there is a possibility of excitement or disorientation. Inside the pet's crate is ideal, but a small laundry room, bathroom, or bedroom are options.
5. Within about 45—90 min, the pet will most likely be fully anesthetized if s/he has not already passed. Check the level of anesthesia safely from a distance, if possible. Using a household item to move the pet to keep you a distance from the aggressive animal provides a good idea of whether or not it is safe to proceed.
6. If the pet is not quite deep enough, the veterinarian can most likely now quickly and safely give an injection of your preferred pre-euthanasia anesthesia combination IM or SQ to complete the induction process.
7. If the pet is deeply anesthetized but still alive, the veterinarian can now provide the final euthanasia injection. Due to the possible hypotension from the pentobarbital, a regular IV injection into a peripheral vein may be difficult. So, the author generally recommends an alternate route, such as Intracardiac,

Intrahepatic, or Intraperitoneal. Although the time to death may be slightly prolonged versus typical euthanasia, in the author's experience, once the final injection is administered, the process does not usually take much longer than that experienced with other sedation/anesthesia methods.

Preparation of "Solid Form" pentobarbital for oral administration.

Because pentobarbital is exceptionally bitter-tasting, preparing the medication in solid form (within gel caps) allows a much better likelihood that the pet will consume the entire dose. This method is helpful:

1. Purchase a bottle of Fatal Plus in powdered form (liquid can be used, but it is messier and much more challenging to work with and store). The powdered form is roughly the same price point as a bottle of liquid and can be obtained from most veterinary suppliers (the author uses MWI Vet).
2. Wearing gloves and a mask is ideal but not necessary. Using a gram scale, measure out the amount of pentobarbital powder needed for the pet. The author's calculations have indicated that 1 g of Fatal Plus powder is approximately equivalent to 2.5 mL of liquid. Therefore, at a minimum, the author would provide 1 g of powder per 25 lbs of pet bodyweight.
3. Preferably, the veterinarian will want to divide this dose into several empty gel caps. The number of caps required will depend on the size gel cap used, which should be adjusted based on the size of the pet and food treat to be used. If you cannot use gel caps, the powder may be placed directly into the food treat(s), but it will require more care to ensure that none is lost and that the pet does not taste the powder and thereby reject the treat.
4. The veterinarian might consider preparing and storing several doses ahead of time to avoid last-minute scrambling when the need arises. Be sure to label and store the medication appropriately.
5. When finished, be sure to thoroughly clean any equipment used in preparing the Pentobarbital to avoid cross-contamination (Smith, 2018).

Pros—can be given orally. The powder can be utilized in capsules or mixed with food/meat. Schedule 2 Pentobarbital can be mixed with food, Schedule 3 Pentobarbital can also be used, but the animal is not as likely to eat it. Powder or liquid can be placed in gel capsules and/or put in food if still eating. May sedate, anesthetize, or euthanize.

   Cons—the Schedule 2 and 3 drugs both taste bad. They are bitter and even with capsules will sometimes not be eaten.

α-2 agonists

Dexmedetomidine has been formulated into an oral paste and can be given for sedation for euthanasia. Sileo® is the name of the paste available.

Dormosedan® (detomidine hydrochloride) (an equine gel product) has also been used off-label in oral sedation dogs and cats. The dose typically used is 0.1 ml/10 lbs for euthanasia only patients.

Being these are newer products (Sileo®) or being used off-label (Dormosedan®), more research needs to be done to assess the efficacy of these products for hospice and euthanasia patients.

Pros—α-2 agonists have reversal agents and can be reversed if needed. The oral formulation is easy to give for stressful situations like thunder and fireworks or aggressive animals. This can be given with food and may sedate well.

   Cons—efficacy of the oral paste and gel in euthanasia patients has varied anecdotally. Medications can also have a reverse effect; see below. An evidence-based study needs to be run.

How medication might make them feel—α-2 agonists can cause restlessness, vomiting, arousal, and increased vigilance. Animals may also be hypersensitive and hyperreactive to sound (Marchitelli, 2015).

Seratonin reuptake inhibitors

Trazadone is a Seratonin 2A antagonist and reuptake inhibitor (SARI) and changes the Seratonin precursor 5-hydroxytryptophan (5-HT2). It can antagonize α-1 adrenergic receptors and reduce blood pressure, so using it in animals as an oral premed may make it less attractive (as hypotension can make venipuncture or identification of veins more difficult during euthanasia). It is used for sedation and behavioral issues in small animals (Plumb, 2015r).

Medication might make them feel—potential adverse effects can include sedation, lethargy, ataxia, priapism, cardiac conduction disturbances, increased anxiety, and aggression. It can cause Serotonin syndrome, primarily when used with other anti-depressant class drugs or those that can affect serotonin. The clinical signs seen in dogs with serotonin syndrome include (in descending order): vomiting, diarrhea, seizures, hyperthermia, hyperesthesia, depression, mydriasis, vocalization, death, blindness, hypersalivation, dyspnea, ataxia/paresis, disorientation, hyperreflexia, and coma (Plumb, 2015r).

Injectable medications
Phenothiazine derivatives

Acepromazine is one of the most commonly used drugs for sedation with in-home euthanasia. Sedation occurs via a dopamine blockade. Injectable acepromazine can be given SQ, IM, or IV. Sedation is enhanced with administration with an opioid and the author recommends using butorphenol (Plumb, 2015a).

> **Dosing**—0.005—0.05 mg/kg IV, IM, or SC, for sedation for euthanasia (Plumb, 2015a), dosing is higher for euthanasia in the author's experience.
>
> Cat—3 mg/cat, Dog 3—30 mg/dog depending on the dog's size usually mixed with other medications. Can be given SQ, IM, IV.

> **Pros**—can place injectable acepromazine in meatball or pill pockets. Will increase dilation of blood vessels and decrease the need for a tourniquet. Has antiemetic and antihistaminic properties (Plumb, 2015a).
>
> **Cons**—not reversible. No analgesic properties. Effects can be variable and aggressive animals may be rousable. Can increase aggressiveness in some animals (Plumb, 2015a). May lower the seizure threshold, though the studies vary in the conclusion of this (McConnell, 2007; Tobias, 2006). It does not taste good, and in the author's experience, animals may reject the food with Acepromazine in it.

Opioids

Opioids are helpful for pain management before euthanasia. Pure μ-agonists are helpful for moderate-to-severe pain.

Partial μ-agonists such as Buprenorphine provide analgesia for mild-to-moderate pain. The benefits of using Buprenorphine include the following: (1) The owner may have doses of it on hand, from a previous vet, (2) It can be given orally or SQ (IM and IV are less commonly used in the home setting), and (3) It can be given before the appointment if they have it on hand. The drawbacks are as follows: (1) It is expensive, especially for larger animals, (2) It takes a relatively long time to get up to adequate plasma levels when given transmucosally, and (3) It may not be as effective if given SQ (Steagall, 2014).

Butorphanol is a μ-antagonist, κ-agonist. It is only utilized for mild pain but can produce moderate sedation and has an additive effect to acepromazine (Plumb, 2015o).

Butorphanol is commonly used for premed sedation for euthanasia. It is moderately expensive and can cause sedation rapidly and briefly help with the pain (Plumb, 2015d). Butorphanol is an analgesic (short-acting in dogs and cats), antiemetic, and antitussive (Plumb, 2015d). Using butorphanol (in combination with Acepromazine) in dogs with Congestive Heart Failure and other respiratory issues, such as tracheal collapse tends to minimize respiratory distress as they start to relax, in the author's experience.

Morphine—Pros—μ-agonist, a powerful sedative, pain medication. Inexpensive.

Cons—can cause vomiting, allergic reaction. Concern for human abuse (Plumb, 2015n).

Hydromorphone—Pros—μ-agonist, a powerful sedative, pain medication. Moderately expensive.

Cons—can cause vomiting. Concern for human abuse (Plumb, 2015i).

Fentanyl—Pros—comes in a patch form, transdermal form. The injectable is very effective and may be used in a comfort kit (Concern for human abuse). Cons—human abuse potential is high. Schedule 2—more paperwork involved (Plumb, 2015i).

Methadone—Pros—μ-agonist and has NMDA antagonist properties. Can be given SQ in patients. Useful for crisis kit. Methadone comes in an oral form but has low bioavailability in dogs. The oral form may be helpful for cats.

Cons—Schedule 2 drug. In the United States, significant expense, relatively inexpensive elsewhere in the world. Like other μ-agonists, it can cause panting, whining, sedation, defecation, constipation, bradycardia, and respiratory depression (Plumb, 2015m).

Oxymorphone—Pros—similar to hydromorphone.

Cons—may cause vomiting, increased intracranial pressure. Like other μ-agonists, it can cause panting, whining, sedation, defecation, constipation, bradycardia, and respiratory depression. Human abuse potential is high (Plumb, 2015m).

Dosing

Morphine—despite variable bioavailability in dogs, the starting oral dose of regular morphine is 1 mg/kg PO q4-6 h. Sustained-release morphine is used in dogs at 2−5 mg/kg PO twice daily.

Injectable—0.5−2 mg/kg IM, SC, or IV (slowly) (Plumb, 2015n).

Cats—0.05−0.4 mg/kg IM, SC every 3−6 h as needed.

Hydromorphone—for dogs—0.1−0.2 mg/kg IV, IM or SC q2-4 h or given as a CRI with an initial dose of 0.05−0.1 mg kg IV and then as CRI at 0.01−0.05 mg/kg/hour (Plumb, 2015i).

Cats—0.05−0.1 mg/kg IV, IM or SC q2-6 h or given as a CRI with an initial dose of 0.025 mg kg IV and then as CRI at 0.01−0.05 mg/kg/h (start at the low end of the range). Monitor body temperature with the use of hydromorphone in cats as hyperthermia may develop (Plumb, 2015i).

Transdermal Fentanyl—**for the control of postoperative pain associated with surgical procedures in dogs** (labeled dose; FDA-approved): 2.7 mg/kg (1.2 mg/lb) using only the syringes/applicator provided and applied topically per the instructions to the dorsal scapular area 2−4 h before surgery. Applied one time only; a single application provides analgesia for 4 days. Do not store the product in the syringes. Not for injection. It cannot be safely dosed in dogs weighing less than 2.7 kg (6 lbs). (Adapted from label information; *Recuvyra*) (Plumb, 2015h).

Buprenorphine—dogs—5−30 μg/kg (0.005−0.03 mg/kg) IV, IM or SC q6-12 h. The bioavailability of transmucosal Buprenorphine in dogs is 35%−50%, it is 5% orally (Plumb, 2015c).

Cats—**to control postoperative pain associated with surgical procedures using the feline-labeled product (*Simbadol*)**; (labeled dose; FDA-approved): 0.24 mg/kg SC once daily, for up to 3 days (Adapted from the label; Simbadol—Abbott Refer to the label (package insert) for additional information.) administer the first dose approximately 1 h before surgery. Do not dispense for administration at home by the pet owner.

a. Extra-label dose: 10−30 μg/kg (0.01−0.03 mg/kg) IM, IV, Buccal (oral transmucosal; OTM) q6-8h (Plumb, 2015c).

Meperidine—dogs—**as an analgesic** (extra-label): dosage recommendations vary, but usually are 3−5 mg/kg (up to 11 mg/kg has been noted) IM or SC. Analgesic duration in dogs usually lasts 30 min to 2 h (Plumb, 2015l).

Cats—not usually recommended in cats.

Continued

> **DOSING—cont'd**
>
> **Methadone**—dogs—dosage recommendations vary but usually range from 0.1 to 1 mg/kg q4-8h IV, SC, or IM.
> Cats—dosage recommendations vary but usually range from 0.05 to 0.5 mg/kg q4-6h IV, SC, or IM (Plumb, 2015m).
> **Butorphanol**—dogs—0.1–0.5 mg/kg IV, IM, SQ. Commonly, 0.2 mg/kg is chosen as a starting dose. Butorphanol provides only mild-to-moderate analgesia (good visceral analgesia); duration of sedative action 2–4 h, but analgesic action may be less than 1 h (Plumb, 2015d).
> Cats—0.1–0.5 mg/kg IV, IM, SQ; provides only mild-to-moderate analgesia (good visceral analgesia); duration of sedative action 2–4 h, but analgesic action may be 1 h or less (Robertson, 2015).

> **How medication might make them feel**—opioids tend to make most animals feel euphoric. Opioids can cause vomiting; butorphanol does not tend to cause vomiting due to NK1 antagonism, though vomiting is listed as a side effect (Marchitelli, 2015).

α-2 agonists

α-2's agonists creates sedation via the agonist effects on alpha-2 adrenoreceptors decreasing Norepinephrine. Sedation can occur within 3–5 min IV and can take up to 15 min IM. They can produce moderate to profound sedation, as well as being proemetic and may trigger urination. They also cause profound vasoconstriction, bradycardia, and decreased respiration and apnea. α-2 agonists should be used with caution or not at all with known seizure patients. Sedation and other effects can be increased with the administration of a μ-opioid (Plumb, 2015e, 2015k).

One of the primary benefits of using α-2 agonists is that they can be reversed.

Dexmedetomidine, xylazine, romifidine, medetomidine, and detomidine HCl are α-2 agonists. Yohimbine HCl is the reversal agent for xylazine. Atipamezole HCl is the reversal agent for all the α-2 agents (Gaynor, 2015).

> **How medication might make them feel**—α-2 agonists can cause restlessness, vomiting, arousal, and increased vigilance. They can also make dogs and cats hypersensitive and hyperreactive to sound (Marchitelli, 2015).

Benzodiazepines

Benzodiazepines' exact mechanism is unknown. It is postulated that benzodiazepines are serotonin antagonists, increase GABA activity, and decrease the release of acetylcholine (Ogbru, 2018; Plumb, 2015s).

The onset of sedation can occur within 1–3 min with IV administration and within 15–20 min with IM administration (with midazolam only). It is primarily metabolized in the liver (Ogbru, 2018).

Consider using a benzodiazepine with seizure patients and patients suspected to have neoplastic brain disease to minimize the possibility of seizures. Benzodiazepines have minimal effects on the cardiovascular and pulmonary systems (Ogbru, 2018).

Common benzodiazepines used in veterinary medicine: alprazolam (Xanax), clonazepam (Klonopin), diazepam (Valium), lorazepam (Ativan), and midazolam (Versed). (Ogbru, 2018).

> **How medication might make them feel**—humans feel relaxed on the benzodiazepines. Benzodiazepines do not cause anesthesia but can help with relaxation and decrease the effects of the NMDA antagonists. The common side effects in humans are sedation, dizziness, weakness, and instability (Marchitelli, 2015).
>
> Other side effects (seen in humans) that may be significant in animals include loss of orientation, headache, confusion, irritability, aggression, and excitement (Ogbru, 2018; Plumb, 2015s).

Anesthetic drugs

NMDA Antagonists-Tiletamine and Zolazepam or Telazol®—this is the proprietary name of Tiletamine (an NMDA antagonist) and Zolazepam (benzodiazepine). There has been a recent generic version of this medication available, called Tizolan®, may also be called Zolatil® outside of the United States. The combination of tiletamine and zolazepam is a fast-acting anesthetic commonly used by in–home euthanasia veterinarians. It can be given SQ, IM, or orally. The oral application will sometimes cause mild-to-moderate drooling (rarely, pawing at the mouth, heavy drooling) because Telazol does taste bad. SQ administration of Telazol can cause other reactions as well, from mild-to-severe fractious behavior, athetosis to pain upon SQ administration. The author recommends premedication with acepromazine and butorphanol 5 min before giving tiletamine and zolazepam SQ, and it will help minimize or make the reaction absent. Another trick is to use the smallest possible needle.

Ketamine is an NMDA antagonist that can be used instead of Telazol. It is less expensive than the Tiletamine and Zolazepam products and can be used along with a benzodiazepine. Ketamine may also produce a reaction, though less frequently than tiletamine/zolazepam. It can be given IM, IV, SQ, and orally (Gaynor, 2015).

> **How medication might make them feel**—the NMDA antagonists induce a cataleptic state and amnesia. They dampen down the function of the cerebral cortex but not the limbic system. There is an altered state of consciousness. People report hallucinations and out-of-body experiences. It is currently unknown if animals feel this way. There can be rhythmic muscle jerking during the excitatory phase of the drug (Marchitelli, 2015).

Alfaxalone—a neuroactive steroid that is also a sedative. Alfaxalone can be used IV, SQ, or IM. It needs to be used with another medication to provide adequate sedation (Plumb, 2015b). However, it may be used as an anesthetic. In this capacity, it is not commonly used in the home setting in the United States but is more common in the clinical setting and outside the United States (Nieuwendijk, 2011).

It can be used with common preanesthetics (Nieuwendijk, 2011).

Etomidate is an imidazole derivative that is not commonly used in the home setting (Aarnes, 2014; Plumb, 2015f).

Propofol—an alkyl phenol-derivative that causes immediate unconsciousness with IV administration. Propofol enhances the effects of GABA. It is in a base of soybean oil, glycerol, and egg lecithin and needs to be given IV (Plumb, 2015p). It is more commonly used in the clinical setting. Sterility is a concern in the home setting, and propofol may be used for euthanasia only. It has the same mechanism of action as pentobarbital and may be used in conjunction with pentobarbital for euthanasia purposes (Plumb, 2015p).

Difficult euthanasias

Euthanasia does not go perfectly every time. The key to each difficult situation encountered during euthanasia is to learn what you could do better for the future and to remain calm in front of the client. Remember that your perception of how the experience went is not necessarily the client's perception regarding how the euthanasia was performed. Setting expectations early and giving families a frame of reference can help walk them through the process. If adverse reactions happen, helping people to understand what the animal is experiencing and what they are seeing can help with interpretation. Supporting the families involved in the euthanasia experience with education makes euthanasia smoother, even when there are adverse reactions. If there is mental illness involved for any of the members of the family, this may complicate the grieving process. Having a mental health professional available to refer to can help. Please see the section on complicated grief for additional information on how to deal with difficult grief situations.

What adverse reactions can be seen with difficult euthanasia? Here is a list of adverse reaction scenarios that can occur during euthanasia.

1. The medication(s) you use to initiate sedation do not seem to be working or may be creating a paradoxical reaction (such as aggression, or disorientation, instead of relaxation). Animals can go through an excitatory phase before the depressive phase of the sedative when they are initially sedated and may start to become restless. In the author's experience, it tends to be associated with their sphincters begin to relax, and they may feel they need to urinate or defecate. Solution: Client can take the cat to the litter box, or take the dog out to urinate or defecate. Or give them either more of the injectable sedation medication or move on to the anesthetic or in the future consider using oral

sedative medication before injectables. You can also give the anesthetic and the sedation together in an SQ injection, but this combination typically will not minimize the pain associated with the anesthetic, which may sting.

2. The dose of medications you use to induce full anesthesia does not anesthetize them or instead makes them appear drunk, aggressive, or disoriented. Solution: use higher dosing for every patient or use a different combination of drugs.

3. Animal acts painful, especially with ketamine or tiletamine and zolazepam. Solution: give a dose of opioid of your choice and a large dose of acepromazine and wait 5-10 min (The author uses Butorphenol and Acepromazine for the first medication combination.) Or begin with oral medications. Phenobarbital, pentobarbital powder, diazepam, gabapentin, and acepromazine are all good oral medications to try if they are eating. You can give the ketamine or tiletamine and zolazepam orally as well.

4. Athetosis reaction to tiletamine or ketamine. Athetosis is defined as repetitive, involuntary, slow, sinuous, writhing movements. (TFD Staff, 2018) Athetosis is due to extrapyramidal dissociation. Solution: Giving the opioid/ace premed or adding an α-2 agonist may help with preventing athetosis reactions. Increasing the dose of ketamine or tiletamine/zolazepam given, or adding a benzodiazapine to the ketamine may also help.

5. Challenges with the administration of the euthanasia solution.

   a. You cannot find a vein, for an IV catheter or butterfly catheter or to administer mediations "off the needle." Solution: Give the euthanasia solution in another location. The animal needs to be anesthetized for organ euthanasia. Consider intraorgan, intracardiac, or intraperitoneal administration. Intraperitoneal administration of euthanasia solution is easy to perform, but it may take additional time and larger volumes of euthanasia solution. Intrarenal is relatively straightforward, as the kidneys are easy to access in small animals and the onset of euthanasia is quick (typically 1−2 min). If your injection inadvertently goes peri-renal it will take longer. Reported times are 1−10 min. Intrahepatic is also straightforward, except on overweight or obese animals, longer needles are needed for intrahepatic injection. Intracardiac also requires longer needles particularly for larger animals, often 2 in. or more. Intracardiac sticks should be considered a last resort with an animal when done in front of owners, as it may be disturbing or confusing to accept seeing this technique. If an intracardiac injection of euthanasia solution is necessary and the caregiver still wishes to be present, the author recommends doing this procedure under a blanket so that the family can focus on the experience.

   b. You cannot find the vein, and you give the euthanasia solution in one of the other areas, and it is taking more than 10−15-min for the animal to pass away. Solution: Administer more euthanasia solution. If administering medications intraorgan, give double the amount that you would have given IV on the first injection.

    c. You give more, and they still do not pass away. Solution: Changing the route by which you give the euthanasia solution (instead of intrarenal, give intrahepatic, etc.).

6. Seizures. The animal has a seizure with any of the medications. Acepromazine often gets blamed for seizures, but many other medications can lower the seizure threshold. The author has had one dog seizure with gabapentin and one with the pentobarbital (halfway through the injection). Tiletamine/zolazapam and ketamine can increase intracranial pressure and should be used in caution with intracranial disease (McConnell, 2007; Plumb, 2015j, 2015q).

7. Dysphoria. Dysphoria can happen with sedation or early anesthesia. It is due to the excitatory phase of sedation. It is more common with opioids (Gaynor, 2015) Solution: Increase the amount of sedation, tranquilization medications, and anesthesia. Consider starting with oral medications, prior to injectable medications.

8. Howling before death. This is very rare. Howling is likely due to dysphoria or an excitatory response to medications. Possible solution: Give sedative first, then anesthetize and then euthanize. This may be disturbing to client's, they may believe their animal is in pain.

9. Agonal breathing, happens prior to the cessation of circulation. Or diaphragmatic twitch, which may happen after the heart has stopped. They look similar, however, have different etiologies. Agonal breathing occurs when the animal is hypoxic and the brain stem stimulates the respiratory mechanism. A diaphragmatic twitch is similar to other muscle twitching. Possible solution: Sedate, anesthetize, and then euthanize. The slower you give medications, the better and the less likely they will have agonal breathing (Marchetelli, 2017).

10. They can have muscle twitching postdeath. Twitching can be seen in a single locale, to whole-body involvement and can last some time (usually a few seconds to several minutes. Extended twitching may be similar to the Lazarus sign in humans. In humans, it has been reported up to 12 h postdeath (Scutti, 2014). Extended twitching post brain death is extremely rare. Possible solution: Education of the family or caregiver about why this happens, that it can be a normal change, though unusual or rare. Normalizing and explaining unusual and rare events that may occur postdeath can help the family with their grief and fears. This may be especially important if you are leaving the animal with the family.

Additional tips and challenging situations to prepare for

1. Remember the caregiver's perception may be different from the veterinarian's perception. Differing perceptions can go both ways. For example, the client may think the euthanasia went horribly, while the veterinarian felt the procedure was routine and went smoothly. An example, a client may be upset that their dog's hips were stretched too far while accessing a vein. And the converse may be true as well, for example, the caregiver may be satisfied with the euthanasia procedure, but the veterinarian feels terrible about taking so long to find a vein. An example is that it took a long time for the pet to go to sleep, it needed additional medication. These are both stressful to the veterinarian but for distinct reasons. In the first scenario, the caregiver is usually upset or traumatized, and in the second scenario, the veterinarian is upset or traumatized by the situation.

   a. Solution: The family's perception may be influenced by fear. One way to ameliorate this fear might be to educate the family on what you are doing before each step. You may also tell them you will explain things that are unusual if they happen to come up. If you feel the procedure is already not going well, it is best to try to maintain a calm and reassuring exterior, continuing to explain each step as you go. If you do not show stress, the caregiver may not realize at all that the euthanasia is not going as planned.

2. It is best not to chase an animal. If an animal is not as sick as the client may have indicated, and they may be inclined to run or hide from a new person in their home.

   a. Solution: Ask prior to arrival or at arrival how the animal feels about strangers. Offer alternatives to giving medication, such as oral adminstration in food for dogs, or telazol or ketamine for cats. If the animal has run away, give the family a short amount of time to retrieve the animal. If the animal is not easily retrievable then the author advises not to wait, but to reschedule.

3. Aggressive animals. If an animal is distressed, scared, or uncomfortable with new people in the home, they may try to bite or run away.

   a. Solution: If the animal has bitten someone, they need to be in quarantine for at least 10 days based on your governing body (or be submitted for rabies testing), and you may have to make another appointment.

   b. Solution: For cats, giving substantial doses of gabapentin (2–500 mg) in food will often help. If you can get them to eat crushed ace, that will be helpful too. You can also give ketamine or tiletamine/zolazepam orally. (They will not likely eat it in food, so you may have to administer orally.) For dogs, giving gabapentin (25–50 mg/L lbs) and acepromazine (3–5 mg/L lb), or Telazol powder (the tablet before reconstitution) or ketamine mixed with food or in a meatball(s). Pentobarbital (liquid or powder) can also be given in a capsule. (Doses are anecdotal, based on author's experience, the younger and more aggressive, the author would increase the doses.) Use foods such as raw hamburger, ice cream, very soft or melted butter, or anything else the owner wants to feed or thinks the dog might enjoy. With aggressive dogs, if the veterinarian is not present in the room or space the dog is in when they are getting the first medications, the dog can relax more readily, instead of having a sympathetic response to the presence of a stranger.

4. Occasionally, people have a tough time being present during the euthanasia and may elect to not to stay in the room or the house during the euthanasia. They

may be concerned, worried, or fearful about what is going to happen and are focused on all that could go wrong. The words we use matter, and although we cannot control the perception of others, we can be thoughtful when choosing the words we use in these situations.

   a. Solution: The author recommends rather than telling people the details of everything that can go wrong, instead consider talking them through situations only if the procedure is not going as planned. Please understand that even if the veterinarian is providing the best explanation, their perception may be more influenced by their own fears or concerns than what you say to them. And they may still want to leave the room or the building if they do not understand or are afraid of any adverse response. Another option, asking them what they would like to know and explaining as questions come up for families. And be ok with them stepping out if that is what they need.

5. Family members who disagree with the euthanasia decision. As discussed in other chapters, you may encounter a family member who is not ready to move forward with euthanasia.

   a. Solution: If you have a mental health professional who can be involved, contact them, hopefully prior to the arrival at the house. Continue to play your role as the veterinarian by giving them their options. Depending on the situation, it may be helpful to give the one struggling with the decision more time as well. Palliative care may be an intermediary solution to give the family member(s) time to process their feelings. Switching the appointment to a palliative appointment with a defined time of trying medication, such as 24, 48 hours can help people sort out feelings, feel like they tried more, and may be able to emotionally handle a decision for euthanasia better. Sometimes with denial, they need more time to process information around the situation, which you hopefully have clarified for them. Occasionally there are also underlying mental health issues and that is why a mental health professional would be helpful to have available for referral. If the family wants to proceed, it is best to make sure that the individual who is hesitant about their decision is still ok to move forward. Leave them information about pet loss support and suicide crisis information. They may never use it, but it is essential to have presented it to the family. Check with the family about their own support, possible mental health support they have available.

6. Clients who ask you to help with the burial.

   a. Solution: Remember in some locations it may be against the law other than in a designated pet cemetery. Check with your local municipality. You may also run into difficulties, mud, rain, and a shallow grave (which will become a problem if the animal is unburied). You will have to consider your legal ramifications of burial and decide whether you want to participate or not.

7. Owners who have been drinking or doing illicit drugs/medications.

   a. Solution: Since the law states impaired owners may not be responsible for their behavior, you will have to decide if you want to proceed. (Check with your local, state, and federal government regulations, or if outside the United

States, check with your regulatory board regarding the laws around decision-making by drug- or alcohol-impaired people). Drug-impaired people can also lack inhibition and may become violent. It is vital to exercise caution under these circumstances. Have a check-in word you can text to your team, or your significant other if you are feeling in danger.

8. Moving large and giant breed dogs after euthanasia with no help from the caregiver available. Note: It is vital to take care of your back while doing this work.

   a. Solution: Bring a spouse, neighbor, or technician to help move. If no one is available, a gurney or a rigid stretcher with wheels can help get an animal to your car. Make sure it fits your particular car.

9. Animals who go into rigor mortis much more quickly than expected. In the literature, this is unusual. The author's experience usually takes 1+ hours for dogs and at least 30 min for cats. (The average time for rigor mortis is 2–6 h for dogs and lasts approximately 36 h) (Brooks, 2016). Rigor mortis occurs because ATP, a bridge between the myosin and actin fibers, stops being produced and "locks" the fibers in contraction. Early decomposition allows the fibers to break down and "relax" the muscle (Brooks, 2016). The Fig. 11.1 shows the basic changes to muscle in rigor mortis.

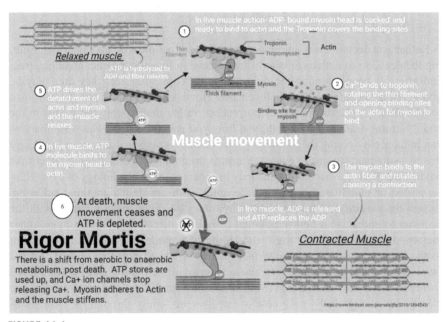

FIGURE 11.1

Rigor mortis.

Created with BioRender.com, Lynn Hendrix ©2021 Álvarez, C. M.-P. (2019). Mechanical and biochemical methods for rigor measurement: Relationship with eating quality. Journal of Food Quality, *1–13.*

Interestingly, in a study on pigs, researchers looked at stress with handling (rough handling vs. gentle handling premortem) in addition to lactate and cortisol levels premortem in relation to rigor mortis. In the study, it was found the higher the lactate levels premortem, the faster they went into rigor mortis (Dokmanović, 2014).

a. Solution: Depending on the scenario, you might consider discussing the potential for early onset rigor mortis in advance if you are leaving the animal with the client. Based on the study on pigs it is evident that gentle handling of our patients may also reduce the risk of this unusual occurrence.

Other unexpected scenarios may happen during difficult euthanasia, which may be unique occurrences or may not be addressed in this text. The hope is that by addressing some of the more commonly reported scenarios, you will be better prepared, even if something that is not in this chapter occurs. The author would like to thank the members of the Veterinarian Palliative Medicine group on Facebook for contributing stories of difficult situations they have encountered, which helped inspire some of the contents of this section. The author would like to thank Dr. Eve Harrison for her edits and contributions to this chapter as well. Future editions may add to the contributions of challenging cases.

Conclusion

A Euthanasia decision is a significant challenge for people who love their pet. Making the decision to euthanize is a difficult decision for most people, creating stress and grief for people around the dying animal. People may feel they are "playing god" ending the life of their beloved pet. However, euthanasia can be reframed for people as the "how" of the dying process, rather than simply the means to the end. "Natural death" is just death, and how you get to death is what veterinarians can influence by giving the animal a gentle death. As veterinarians, we can achieve this by using medications to guide the animal through a peaceful passing rather than having to endure the discomfort that may be inherent in the physiology of dying. Unsupported or unpalliated death may be quick with apparently minimal suffering, though the majority of the time, that is not the case. Supporting a family with the decision to euthanize a beloved animal can be multifactorial. Among many other factors, the disease process itself, the ability to provide and administer treatment to the animal, physical and emotional quality of life of both the animal and the owner(s), the animal's will to live, the autonomy of the animal, and respite for the owner all factor into the decision to euthanize an animal. Our ability to communicate clearly and thoughtfully and guide a caregiver or family through the process of euthanasia of a beloved animal can be a beautiful and moving experience when done with the proper education and sensitivity.

References

Aarnes, T. (2014). In *Anesthetic plans: From premed to recovery (Atlantic coast veterinary conference proceedings)*. Retrieved from Veterinary Information Network.com https://www.VIN.com/VIN.

Álvarez, C. M.-P. (2019). Mechanical and biochemical methods for rigor measurement: Relationship with eating quality. *Journal of Food Quality*, 1–13.

Brooks, J. (2016). Postmortem changes in animal carcasses and estimation of the postmortem interval. *Veterinary Pathology*, 929–940.

Dokmanović, M. B. (2014). Relationships among pre-slaughter stress, rigor mortis, blood lactate, and meat and carcass quality in pigs. *Acta Veterinaria*, 124–137.

Gaynor, J. S. (2015). *Handbook of veterinary pain management*. St. Louis: Mosby/Elsevier.

Leary, S.e. (2018). *AVMA guidelines for the euthanasia of animals*. Retrieved from AVMA.org https://www.avma.org/KB/Policies/Pages/Euthanasia-Guidelines.aspx.

Marchetelli, B. (2017). In *IAAHPC annual conference*. Seattle, WA: IAAHPC.

Marchitelli, B. (2015). How exactly does that drug work?. In *IAAHPC* (p. 7). San Diego: IAAHPC.

McConnell, J. K. (2007). Administration of acepromazine maleate to 31 dogs with a history of seizures. *Journal of Veterinary Emergency and Critical Care*, 262–267.

Merriam-Webster Dictionary. (June 10, 2018). *Euthanasia*. Retrieved from Merriam-Webster.com: https://www.merriam-webster.com/dictionary/euthanasia.

Nieuwendijk, H. (March 2011). *Alfaxalone (Alfaxan®)*. Retrieved from Veterinary Anesthesia & Analgesia Support Group: http://www.vasg.org/alfaxalone.htm.

Ogbru, A. M. (2018). *Benzodiazepines*. Retrieved from RXList.com: https://www.rxlist.com/benzodiazepines/drugs-condition.htm.

Plumb, D. (July 12, 2015a). Acepromazine. In D. Plumb (Ed.), *Plumb's veterinary drug handbook*. Stockholm: PharmaVet, Inc.

Plumb, D. (2015b). Alfaxalone. In D. Plumb (Ed.), *Plumb's veterinary drug handbook*. Stockholm: PharmaVet, Inc.

Plumb, D. (2015c). Buprenorphine. In D. Plumb (Ed.), *Plumb's veterinary drug handbook*. Stockholm: PharmaVet, Inc.

Plumb, D. (2015d). Butorphanol. In D. Plumb (Ed.), *Plumb's veterinary drug handbook*. Stockholm, Wisconsin: PharmaVet, Inc.

Plumb, D. (2015e). Detomidine. In D. Plumb (Ed.), *Plumb's veterinary drug handbook*. Stockholm, WI: PharmaVet, Inc.

Plumb, D. (2015f). Etomidate. In D. Plumb (Ed.), *Plumb's veterinary drug handbook*. Stockholm: PharmaVet, Inc.

Plumb, D. (2015g). Euthanasia agents with pentobarbital. In D. Plumb (Ed.), *Plumb's veterinary drug handbook* (8th ed.). Stockholm, Wisconsin: PharmaVet, Inc.

Plumb, D. (2015h). Fentanyl. In D. Plumb (Ed.), *Plumb's veterinary drug handbook*. Stockholm: PharmaVet, Inc.

Plumb, D. (2015i). Hydromorphone. In D. Plumb (Ed.), *Plumb's veterinary drug handbook*. Stockholm: PharmaVet, Inc.

Plumb, D. (2015j). Ketamine. In D. Plumb (Ed.), *Plumb's veterinary drug handbook*. Stockholm, WI: PharmaVet, Inc.

Plumb, D. (2015k). Medetomidine. In D. Plumb (Ed.), *Plumb's veterinary drug handbook*. Stockholm, WI: PharmaVet, Inc.

Plumb, D. (2015l). Meperidine. In D. Plumb (Ed.), *Plumb's veterinary drug handbook*. Stockholm: PharmaVet, Inc.

Plumb, D. (2015m). Methadone. In D. Plumb (Ed.), *Plumb's veterinary drug handbook*. Stockholm: PharmaVet, Inc.

Plumb, D. (2015n). Morphine. In D. Plumb (Ed.), *Plumb's veterinary drug handbook*. Stockholm: PharmaVet, Inc.

Plumb, D. (2015o). Pharmacology of narcotic (opiate) agonist analgesics. In D. Plumb (Ed.), *Plumb's veterinary drug handbook*. Stockholm, Wisconsin: PharmaVet, Inc.

Plumb, D. (2015p). Propofol. In D. Plumb (Ed.), *Plumb's veterinary drug handbook*. Stockholm: PharmaVet, Inc.

Plumb, D. (2015q). Telazol. In D. Plumb (Ed.), *Plumb's veterinary drug handbook*. Stockholm, WI: PharmaVet, Inc.

Plumb, D. (2015r). Trazadone. In D. Plumb (Ed.), *Plumb's veterinary drug handbook*. Stockholm, Wisconsin: PharmaVet, Inc.

Plumb, D. (2015s). Valium. In D. Plumb (Ed.), *Plumb's veterinary drug handbook*. Stockholm: PharmaVet, Inc.

Robertson, S. A. (2015). Cat-specific considerations. *Handbook of Veterinary Pain Management* (3rd, pp. 493−516). Elsevier, INC.

Scutti, S. (December 15, 2014). *What a forensic scientist doesn't tell you: 7 postmortem responses of a dead body*. Retrieved from Medical Daily https://www.medicaldaily.com/what-forensic-scientist-doesnt-tell-you-7-postmortem-responses-dead-body-314404.

Smith, A. (2018). Email from Dr Anthony Smith. CA, USA.

Steagall, P. (2014). A review of the studies using buprenorphine in cats. *Journal of Veterinary Internal Medicine*, 762−770.

TFD Staff. (August 2, 2018). *Athetosis*. Retrieved from Medical Dictionary-The Free Dictionary.com: https://medical-dictionary.thefreedictionary.com/athetosis.

Tobias, K. (2006). A retrospective study on the use of acepromazine maleate in dogs with seizures. *Journal of the American Animal Hospital Association*, 283−289.

Wilson, J. (September 4, 2017). *What is the difference between sedation and general anesthesia?*. Retrieved from News-Medical Life Sciences https://www.news-medical.net/health/What-is-the-Difference-Between-Sedation-and-General-Anesthesia.aspx.

Respectful aftercare of the beloved pet

Lynn Hendrix, AA, BA, DVM, CHPV [1,2,3,4]

[1]*Owner, Veterinarian, Beloved Pet Mobile Vet, Davis, CA, United States;* [2]*Former Board of Directors, IAAHPC, Chicago, IL, United States;* [3]*Consultant, Hospice, Palliative Medicine, End of Life, VIN, Davis, CA, United States;* [4]*President, Founder, World Veterinary Palliative Medicine Organization, Davis, CA, United States*

One of the more difficult aspects of veterinary hospice and palliative medicine is how to care for the body after euthanasia or palliated death from the disease. It may be helpful to discuss body care wishes prior to death. Recording the wishes of the family in the medical record can help the team focus on the family's emotional needs at the time of the death without having to have the conversation again. The family should have the names and phone numbers of crematoriums in the packet of information you leave with them, for an emergency or sudden death occurs.

If you are starting your practice and are looking for a cremation service, it is important to know what they do, how they do it, and to visit each one before you chose. Ask for crematorium records, talk to staff members and other veterinarians about their experiences, and check their reviews online (remember that people who are leaving these are grieving). Visit the crematorium you choose frequently and without warning. Make sure you are comfortable with what they do, how they do it, how they return the cremains to you or the family, what they return cremains in, if they do pawprints or not, and how quickly they return to you or to your families. Think about what you would like them to be able to do for you. Do they have a burial option for people who choose not to cremate? For most families, having their beloved animal's cremains back quickly is preferred, though this author has had people who are not ready to receive them back for some time (be cognizant of how long they may need). Consider whether you want to deliver ashes back to your clients, or if you want to have the crematorium to pick up and deliver, or have a delivery service.

Burial: Burial may be an option available for some people. A pet cemetery may be another option for people who do not want cremation. Home burial may or may not be an option. The author strongly recommends finding out what your local laws allow. If the animal was euthanized, there may be additional regulations for burial. In many locales, it may be against the law. Check with the city or county regulatory board for further information, and many regulations are available online.

In general, in locations that do allow burial, they often require a 6-foot-deep burial plot. This helps to prevent the body from being dug up and eaten, which can be a problem if they have been euthanized, due to the pentobarbital or other medications used. The euthanasia solution continues to be toxic to pets and wildlife and can cause secondary poisoning or death. There may be large fines levied against people whose animal may have caused secondary poisoning. There can also be fines levied against the veterinarian, so it is important to stress the seriousness of the depth of the burial site and the legality of burial. There are newer euthanasia techniques being explored in large animals that may be useful in small animals which are going to be buried. Intrathecal lidocaine or IV Magnesium may be options in the future that would not put wildlife at risk. More research needs to be performed before this becomes common practice.

Fire-based cremation: Fire-based cremation is the most common way for animal body disposition in the United States. There are several versions of what can be done for families, and you may be or not be aware of them. Fire-based cremation removes all the soft tissue via very hot fire (1400−1800°F, 760−982°C) and reduces it to bone material only. The bone is further reduced with a machine that pulverizes it to small particles. Pacemakers and bone implants are also remaining with fire-based cremation. Pacemaker batteries can explode, so it is important to let the crematorium know if they have a pacemaker, so that they can be prepared (Cremation Resource staff, 2018).

With cremation services, consider how the cremains are going to be returned to the client Are they in a box or another container? Is it sealed? Are the clients able to open the container if they choose to do so? Do they provide a scatter tube or some other means of scattering? Are they returned directly to the client, are they mailed, and what are they returned in (packaging vs. urn)? Do they have other urns to choose from? Do they have jewelry type urns? Will they do pawprints for the client? What kind of pawprints are they providing? Is it something you could do? Are they open to having a coffin? Will they allow witnessed cremation?

Types of cremation

Communal (or group) cremation—is a multiple body cremation. The cremains are not usually returned to the family but scattered somewhere else. There is comingling of ashes with this type of cremation. Find out how the scattering occurs, the location, and visit if you are able.

Partitioned private cremation—With partitioned private cremation, there is more than one animal in the crematorium at one time, but they are separated either by space or by barriers. Some newer crematoriums may have an individual chamber in the same machine (which would be considered single private cremation), however other machines have a single burner and incomplete walls separating the bodies. It is a good idea to find out what the cremation service does with their partitioned private cremations. There may be comingling of ashes. The cremains should be returned to you in a timely fashion or directly to your client.

Single private or individual cremation—With individual cremation, there is a single animal in the crematorium at one time. There may be multiple individual chambered crematoriums. Some crematoriums call this ultraprivate cremation. There is no commingling of ashes with this type of service. If you want to make sure your clients are getting their animals back, this type of service may provide that reassurance.

Witnessed cremation—Some crematoriums may allow witnessed cremation. Witnessed cremation can be significant to some people, for personal, cultural or religious reasons. Allowing to witness a beloved pet's cremation, gives many people peace of mind and increases the trust of both client and veterinarian with the crematorium.

Water-based cremation—Water based cremation goes by many names, aquamation, green cremation, and alkaline hydrolysis. Alkaline hydrolysis uses water and a couple of salts to degrade the soft tissues from the bone. The bone remains at the end of the process. Alkaline hydrolysis is legal in most states in the United States for pets. Check with your state water board for more information. The systems come with low-pressure and high-pressure tanks. They provide the same service; the low-pressure systems take longer to process the body and cost less than the high-pressure system. The high-pressure system can go as quickly as the flame-based cremation. The effluent that is left is void of virus, bacteria, and prions which are degraded with the alkaline process (Murphy, 2009; Lemire, 2016). As with fire-based cremation processes, the bones are then processed into a powder that tends to be finer than with fire-based cremation and with about 20% more bone available (Cooney, 2016).

Either of these systems could be considered if you were planning on adding a cremation service to your business.

Occasionally, you may have people who would prefer something besides the standard cremation or burial. Veterinarians may want to have knowledge of other options, even if they do not directly provide them.

Taxidermy—With taxidermy, the animal is skinned, the skin is tanned, and then placed on a model in a position of the client's choice. There are glass eyes placed, plastic tongues; however, the fur is very soft after the process. The goal is to make the mount as lifelike as possible (The Editors of Encyclopedia Britannica, 2018).

Freeze drying—Freeze drying is a type of taxidermy. The body is left intact and dehydrated in a large dehydrator. The animal appears very life-like after processing and the fur is still soft. There is no model underneath the skin (Johnson, 2018).

Donation of the body to a veterinary university—If you have a veterinary university or veterinary technician school nearby, they may have a body will program. They may have rules for the type and size of the animal that they would take. The client will want to make prior arrangements if possible with the university so that they are prepared to take the body. The university may not return any bodies.

Rendering—Rendering is a type of body disposal that processes the body by grinding the body and utilizing it for fertilizer or for animal feed. It is not legal to use euthanized animals for animal feed in the United States. There is a drying process, drying out the bodies before grinding. This process is usually used for fertilizer. There is also a wet processing, often used with farm animals usually utilized for animal feed. The body is turned into a "stew-like" process and processed into food products. This is not human-grade food. The author does not recommend rendering plants as your form of body disposal unless you are very clear with clients that what is happening with their beloved pet's body (EPA, 1995).

Necropsy—Occasionally, families want to know what happened to an animal who dies, what disease process was going on, if they had not had it worked up prior to your involvement, and will ask for a necropsy. Veterinarians can perform necropsy themselves or send it to a lab, or if you have a university or lab nearby, they may help. Necropsies can help the peace of mind for some clients that they chose euthanasia wisely; however, if the necropsy does not turn up gross disease, that may be a challenging conversation.

Rituals around body care

This section will list various tools and helpful rituals around the after care of the body. **Candles**—people may choose to use candles around the dying process, and it can be a tradition to light a candle for the deceased.

Funerals—Funerals are different than memorial services. Funerals involve a body, possibly a casket, open or closed, and the body may lie in state. Funerals may be held at a church or a memorial home and are much more common for humans than for animals. However, there are some religious houses of worship that may have a funeral service for animals. Check with your local religous houses.

Pet memorial services—There are pet memorial businesses that are starting to pop up around the nation. A pet memorial may resemble a furneral without having a body or casket present. These would be a place were the family could memorialize their pet, and include people who may have been affected by the pet's presence in their lives. Look in your local area. They may be attached to a crematorium, pet cemetery, or other aftercare services.

Herbs/incense

There may be many herbs and incense that people might use with body care. These are a few that may be used. Catnip—may be used to help relax cats before euthanasia but can also be used postdeath as a symbol (Weise, 2018).

Sage—may be used for many traditions, can be present in the house, or burned and smudged.

Incense-there are distinct types of incense, examples of incense can be Frankincense, Myrrh, Myrtle, and Sandalwood, which may be used for rites of passage (Weise, 2018).

Crystals

Crystals may signify a belief or energy that the person needs or feels the animal may need (Weise, 2018). Clients may place crystals on their animal for cremation or prior to burial. An example is rose quartz which may signify love.

Personal items of animal

Collars, a favorite toy or blanket, may be used during euthanasia or death and sent with animals to the crematorium or held onto for an alter or funeral/memorial service.

Religious and cultural traditions

You may be asked to participate in a variety of religious or cultural traditions when going into people's homes. Being open and educated on different traditions will help you support families with diverse cultures and religions. The list is not comprehensive but remember that there are lots of distinct ways of providing care and support for people. These are traditions for human death, and pet death may be viewed differently; however, as more families see their pet as an extension of family, those traditions may be upheld. Remember these are very general to give you an overview and based on the traditions for human death and not every religion or culture view animals in the same way as humans. In the author's experience being open to the experience, if you are allowed to participate, can strengthen your human experience.

Christianity—note, there are many different specific traditions not covered here.

Belief—there is heaven and hell for humans (Belief Net staff., 2018).

Body care—prayer may be said, with humans, often a priest or pastor is involved, there may be an open or closed casket.

Necropsy is acceptable.

Cremation is generally acceptable.

Body preparation—may not need preparation for many traditions, except if they are going to have an open casket ceremony.

Viewing—not necessary for many traditions (Everplans staff, 2018).

Catholic

Belief—They believe in heaven, hell, and purgatory for humans (Belief Net staff., 2018).

Body care—may want a priest to be involved. May want to say a prayer.

Necropsy is generally acceptable.

Cremation—historically has been unacceptable, more recently, has been more accepted.

Body preparation—may want to have the body lie in state for a day or more.

Viewing—with humans, it is traditional to have a viewing of the body. Maybe not as traditional for pets (Everplans staff, 2018).

Judaism

Belief—with humans, that death will lead to rebirth in a world to come (Belief Net staff., 2018).

Body care—traditional to bury within a day of death for humans.

Necropsy—generally not acceptable for humans, maybe unacceptable for pets.

Cremation—It depends on the orthodox of the person. Very orthodox and traditional may not allow cremation, reformed folks may allow.

Body preparation—may want to wash and prepare the body. May be different for animals.

Viewing—no viewing (Everplans staff, 2018).

Muslim

Body care—for humans should be buried as soon as possible.

Necropsy is generally not accepted as it is considered a desecration of the body. Cremation is forbidden for humans.

Body preparation—They may want to do something to prepare the body. Washing and shrouding are how they prepare for humans, they may want to keep the body to prepare it, and they may want to keep it for burial.

Viewing—There is no viewing (Everplans staff, 2018).

Hinduism

Belief—For humans, death is a part of the continuing cycle of life, death, and rebirth. They may believe the soul transfers to another body after death (Belief Net staff., 2018).

Body care—For humans, they may not want to touch the body immediately after death, it is seen as impure.

Necropsy is acceptable.

Cremation is acceptable.

Body preparation—they may want to care for the body after death some time later.

Viewing—may want to have a viewing. It is brief in the Hindu tradition (Everplans staff, 2018).

Buddhist

Belief about death—For humans, death is a part of the continuing cycle of life, death, and rebirth. The soul transfers to another body after death (Belief Net staff, 2018).

Body care—the body needs to stay for some time period, as Buddhists believe the soul does not leave the body right away. Chanting, prayers may be said.

Necropsy is acceptable.

Cremation is acceptable.

Body preparation—the body must be cold before preparation.

Viewing—A wake, celebration of life, maybe performed (Everplans staff, 2018).

Indigenous peoples—traditions may be as varied for different culturals.

Body care—varies, burial may be preferred.

Necropsy is unknown.

Cremation—some traditions allow.

Body preparation—varied.

Viewing—varied (Encyclopedia of Death and Dying, 2018).

Pagan

Belief—It is a part of the continuing cycle of life, death, and rebirth.

Body preparation—may want to wash the body, and smudge with scented oil, incense

(Belief Net staff., 2018).

Body care may be as varied as there are humans on this planet. It may even be varied among households. Meeting people where they are emotionally and culturally can provide you with some wonderful and varied experiences around the care of the body. In the author's experience, most people choose cremation services of some kind, or burial. But, the author has seen many different traditions as well and try to help people achieve their body care goals. The traditions and rituals we hold are a significant part of the grieving process.

References

Belief Net Staff. (2018). *Transition rituals*. Retrieved from Beliefnet.com.

Cooney, K. (2016). *Informal interview with Kathy Cooney* (L. Hendrix, interviewer).

Cremation Resource Staff. (2018). *How is a body cremated?*. Retrieved from Cremation Resource.org http://www.cremationresource.org/cremation/how-is-a-body-cremated.html.

Encyclopedia of Death and Dying. (2018). *Native American religion.* Retrieved from Encyclopedia of Death and Dying http://www.deathreference.com/Me-Nu/Native-American-Religion.html.

EPA. (September 1995). *Meat rendering plants.* Retrieved from EPA.gov https://www3.epa.gov/ttn/chief/ap42/ch09/final/c9s05-3.pdf.

Everplans Staff. (2018). *Funeral traditions of different religions.* Retrieved from Everplans https://www.everplans.com/articles/funeral-traditions-of-different-religions.

Johnson, M. (July 6, 2018). *For pet owners who just can't say goodbye, there's always freeze-drying.* Retrieved from Mother Nature Network https://www.mnn.com/family/pets/stories/for-pet-owners-who-just-cant-say-goodbye-theres-always-freeze-drying.

Lemire, K. R. (2016). Alkaline hydrolysis to remove potentially infectious viral RNA contaminants from DNA. *Virology Journal, 88.*

Murphy, R. S. (2009). Alkaline hydrolysis of mouse-adapted scrapie for inactivation and disposal of prion-positive material. *Journal of Animal Science*, 1787−1793.

The Editors of Encyclopedia Britannica. (2018). *Taxidermy.* Retrieved from Britannica.com: https://www.britannica.com/science/taxidermy.

Weise, M. (April 26, 2018). *Pet life celebration ritual.* Retrieved from Pet Helpful https://pethelpful.com/pet-ownership/pet-life-celebration-ritual.

Dealing with compassion fatigue, burnout, and impostor syndrome

13

Lynn Hendrix, AA, BA, DVM, CHPV [1,2,3,4]

[1]*Owner, Veterinarian, Beloved Pet Mobile Vet, Davis, CA, United States;* [2]*Former Board of Directors, IAAHPC, Chicago, IL, United States;* [3]*Consultant, Hospice, Palliative Medicine, End of Life, VIN, Davis, CA, United States;* [4]*President, Founder, World Veterinary Palliative Medicine Organization, Davis, CA, United States*

The veterinarian, Dr. Sophie Yin died in 2014. She was a world-renowned veterinary behaviorist, who created science-based, paradigm-changing behavioral programs to help animals get through their day in better ways. Dr. Yin created Low-Stress Handling, the first program to help veterinarians reduce stress for animals during veterinary visits. She was featured on several television shows, spoke at conferences worldwide, and had written many books. She was well-loved and respected in the profession. And yet … internally, she struggled.

Suicide has hit our profession harder than most professions. Suicide may occur because of overwhelming stressors, external problems, and internal challenges that can contribute to mental illnesses, including depression and anxiety. Compassion fatigue became a buzzword in veterinary medicine when the death of Sophia Yin and other veterinarians in the country started hitting the national news in 2014. So, what does compassion fatigue mean? Who does it affect? Are animal hospice or palliative veterinarians or team members more prone to compassion fatigue? How is compassion fatigue different from burnout? How does impostor syndrome contribute to burnout and compassion fatigue? How can we get through our difficult days?

The difference between compassion fatigue and burnout

Burnout was first described in 1974 by American psychologist Herbert J. Freudenberger. He identified three components of burnout: emotional exhaustion, depersonalization, and reduced personal accomplishment (Fig. 13.1) (Coles, 2017).

Burnout can be multifactorial with both endogenous and exogenous factors. Endogenous factors may include having excessive personal expectations, tendencies toward perfectionism, and habitually taking on increasing work, despite getting less and less rest. People who struggle with burnout may have dysfunctional coping skills, such as alcohol or medication dependency. They may struggle with boundary setting and coping with impostor syndrome (Mealer, 2021).

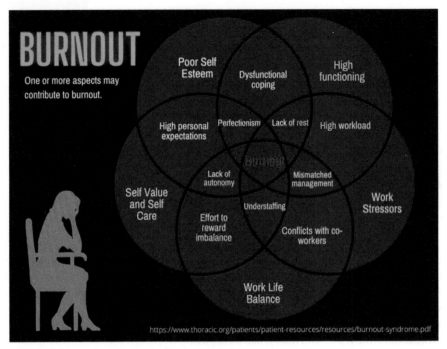

FIGURE 13.1

Possible contributory factors in burnout.

Lynn Hendrix ©2021.

Exogenous factors can include work overload, lack of autonomy, diminishing rewards, loss of community and teamwork, lack of equity, as well as differences in values between management and individuals. The individual may take on more work during the working day and having additional cases added to the day are everyday situations in veterinary medicine. Management may try to accomodate every case that comes in or calls the hospital or clinic, whereas the team may be overloaded with cases during the day. Given the endogenous factors, this can create an internal conflict with the individual team member. Lack of autonomy may include not being permitted to make individual decisions in your day, lack of trust, or lack of management support. Loss of community and teamwork may occur in situations with understaffing, mismatched management styles for the individual veterinarians' needs, and may lead to conflicts amongst coworkers as a result. There may be a lack of work/life balance, creating additional stresses on the veterinarian (Gaither, 2018).

The Maslach Burnout Inventory is commonly used to assess burnout experienced by professionals. Summarized, the Maslach Burnout Inventory looks at Emotional Exhaustion, Depersonalization factors, and Personal Accomplishment (Mealer, 2021).

If you feel like you might be burnt out, you can do a Maslach Burnout Inventory online to help you start on a path of improvement (Fig. 13.2).

Freudenberger and Gail North also identified 12 stages leading up to burnout (Coles, 2017). These stages correspond to both internal and external contributors

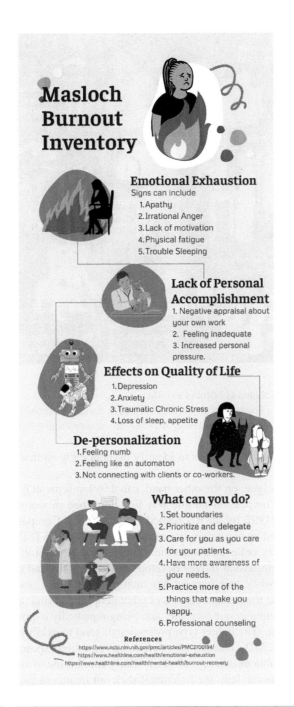

FIGURE 13.2

Maslach Burnout Inventory and how you can improve burnout.

Lynn Hendrix ©2021. Kaschka, W. P. (2011). Burnout: A fashionable diagnosis. Deutsches Arzteblatt International, 781−787. doi: ;https://doi.org/10.3238/arztebl.2011.0781; Prinz, P. H. (2012). Burnout, depression and depersonalisation—psychological factors and coping strategies in dental and medical students. GMS Zeitschrift fur medizinische Ausbildung, Doc 10.

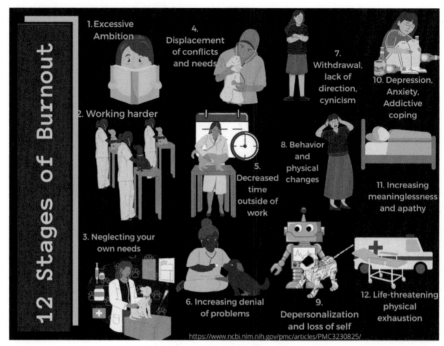

FIGURE 13.3

Freudenberger's 12 stages of burnout in order.

Created on Canva by Lynn Hendrix ©2021. Kaschka, W. P. (2011). Burnout: A fashionable diagnosis. Deutsches Arzteblatt International, 781–787. doi: https://doi.org/10.3238/arztebl.2011.0781.

to burnout and help veterinarians to identify burnout early so that they can change course (Fig. 13.3).

Compassion fatigue, on the other hand, can develop separately from or in addition to burnout. Compassion fatigue was first described in women, and the term came into use in 1992 by an RN named Carla Joinson. Compassion fatigue has also been described as secondary traumatic stress disorder (STSD) by Dr. Charles R Figley. Dr. Figley believed compassion fatigue may be as problematic as PTSD (Figley, 1995). Compassion fatigue develops due to empathy and compassion overload specifically, while true burnout has multiple etiologies (Coles, 2017). Being exposed once to the trauma and distress of other people can bring up feelings around past or present trauma in our own life, and being repeatedly exposed may result in compassion fatigue. The helper-type professionals tend to exhibit a high degree of empathy, and those MDs, nurses, and veterinarians are often exposed to higher levels of distress and trauma of other people daily. Early recognition of signs of burnout or compassion fatigue can help the individual seek out treatment early. These are the five stages leading toward compassion fatigue, which also overlap with the 12 phases of burnout (Mescia, 2004) (Figs. 13.4 and 13.5).

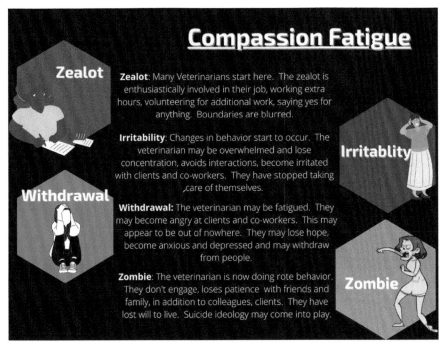

FIGURE 13.4

Stages to compassion fatigue.

Created on Canva by Lynn Hendrix ©2021. Mescia, N. D.,G. J. (2004). Understanding compassion fatigue.
Retrieved from Florida Center for Public Health Preparedness http://www.fcphp.usf.edu/courses/content/ucf/
ucf_manual.pdf.

The most common scale used to quantify compassion fatigue is the ProQoL (Cocker, 2016). This scale can be found online for free at https://proqol.org/. Another scale created by Brian E. Bride is the Secondary Traumatic Stress Scale. If you are scoring high on these scales, please seek out professional help (Fig. 13.6).

Veterinarians and veterinary team members have a higher percentage of people than other professions inclined to anxiety and depression, and suicide (Nett, 2014). A survey study reported in 2016 showed stressors might include decreased job satisfaction, and more hours worked. It also found that the less prepared they felt they were for the job, the higher the likelihood of compassion fatigue (Dicks, 2016). The survey identified women as more likely to be identified with compassion fatigue than men. Working in the companion animal field and caucasian veterinarians were associated with higher rates of compassion fatigue than were food animal/equine vets or veterinarians of color. Younger clinicians were also more prone to higher scores in compassion fatigue (Dicks, 2016).

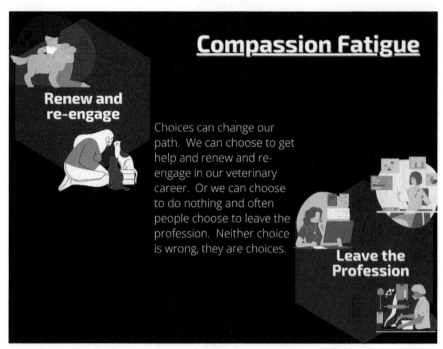

FIGURE 13.5

Choices that we have with compassion fatigue.

Created on Canva by Lynn Hendrix ©2021. Mescia, N. D.,G. J. (2004). Understanding compassion fatigue.
Retrieved from Florida Center for Public Health Preparedness http://www.fcphp.usf.edu/courses/content/ucf/
ucf_manual.pdf.

Table 3. Secondary Traumatic Stress Scale
The following is a list of statements made by persons who have been affected by their work with traumatized clients. Read each statement, then indicate how frequently the statement was true for you in the past *seven days*.

	Never	Rarely	Occasionally	Often	Very Often
	1	2	3	4	5
1. I felt emotionally numb.					
2. My heart started pounding when I thought about my work with clients.					
3. It seemed as if I was reliving the trauma experienced by my client.					
4. I had trouble sleeping.					
5. I felt discouraged about the future.					
6. Reminders of my work with clients upset me.					
7. I had little interest in being around others.					
8. I felt jumpy.					
9. I was less active than usual.					
10. I thought about my work with clients when I didn't intend to.					
11. I had trouble concentrating.					
12. I avoided people, places or things that reminded me of my work with clients.					
13. I had disturbing dreams about my work with clients.					
14. I wanted to avoid working with some clients.					
15. I was easily annoyed.					
16. I expected something bad to happen.					
17. I noticed gaps in my memory about client sessions.					

Copyright 1999, Brian E. Bride.

NOTE: "Client" is used to indicate persons with whom you have been engaged in a helping relationship. You may substitute another noun that better represents your work, such as consumer, patient, recipient and so forth.

FIGURE 13.6

Secondary Traumatic Stress Scale ©1999 Brian E. Bride.

Used with permission from Brian E. Bride 2021 Coles, T. (October 27, 2017). Compassion fatigue and burnout:
History, definitions and assessment. *Retrieved from Veterinarian's Money Digest https://www.vmdtoday.com/*
journals/vmd/2017/october2017/compassion-fatigue-and-burnout-history-definitions-and-assessment.

What can you do to change your path?
Begin with a daily self-care plan

Making the time to care for yourself, so you can be the best you can be for your patients, your clients, and you can be a challenge. If you do not renew and refill, you will not be fully there for yourself or fully there for them. Making time for self care is a conscious daily task until it becomes a habit. It will take a shift in mindset, a shift from your norms, and a shift from your current habits. Your self-care plan may include the following:

Recognition

- Awareness of the problem is your first step. Recognition of your body and mind that you have reached a limit or are overwhelmed is your first step.
- Identify the external stressors. What is making you stressed? Is work increasing your workload? Are you burnt out at work? Do you have additional home stress from family or friends? Are you doom scrolling on social media? Do you live in a high-crime area or a location of war?
- Identify internal stressors. What was it about that case or multiple cases that caused your stress? How did each case make you feel? Did you tense up, cry, get angry at that client, even if you didn't verbalize it? Are you internalizing your feeling through the day because you are not allowed to express them at work? How does your body feel when it is stressed? Are you finding that you are getting angry, stressed, crying more frequently at work or at home? Are you getting physically ill? Have you been diagnosed with a chronic issue? Do you have apathy and just do not care anymore? Are you starting to feel tense reading this?
- Make a list of your stressors to recognize and acknowledge them.
- Numbing feelings with medications or alcohol, food, or other unhealthy coping methods may help temporarily but will not help in the long term. Dealing with feelings as they come up and acknowledging the good, bad, and ugly feelings is the throughway to move through compassion fatigue and burnout. Being overwhelmed with feelings can be very uncomfortable, and we tend to revert to what worked with coping when we were overwhelmed as children. This work takes time, daily work on change and you do not have to be perfect on day one. Get professional help, a coach, or a counselor to help you sort out feelings. (AIS Staff, 2020)

Equilibrium

- If you are experiencing stress, fatigue, burnout, or compassion fatigue, your next step may be to stop what you are doing and move away from the stressors. Take time off from work. If you cannot take the entire time off, take mini escapes, even throughout a day. These mini escapes are not taking a bathroom break, or sitting for five minutes to consume food. They are taking a walk around the block, driving to a park nearby to eat. Taking a dog for a walk, or playing with kittens, going for a horseback ride, preferably away from your place of business.

- Recenter yourself. Recentering yourself can mean getting more sleep and eating healthier foods, but it may also mean taking time to meditate, to exercise, and remove yourself from the stressors. Recentering yourself is only a step. There is more work to be done before placing yourself back into work stressors.
- Find quiet time to sit with uncomfortable feelings. Acknowledge any grief or sadness in your life, whether it is anticipatory, in the past, or in the present (This can be difficult to do, just like anything new). If you can, go to a favorite space, for example, the ocean, a lake, the mountains, on a hike, or turn a space in your house into a "spa" room. Create a space that is sacred and where you can feel safe. Remove clutter not only from the room but from your head while your in this space. This again takes time and practice.
- Start recognizing small things that make you feel joy. Joy is an internal feeling as opposed to happiness, which is external. Individuals can appear happy, but have deep sorrow and grief that they carry with them. This step is for searching those internal feelings of joy. Those small wins at home and work are particularly important. Acknowledge a lovely client or coworker who made your day better, a thank you card, or a gift you received. Make a list of things that bring you joy.
- Identify things or situations that made you laugh daily. Reflect on those events at the end of the day. This can be a good meditation.
- Recognize what replenishes or restores you each day. Practice this step daily. Write them down if you need to see them daily. These can change over time.
- Learn to ask yourself if you have control over a situation or not. We may want to control everything and need to start acknowledging what we can and cannot control. Focus on "What is" and not "What if's."
- Start shifting your focus and language on how you see problems and stressors. Changing the language can change how we feel internally about external situations. Using positive internal language can change your brain. For example, using words like—challenge-instead of—problem, or joy instead of happiness.
- Write a personal mission statement. Define your personal and professional goals. If you are the kind of person who likes checklists, create a timeline and a checklist. Reevaluate every few months as you progress. Your goals may change over time.
- Finding your passion! While you may be in a job at a brick and mortar at this moment, you picked up this book for a reason. Maybe end-of-life care for veterinary patients is your passion. Maybe, you discover that you would prefer a different type of house call practice along your journey. Maybe you want to work in other ways as a veterinarian or even explore a different field. If you have made it to this section, know that finding your passion, building on your life journey will help you find compassion satisfaction (AIS Staff, 2020).

Community and connection

- Being social creatures, connecting with people and pets can help us generate joy by changing our neurotransmitter and hormonal release (Dfarhud, 2014). Seeing animals and their people in their homes can be a much more intimate and social connection with both pet and client than seeing patients every 15 or 30 minutes.
- Can you think of a family member or friend you can call that will help support you? Call them daily if you can. If you have more than one, you have more support. Reach out to trusted colleagues, family members, or friends.
- Find professional help to make additional connections. Recognizing that you have compassion fatigue or burnout is the first step. Mental health professionals may be essential to helping veterinarians through their compassion fatigue. If you have a mental health professional that helps you with your service, ask if they feel comfortable helping you and your staff with compassion fatigue if it arises. Finding a mental health professional who focuses on compassion fatigue can give specific tools to help veterinarians and staff to deal with compassion fatigue.
- Find community connections, other veterinarians who share similar stories. In-person connections improve our resilience and joy (AIS Staff, 2020).

Strengthening resiliency

Improving resiliency is discussed in the literature to get through our daily stressors. Veterinarians are already resilient. We have been through a lot to get where we are and could give master classes on resiliency. This list may speak to some, to help you build tools and skills to work on daily. According to the ACEVO, these are some steps you can take to strengthen resiliency (ACEVO Staff, 2018). The following is a modified list from their website.

1. Using touch during times of stress can help release oxytocin and can help decrease your stress levels. These are some techniques they suggest.
   a. Placing your hand on your heart and deep breathing.
   b. Being held by someone trusted, being near someone trusted, or thinking about someone trusted.
   c. Massage, even massaging your own hands or feet, can help.
2. Being aware and adjusting body posture. Power poses and smiling can help change our neurochemistry.
3. Affecting a positive attitude and focusing on gratitude. Keep your attention on the positive things that have happened that day and what you are grateful for during the day. Concentrate on them for at least 30 seconds.
4. Compassionate self-talk.
   a. Pausing in moments of stress and acknowledging that something stressful is occurring.
   b. Saying out loud statements like, "This is painful, upsetting."
   c. And then follow it up with positive self-talk such as "I am here for you," "You are special, sacred, or ok." "It is ok for me be to stressed about this".

5. Creating a positive portfolio.
   a. Asking for written positive feedback. This can be in the form of postcards, or cards, emails, tweets, or other social media from your friends and family. Then, put them on a sheet of paper to read every day.
   b. Making a binder of Thank You Letters from your clients.
   c. Freestyle journaling, or writing in gratitude journals.
   d. These can help "rewire" our self-talk.
6. Mindfulness-helping you find the gift in the mistake.
   a. Acknowledge what happened.
   b. Acknowledge what you did at the moment.
   c. Acknowledge the "cost" to you.
   d. Look for the lesson. This can be difficult to do when we are depressed, anxious, or grieving. It is ok to find a lesson later.
   e. And then consider what you might have done differently.

Changing our mindset and improving your life is your journey, as unique as you are, take ownership of your life. It is important to remember that failure happens to everybody. We all have bad days, and we try to keep them from turning into bad years.

Embracing spirituality

Spirituality does not have to involve an organized religion, though if you have one, leaning on your religious community can also help you get through a crisis and help you replenish your wellbeing. Organized religion can support you with connections to people. You can also find your way to connect, to the planet, to yourself, and to others with similar beliefs.

Boundary setting

Setting boundaries are a powerful tool to prevent burnout and compassion fatigue. Setting your boundaries early is a crucial step for those providing veterinary palliative and hospice care. Boundaries can help you establish a healthy relationship with the families of your patients. Veterinarians need to begin with clear expectations for clients. Knowing what your boundaries are before you see clients can help you set expectations for clients. Write a list of what expectations you want to develop. Put your boundaries in writing, place them on your website, tell people on the phone, in person, and hand them to clients in writing that you leave with them at the first meeting. You can have them sign off on acknowledgment of these boundaries. Veterinarians can connect intimately with palliative families. You do not have to be 24/7 to do this work. So defining what your hours are, and your availability is is crucial. While many families will observe boundaries, there may be connections with some people who have emotional, social, cultural, and mental health issues where boundaries can become blurred.

Setting personal boundaries may be hard for some veterinarians. Veterinarians may work long hours and often care for each patient as though it was their pet. As discussed earlier in the chapter, compassion fatigue can set in for any veterinarian, and lack of personal boundaries plays a crucial role. So here are some ideas for boundaries setting for the housecall practice.

Think about the following boundaries:

1. You can start with simple boundaries, such as the hours, days you are available. Scheduling everything in your life, not just the clients, but your family time (which is very important), meetings, getting gas, going to the bank, or post office … anything that you need to do to make your personal time as important as "work" time. This can be challenging for some people. When starting your business, you can be flexible with your time, however, as you get busy you will want to define your boundaries, so starting at the beginning can get you past that uncomfortable feeling and make it a habit.

2. Consider how would you like to receive communication? Is it ok for clients to text you, email you, call you? Can you redirect them to a website, a team, or an online scheduler to minimize your additional time on the phone?

3. If you have palliative or hospice clients, what do you recommend for them to do if you are not available? Do they have emergency information, a crisis kit? Instructions on what to do if they have an emergency?

4. You DO NOT have to practice 24/7 to be a hospice or palliative vet. Please do not feel like you have to be available all the time for clients. It is not sustainable for a sole practitioner to be available all the time. However, you do want palliative clients to have a plan in case you are not readily available. A crisis kit is another way to create that boundary, empowering the client to give medication to sedate their pet, help to ameliorate acute pain, seizures, bleeding, etc.

5. How are you going to follow up with clients? How often are you going to follow up? Are you going to call or do it in writing? Are you going to have in-person or telemedicine follow-ups? Are you following up with your colleagues who may have referred you? How are you following up with them? Are you sending emails, letters?

6. How do you want to schedule appointments? Via phone calls, email, online appointment scheduler? Are you going to have team members?

7. How are you going to handle being overwhelmed with appointments? (a good problem to have but this can be emotionally draining). Being overwhelmed with appointments may not occur for a while. However, this is a consideration to think about as you are writing lists.

8. What will you do if you have grief from personal loss (a pet, a family member, a friend loss)? You will want to consider that your clients will be going through this as well and prepare written resources for clients to help support them. Have a plan for your losses, how are you going to take time away from the business, how are you going to contact clients?

9. How are you going to schedule days off? Initially, days off may be a natural flow of the business, but it may become more difficult to set that boundary as you grow.

10. Are you going to cancel personal plans to help a client? If you cancel personal plans, are you going to regret it later? Are you going to charge extra for after-hours appointments (the author strongly recommends this if you choose to help people after hours). Remember, no one goes to their death bed wishing they worked more. They wish they had spent more time with friends and family. Do you have small children? How much do you want to be away from them? Consider these as you are developing your plan.

11. When you get very busy, when will you hire someone to answer phones? Is this in your business plan? Consider placing it in your business plan.

12. How are you going to handle cultural differences? Political differences?

Some warning signs of boundaries being breached may be the following:

1. Clients who do not listen to your rules. For example, they may leave messages when you are not working or on vacation and expect calls to be returned. Clients who expect you to drop what you are doing to assist them.

2. Clients who use emotional manipulation, sadness, guilt, anger, or passive-aggressive commentary to engage you.

3. Clients wanting to know where you live, your personal phone number (remember some people will call because they have a direct line to a veterinarian, and they can bypass a receptionist or tech). (The author strongly recommends having a secondary VoIP phone system, so clients cannot directly contact you on your personal phone number.)

4. Clients with whom you share meaningful personal information may overreach your personal boundaries into your professional life. It may be easy to do, as you meet clients in their homes and can connect strongly with some people.

5. Clients who want to socialize or connect on social media outside of care (Barbour, 2021).

What can you do if clients overstep your boundaries?

1. Set clear expectations early. For those clients who overstep, correct the problem quickly. Remind them of your hours or how to contact you. Engage an auto-send on your phone text, email for after-hours, or on vacation can help until you have a team to respond for you. When you have a team, they should only answer the phone, text, email during business hours. These expectations should be in writing on your website and the paperwork you would leave with a client. It also helps to say it at appointments, though they may not always remember if you say it.

2. You can still have empathy and compassion while correcting a boundary overstep.

3. Check-in with colleagues regarding possible boundary overstep and get support.

4. Recognize when you might have signs of burnout, compassion fatigue, or personal conflict with a client that is separate from a boundary overstep.

5. Have professional counselors available for you or your team members if you are overwhelmed or feeling burnout or compassion fatigue (Barbour, 2021).

Coping skills

Having healthy coping skills for the daily stressors can help during stressful times. Coping skills have often been regressed to drinking a glass of wine or smoking. However, those are ways of medicating a hurt, coping skills learned early in our lives and socially acceptable and yet do not address the deeper issues that stifle us from moving through stress. Unhealthy coping skills can lead to burnout and can contribute to compassion fatigue.

The Positive Psychology Program has put together a comprehensive list of coping skills that the veterinarian can practice daily to help get through difficult days, weeks, or longer. These coping skills are from their website used with their permission and have been slightly modified to address specifics for veterinary medicine (PPP Staff, 2018). The Positive Psychology Program is an excellent resource for more support and tools to help the veterinarian get through a day.

Diversions

Healthy diversions can involve changing our thinking by diverting our attention. Physical changes in our body can change our perspective and gives our brain something else to do. Here are some examples from the Positive Psychology Program.

- Write, draw, paint, photography
- Play an instrument, sing, dance, act
- Take a shower or a bath
- Garden
- Take a walk, or go for a drive
- Watch television or a movie
- Watch cute kitten videos on YouTube
- Play a game
- Go shopping
- Clean or organize your environment
- Read
- Take a break or vacation

Social/interpersonal coping

We can also divert our brain by being social with another. Socializing can be accomplished with a friend, family member, or pet. Taking a dog for a walk, playing with a cat, or calling a friend can be very helpful. These are additional ideas around social and interpersonal diversion from the Positive Psychology site.

- Talk to someone you trust
- Set boundaries and say "no"
- Write a note to someone you care about
- Be assertive
- Use humor
- Spend time with friends and family

- Serve someone in need
- Care for or play with a pet (outside of the veterinary hospital)
- Role-play challenging situations with others
- Encourage others
- Join a support group

Cognitive coping

Engaging your brain in specific tasks can also help. Ideas are from the Positive Psychology website.

- Make a gratitude list
- Brainstorm solutions
- Lower your expectations of the situation
- Keep an inspirational quote with you
- Write a list of goals
- Take a class
- Act opposite of negative feelings
- Write a list of pros and cons for decisions
- Reward or pamper yourself when successful
- Write a list of strengths
- Accept a challenge with a positive attitude

Tension releasers

Tension occurs when we are stressed. Our body can hold tension. Have you ever had a tension headache or noticed your shoulders are in a shrug position when you consciously relax them? Those are examples of tension we hold in our bodies. We can release tension with exercise, yoga, meditation, crying, laughing out loud, taking a bath, or eating.

Spiritual

Spiritual practices can also be a way to relieve stress. Suggestions from the Positive Psychology Website.

- Pray or meditate
- Enjoy nature-take a walk
- Get involved in a worthy cause
- If you have a church, synagogue, mosque, temple, altar, monastery, or meeting house, or another place of spiritual support, visit and rejuvenate.

Setting limits

Setting limits for yourself can significantly change your life and stress level. Learning to say no to some things, prioritizing yourself first can be the first step. Changing your mindset takes practice, and it is easy to slip back into old habits, so be aware it can happen. Using your calendar to mark times for you as though you were an appointment and then following through with that is a straightforward way to make sure you have limited your time taking on appointments and seeing family and friends. Or just being present, or exercising, meditating, or doing the best coping skill for you.

Coping skills help you get through each day. Healthy coping skills may include the following:

- Meditation and relaxation techniques
- Having time to yourself
- Physical activity or exercise
- Reading
- Spending time with friends
- Finding humor
- Spending time on your hobbies
- Spirituality
- Spending time with your pets
- Getting a good night's sleep
- Eating healthy

Unhealthy coping skills may include the following:

- OTC or illicit medications/drugs
- Excessive alcohol use
- Self-mutilation
- Ignoring or bottling up feelings
- Working too much
- Avoiding your problems and using medication/drugs or alcohol to avoid feelings
- Denial of the challenges in your life (NAMI Staff, 2021)

Impostor syndrome

This chapter would be incomplete without a discussion on impostor syndrome. Impostor syndrome occurs frequently within populations of intelligent, successful people. People experiencing impostor syndrome internally believe they are fooling everyone around them and that maybe they are not as accomplished as they may be assumed to be. Although initially studied in women, impostor syndrome can occur with both men and women. When first identified, systemic racism and sexism were not a recognized component, though both may contribute to the internal feelings that arise (Tulshyan, 2021b).

A study on burnout and imposter syndrome in medical students showed that ½ of the women and ¼ of the men had impostor syndrome. It may also be associated with burnout, cynicism, emotional exhaustion, and depersonalization (Villwock, 2016). Imposter syndrome starts in early childhood in learning how to cope in the environment of criticism and with an emphasis on overachievement. Veterinarians of color and female veterinarians may be more susceptible to impostor syndrome (Weir, 2013).

Valerie Young (Author of The Secret Thoughts of Successful Women: Why Capable People Suffer From the Imposter Syndrome and How to Thrive in Spite of It) categorizes it further (Fig. 13.7) (Wilding, 2017):

1. The Perfectionist—The perfectionist sets very high goals for themselves (and often for others as well). When they do not reach a goal, they berate themselves (or others) for it. These people tend to be the micromanagers, or the manager who does everything themselves and cannot delegate to other team members. They are the "control freaks," those who want to control everything but, of course, cannot.

2. The Superwoman/man—These folks believe they have what it takes to push themselves hard and do more and more. They stay later, work harder, do not have a life outside of work, go home exhausted only to return to the office the very next day. This type of person tends to focus on external validation, often being validated by the work itself, rather than by an internal satisfaction of their work.

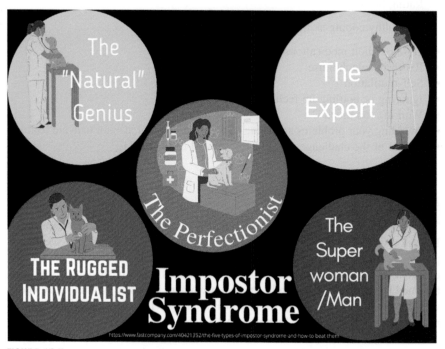

FIGURE 13.7

Imposter syndrome—anyone can feel this way and still be an accomplished veterinarian.
Lynn Hendrix© 2021. Wilding, M. (May 18, 2017). The five types of impostor syndrome and how to beat them. Retrieved from Fast Company https://www.fastcompany.com/40421352/the-five-types-of-impostor-syndrome-and-how-to-beat-them.

3. The Natural Genius—The natural genius judges themselves based on their success versus their ability or effort. They must get things right on the first try, or they consider themselves not successful. The people who fall into this category may have been the kid considered the "smart" person in their family.
4. The Rugged Individualist—The person who never wants to ask for help is the Rugged Individualist. They do not ask for help because they do not want to look dumb or foolish. Their self-worth may be based on their ability to accomplish a task, and if they are not able to do so on their own, they feel like an impostor.
5. The Expert—This person feels like they have fooled someone into hiring them. This type is concerned about being inexperienced or not knowledgeable enough. (Wilding, 2017). However, when anyone starts a new job, there is a learning curve.

How can one move through impostor syndrome?

Acknowledging impostor syndrome is the first place to start.

1. Recognize the feeling that you are pretending and that it is affecting you. Name the feeling.
2. Have colleagues and team members remind you that you have done the work to justify you being there when you are feeling this way. No one is perfect, and everyone is on a journey. Remember, your day one of a job is far different than your last day at a job.
3. Remove emotions from factual information. If you have just obtained your DVM, you deserve to have your degree. If you just signed papers to start your practice, you have worked hard to get there. There is always more to learn, we are on a journey, but acknowledge what you know.
4. Understand there are going to be times where self-doubt is appropriate.
5. Focus on your positive accomplishments. You know what you know, and now you know what you do not know.
6. Learn from your mistakes. Mistakes can often be our best teacher, not something to be feared.
7. Develop new strategies to understand when feelings of self-doubt come up. Read up on a subject you struggle with or feel unsure about. Talk with colleagues, engage on social media to help you know you are not alone in your feelings (Persky, 2018).
8. Acknowledge when it is the environment you are in, the team you work with, the culture of the workplace that may be contributing to your feeling less than. Work culture plays a bigger role in our feelings than we may acknowledge (Tulshyan, 2021b).
9. If you are a leader at your practice, learn more about systemic racism, and sexism and homophobia and practice ways to improve your work culture (Tulshyan, 2021a).

Conclusion

Burnout and Compassion Fatigue can affect veterinarians to a high degree. We are empathetic, compassionate people who are highly driven to succeed. Burnout occurs outside of empathy; compassion fatigue occurs because of our empathy. Both are multifactorial, and many of the factors overlap. Compassion fatigue is a misnomer, and it is a secondary traumatic stress disorder related to PTSD. People suffering from STSD (should be formerly known as compassion fatigue) need to seek out help. Burnout may also need professional help to heal.

Setting personal boundaries for your practice can help alleviate some of the stress involved in end-of-life care. Remember what your priorities are. If you are unsure, write them down and put them somewhere where you will see them frequently. Move your goalposts as you need to and move them as you shift your mindset. Do not get to the point of burnout or, worse, compassion fatigue (which is a secondary traumatic stress disorder).

Impostor syndrome can also contribute to the frame of mind of not feeling worthy. Systemic racism and sexism and homophobia in our work cultures can contribute to our feelings of being an imposter. Looking for leaders that create cultures of equity that support our sense of self.

Compassion fatigue and impostor syndrome can also contribute to depression and anxiety. Getting professional support can get you back on track and feeling more confident. You are not alone. Many colleagues suffer from anxiety, depression, burnout, secondary traumatic stress disorder, compassion fatigue, or impostor syndrome. If you are a veterinarian reading this book and you feel like have compassion fatigue, impostor syndrome, burnout, anxiety, depression, please reach out to us on Facebook https://www.facebook.com/groups/worldvetpalliativemedicine/.

References

ACEVO Staff. (2018). *Techniques for strengthening resilience*. Retrieved from ACEVO.org.uk https://www.acevo.org.uk/techniques-strengthening-resilience.

AIS Staff. (2020). *Compassion fatigue*. Retrieved from The American Institute of Stress https://www.stress.org/military/for-practitionersleaders/compassion-fatigue.

Barbour, L. T. (2021). Professional-patient boundaries in palliative care. *Palliative Care of Network of Wisconsin.* https://www.mypcnow.org/fast-fact/professional-patient-boundaries-in-palliative-care/.

Cocker, F. (2016). Compassion fatigue among healthcare, emergency and community service workers: A systematic review. *International Journal of Environmental Research and Public Health*, 618.

Coles, T. (October 27, 2017). *Compassion fatigue and burnout: History, definitions and assessment*. Retrieved from Veterinarian's Money Digest https://www.vmdtoday.com/journals/vmd/2017/october2017/compassion-fatigue-and-burnout-history-definitions-and-assessment.

Dfarhud, D. M. (2014). Happiness & health: The biological factors- systematic review article. *Iranian Journal of Public Health*, 1468−1477.

Dicks, M. B. (November 29, 2016). *Chipping away of the soul: New data on compassion fatigue and compassion satisfaction in veterinary medicine.* Retrieved from DVM 360 https://www.avma.org/PracticeManagement/BusinessIssues/Documents/2016-Nov-29_C hipping-away-of-the-soul_New-data-on-compassion-fatigue_and-compassion-satisfactio n_in-veterinary-medicine.pdf.

Figley, C. (1995). *Compassion fatigue: Coping with secondary traumatic stress disorder in those who treat the traumatized.* New York, NY: Brunner/Mazel.

Gaither, C. (August 22, 2018). *6 major job/employee mismatches which cause job burnout.* Retrieved from NC Professionals Health Program https://www.ncphp.org/6-major-jobemployee-mismatches-which-cause-job-burnout-by-clark-gaither-md-faafp/.

Kaschka, W. P. (2011). Burnout: A fashionable diagnosis. *Deutsches Arzteblatt International*, 781−787. https://doi.org/10.3238/arztebl.2011.0781

Mealer, M. M. (2021). *What is burnout syndrome?* Retrieved from American Thoracic Society https://www.thoracic.org/patients/patient-resources/resources/burnout-syndrome.pdf.

Mescia, N. D.,G. J. (2004). *Understanding compassion fatigue.* Retrieved from Florida Center for Public Health Preparedness http://www.fcphp.usf.edu/courses/content/ucf/ucf_manual.pdf.

NAMI staff. (2021). *Resource toolkit.* Retrieved from NAMI.org https://www.nami.org/Home.

Nett, R. W. (2014). *Notes from the field: Prevalence of risk factors for suicide among veterinarians — United States, 2014.* Retrieved from CDC.gov https://www.cdc.gov/mmwr/preview/mmwrhtml/mm6405a6.htm?s_cid=mm6405a6_e.

Persky, A. M. (2018). Intellectual self-doubt and how to get out of it. *American Journal of Pharmaceutical Education*, 6990.

PPP Staff. (2018). *Coping skills.* Retrieved from Positive Psychology Program.com https://positivepsychologyprogram.com/.

Prinz, P. H. (2012). Burnout, depression and depersonalisation−psychological factors and coping strategies in dental and medical students. *GMS Zeitschrift fur medizinische Ausbildung.* Doc 10.

Tulshyan, R. B. (July 14, 2021a). End imposter syndrome in your workplace. *Harvard Business Review*, e.

Tulshyan, R. B. (February 11, 2021b). Stop telling women they have imposter syndrome. *Harvard Business Review*, e.

Villwock, J. A.,S. L. (2016). Impostor syndrome and burnout among American medical students: A pilot study. *International Journal of Medical Education*, 364−369.

Weir, K. (November 2013). *Feel like a fraud?* Retrieved from American Psychological Association https://www.apa.org/gradpsych/2013/11/fraud.

Wilding, M. (May 18, 2017). *The five types of impostor syndrome and how to beat them.* Retrieved from Fast Company https://www.fastcompany.com/40421352/the-five-types-of-impostor-syndrome-and-how-to-beat-them.

Personal safety and difficult home visits

Lynn Hendrix, AA, BA, DVM, CHPV [1,2,3,4]

[1]*Owner, Veterinarian, Beloved Pet Mobile Vet, Davis, CA, United States;* [2]*Former Board of Directors, IAAHPC, Chicago, IL, United States;* [3]*Consultant, Hospice, Palliative Medicine, End of Life, VIN, Davis, CA, United States;* [4]*President, Founder, World Veterinary Palliative Medicine Organization, Davis, CA, United States*

Veterinarians encounter difficult clients in general brick and mortar practices and house call practices are not immune. Palliative or hospice veterinarians deal with highly emotional people and may encounter a difficult home visit. Emotions around grief may involve anger, especially if the euthanasia do not go well at least from their perspective. (Grief and the grief process, including denial, is discussed in Chapter 9, Grief Support.) A veterinarinan trained in end-of-life care may help alleviate the fears and distress of losing a pet with support of the caregiver with education and decision making. However, even if you may only provide euthanasia services and may only be there for the final visit, and being empathetic can be essential to help defuse a situation. Expanding your education in human psychology and behavioral coursework in human psychology can bolster your strengths. The University of Tennessee has a program on Veterinary Social Work.

If getting extra degrees is not appealing, advancing excellent listening and communication skills can help minimize contentious behavior. There are many excellent communication courses that you may ascertain online, in conferences, at some veterinary schools. Boundary setting can also help these situations. Training in self-defense and martial arts may help make you more comfortable going into more challenging households. It is recommended to get weapon training if you decide to carry a weapon. This chapter is about planning for what to do if you get into a situation that may be difficult, not just in terms of personal safety but what to do if a person is suicidal oryou have a hard time connecting with, cancellations and finally, firing clients that cross boundaries.

Personal safety

Since personal safety is a primary issue for house call veterinarians, we will begin with these issues. Your personal safety supersedes the appointment. Get out of a situation if you are feeling threatened at all. Listen to your inner voice. Before you are in a threatening situation, you want to plan action if things change rapidly—plan for the worst and always hope for the best. Think about the following questions. What are you going to do if someone is angry at the door? Or becomes angry during the appointment? How are you going to stop or slow an angry person? What are you going to do if someone comes at you, is physically threatening you? If someone has a weapon? If you are on the ground and they are standing above you? What if you do not feel comfortable on the phone, in person, if they have a weapon? What would your plan be? Do you plan on carrying some sort of weapon? Mace, pepper spray, gun? (The author wants to mention here that an angry, adrenalized man can overpower a women and use the weapon against them). Have you had any self-defense training? Do you know how to get out of zip ties, handcuffs?

These are very scary topics. And let me reassure you and tell you it is unlikely that you encounter these problems, but reports on listservs/social media underscore the danger. There are veterinarians who have been attacked and luckily got away. And occasionally, we do hear about someone who did not, which is why we need to discuss this topic as disconcerting as it may be. It is better to be prepared and never use the plan than to find yourself in a crisis without a plan.

Phone contact

Assessing your safety begins with your first phone contact. Listening to where people have been in the process of their animal's disease, which vets they have seen, what has been done so far, what medications the animal is on, what they understand about the disease, and what they believe are their options are just part of the conversations that you could have on the phone. Listening to the underlying fear, what the clients are concerned about, what they are afraid of, their goals, and their previous experiences with death and dying and euthanasia are principal issues that also may come up on the phone. These may need to be gone over again in the home visit, especially if there is more than one family member and anyone who disagrees with the decision for treatment or euthanasia.

An angry call

Anger, rational or irrational, may arise on a phone call. Rational anger can exist with grief if they feel frustrated about the dying process, have not felt supported, or have been told they "Have to" euthanize their beloved pet. They may use phrases like, "my vet told me I HAVE to euthanize my pet," or angrily say, "I hate all vets." With rational anger, finding out more about what has been happening in their life can help diffuse the anger.

Occasionally, you will get calls that just do not feel right. Something tells you the person on the other end is not having rational anger. There may not be anything they specifically said (or maybe there is) but honor your feeling if you get such a feeling.

With irrational anger, the anger will be difficult to diffuse. If you feel threatened during a phone call or their anger is not rational on the phone, decline the appointment. You are booked, busy, out of town, it does not matter excuse what you use, do not go if you are feeling weird about the phone contact at all.

If you decide to go, make sure you tell people where you will be, how long you plan on being there, and a check-in time. Even a check-in phrase that you can text someone to let them know you are ok or that you are not. Make it one word and something that would not get the client's suspicions up, like green for all clear and red for I am in trouble. There are also apps you can use on your phone or some mobile watches that can track you. Have a plan for getting out of the house if things get uncomfortable or dangerous, which will be covered later in this chapter.

An example of a call that sounded dangerous

I had a guy call me once who wanted to take me off-grid … his words. He wanted me to drive an hour to a remote location and then get in his car alone with him and go another hour to another even more remote location. NOPE! And this was early in my business, and I hated turning away people. But this scenario just screamed, I am going to be hurt, or worse … So trust your instinct.

Drug-seeking phone calls

Drug-seeking behavior can often be elicited over the phone. Drug seekers may be overt in their drug-seeking. They may ask you to bring specific injections or pills by name or product before you have ever seen their pet. Typical drug-seeking behavior is listed in the infographic (Fig. 14.1). Contact the DEA if you have further questions about potential drug-seeking behavior.

These phone calls can be easy to decline and if you go to their house, do a thorough exam if you can of the house, looking for drug paraphernlia. Be cautious with prescribing medication and make sure you have any prescription well documented. Avoid leaving a prescription pad in an area that someone could get a hold of it. With the opioid crisis in the United States, it may be more challenging to prescribe opioid-type medications for animals, so be cautious.

Arriving at the house

Safety plans commence from the moment you get out of your car and walk up to the door. Start mentally planning your escape routes: where the doors, windows, and gates are. Are they locked? Are there chairs nearby? It can be a quick visual survey of the area. Most houses you will visit are lovely, neat, and orderly. Occasionally, you will find one that has limited space, stacks of papers, or even a hoarding house,

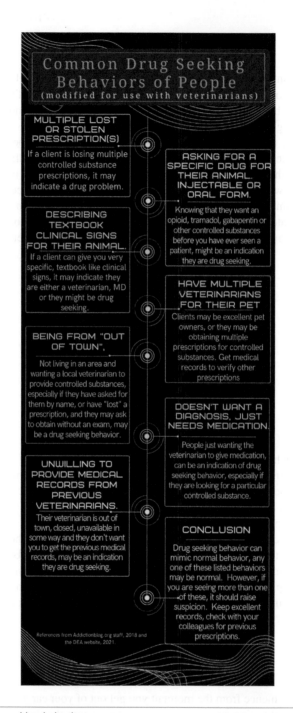

FIGURE 14.1

Common drug-seeking behaviors.

Created by Lynn Hendrix DVM, CHPV ©2021 Addictionblog.org Staff. (2018). How to tell if someone has drug seeking behavior. *Retrieved from Addictionblog.org http://addictionblog.org/FAQ/identifying-addiction/how-to-identify-drug-seeking-behavior/; DEA Staff. (1999).* Don't be scammed by a drug abuser (from 1999 brochure). *Retrieved from DEA Diversion Control Division https://www.deadiversion.usdoj.gov/pubs/brochures/drugabuser.htm.*

where you can barely fit through the door. Outdoor yards may be the same way. Sometimes the house or yard smells of urine or feces, or is filled with urine or feces, body odor, or even scented candles or incense or cigarette smoke (or other drugs) inside the home can be overwhelming. Suggesting a different space out in the backyard or on a balcony may help overcome some of these challenges, but can limit your escape route, so be cautious. While these are not necessarily overt safety issues, they can contribute to your overall well being.

Getting to the animal can also sometimes be challenging. If the animal is feral, having it contained is essential, preferably in a cage, or kennel if it is small, in another room if it is a bigger aggressive dog. With cats or small dogs, giving them meds orally in some yummy food, Churu®, ice cream, peanut butter, butter (something to lick) or with a bit of maple syrup (Thank you to Tiffany Ma DVM from Compassion Pet Hospice in Castro Valley, CA, for the suggestion, she suggests 0.1 mL of each syrup/Telazol to avoid drooling). Offering food when giving an injection can help minimize the stress of the injection m. With aggressive dogs, the author will often give oral medication to the owner in treats and let them feed them after a quick view of the healthy animal. Though it is not optimal, but if a glimpse of a stranger can set them off, getting them relaxed first will make the euthanasia go much more smoothly and quickly. Aggressive animals are not good candidates for hospice and may not be great candidates for palliative care, though house call veterinarians may be able to euthanize them.

Lighting can be another concern. A darkened room or nighttime can create a significant challenge in examining an animal or giving medication. It may also be a concern for safety as your eyes adjust. A trick the author uses is the flashlight on a smartphone. For euthanasia you can keep the lighting under a blanket and that makes the animal and the owner comfortable while still being able to see. Other veterinarians get a headlamp. The author does not like headlamps. They are too bulky, and having something on your head that will blind the client and possibly the pet when looking at them and is not creating a comfortable space, but it is another way to help light up the space you need.

Physical abuse

If you do go to a house and things become physical, or you are physically threatened in any way, if you do not feel safe, leave the house. It is vital to get your physical body out of the house. Physical abuse can include inappropriate touching, hitting, showing, using a gun, knife, or another weapon, and sexual assault. Make an excuse to get yourself out of the house, get something from your car, or say you must take a phone call because it is an emergency. Even if you must leave your stuff behind, get out of the house. Call the police as soon as you feel safe. Leave your key and your phone in your purse and grab them when you are headed back to your car. Or have them in a pocket, so they are already with you. Do not worry about leaving controlled drugs behind. Controlled drugs left at a house are an excellent reason for the police to show up.

Angry and emotionally abusive clients

Know that anger is part of the grieving process, and as such, a house call veterinarian may run into the occasional angry client. Or someone who does not agree with the rest of the family and is angry that the family called you out. Or they may have a mental illness. Or they just may be angry about the situation. Whatever the reason, knowing how to assess and handle anger is key to successfully dealing with anger.

1. As difficult as dealing with angry people may be, starting with a calming, soothing voice can help to diffuse anger. Think about an animal who is terrified or aggressive. People can react the same way as an aggressive dog to a soothing voice.
2. Utilize your listening skills. What are they angry about? Are they projecting anger onto you because you happen to be there, or was something you said that may have untentionally caused an angry response?
3. Use empathy statements. For example, "sounds like you had a rough day," or "it would be hard to make this decision."
4. Talk through solutions. For example, how would you like to proceed? What would make you feel better about this decision? Would you like to discuss other options for care?
5. Take time as you speak with an angry person, unless they are escalating their behavior. You probably do not come down from anger quickly, and neither do other people, so realize that it may take time for the neurochemical changes in the brain to dissipate.
6. Try not to judge or push an opinion on an angry person. Endeavor to understand their perspective.
7. If all else fails, walk away. Of course, walk away if the client is threatening you in any way (Martin, 2018).

Case example

"Here is an example of a case that didn't sound bad over the phone, didn't seem bad when I first got there, but the case devolved to anger as we went along.

A woman called me to euthanize her brother's dog. Her brother was disabled, had just taken the dog to a vet who had diagnosed a mass on the spleen, and the dog had a bleed. When I arrived at the mobile home park, I was greeted angrily by a very large man with several obvious infirmaries. He growled a greeting at me through clenched teeth and wouldn't look me in the eye. His sister and I did the paperwork, and then he literally threw his money at me for the bill, standing over me sitting on the floor, glaring. If his sister hadn't been there, I would have worried about being assaulted.

Had I taken him at face value and just reacted, the situation could have escalated. But I knew that this was likely a grief reaction and not a personal reaction toward me but the situation. I empathized with him. I knew if it were my dog, I would be upset that I was having to decide on euthanasia without really processing what was happening physically with the dog, having just been diagnosed. He didn't really have time to process the information. I also knew that part of the grief response is anger. I tried to use empathetic statements, like "it sounds like you have had a tough day, and it must be difficult losing your dear friend". Nothing I said made a difference in the level of anger on that day. However, when I came back a couple of weeks later, he was profusely apologetic and told me he knew that I cared about him and his dog and burst into tears and hugged me. Understanding, empathy, and listening can go a long way."

Most of the time, people appreciate house calls for end-of-life care and can maneuver the difficulties of anticipatory grief and postdeath grief. However, some aspects of house call palliative care or euthanasia can become difficult or dangerous. The author strongly recommends taking ongoing martial arts training to learn more about self-defense and what to do when or if violence escalates.

Weapons in the home

There have been rare reports by house call veterinarians who have gone into houses with a gun or knives or swords out in the open or have been brought out during the conversation. If this happens to you, it is better to plan what you are going to do. If you do not feel comfortable, you do not have to stay in a situation that makes you uncomfortable. If the situation is dangerous, find a diplomatic way to leave, have a particular word that you say or text, or a staff member can indicate the situation is no longer safe. Make an excuse to go out to your car, say you need to retrieve something you did not bring in. There are lots of ways to get out of the house. Once you drive away, you should call the police if you feel threatened. Veterinarians and their team need to have a written rule about what to do in their employee manual when confronted with this situation (Fig. 14.2).

When families disagree

What do you do when families disagree on treatment or euthanasia? Having families who disagree can be tricky to find yourself in the house call setting. In a perfect world, we would have a social worker or another mental health professional who could help us delve into the differences of opinion with families. One solution would be to consider adding one to your practice or at least have a referral in the beginning. One of the tools that the author has found helpful was to develop a basic advanced

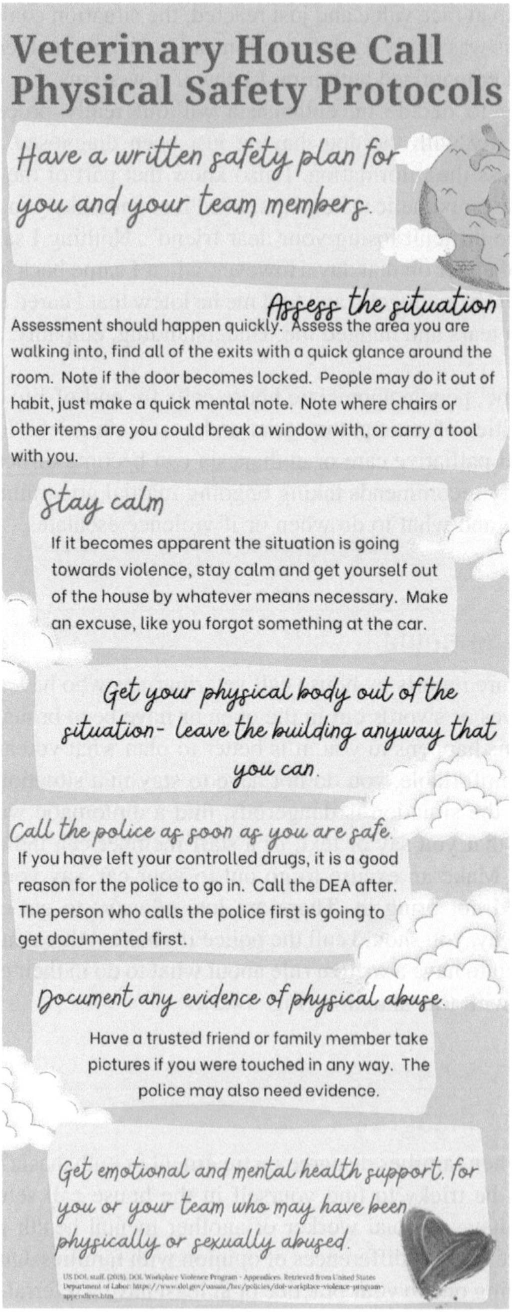

Veterinary House Call Physical Safety Protocols

Have a written safety plan for you and your team members.

Assess the situation

Assessment should happen quickly. Assess the area you are walking into, find all of the exits with a quick glance around the room. Note if the door becomes locked. People may do it out of habit, just make a quick mental note. Note where chairs or other items are you could break a window with, or carry a tool with you.

Stay calm

If it becomes apparent the situation is going towards violence, stay calm and get yourself out of the house by whatever means necessary. Make an excuse, like you forgot something at the car.

Get your physical body out of the situation- leave the building anyway that you can.

Call the police as soon as you are safe.

If you have left your controlled drugs, it is a good reason for the police to go in. Call the DEA after. The person who calls the police first is going to get documented first.

Document any evidence of physical abuse.

Have a trusted friend or family member take pictures if you were touched in any way. The police may also need evidence.

Get emotional and mental health support, for you or your team who may have been physically or sexually abused.

US DOL staff. (2018). DOL Workplace Violence Program - Appendices. Retrieved from United States Department of Labor: https://www.dol.gov/oasam/hrc/policies/dol-workplace-violence-program-appendices.htm

FIGURE 14.2

Veterinary house call physical safety protocols.

Lynn Hendrix ©2021 US DOL Staff. (2018). DOL workplace violence program - appendices. Retrieved from United States Department of Labor https://www.dol.gov/oasam/hrc/policies/dol-workplace-violence-program-appendices.htm.

directive that the people could discuss and fill in point by point about what is important to each individual. Do they agree on euthanasia? What would they find as critical criteria, less critical, deal breakers for each individual, can they come to some compromise or understanding of another individuals perspective? What is vital to each individual in terms of medical interventions? What is essential to their personal quality of life? Putting it in simple terms for families can help support their decision making, what do they want to see their animal be able to do? What do they not want them to go through? List criteria. Same with the family quality of life, what do they find necessary, what are they having a hard time doing?

Emotional and verbal abuse

You may not run into physical abuse in your practice; however, emotional and verbal abuse may occur and may be more common than physical abuse. It is not ok for you to accept verbal or emotional abuse either. Just like physical abuse, you can get your physical person out of the situation so that it does not escalate into a physical situation. These are some suggested safety protocols for verbal and emotional abuse (Fig. 14.3).

Complicated grief

Hopefully, you never run into a complicated grief situation, although they are likely more common than are reported. As defined, complicated grief is longer and felt more intensely through time than is typical and reintegration back into life may be impaired (Shear, 2011). Complicated grief can also occur when the person has a complex bond with an animal or the bond may encompass other circumstances in their life. The author has met people whose only friend is the animal that is dying, or the animal belonged to a relative or friend that had passed. More profound situations may be animals that have helped the person through a tough time, sexual abuse, domestic abuse, cancer or other chronic disease and posttraumatic stress syndrome. These clients may not discuss these more in-depth relationships with a short appointment, but may come up more frequently with house call veterinarians doing end-of-life care. It may take some extensive and sensitive questions to help elicit the information and to include a social worker or counselor to help them through the compounded grief they may develop.

Complicated grief can come up in difficult home visits when clients have had other recent losses, have a terminal illness, or are dying themselves. You can also have clients who have a mental illness, though the mental illness is not always apparent when you arrive at an appointment. There can be some clues that you may need additional mental health for them help these clients.

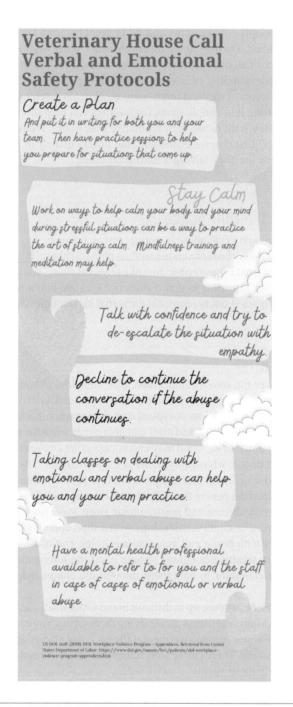

FIGURE 14.3

House call verbal and emotional safety protocols.

Lynn Hendrix ©2021.

> Warning signs of mental illness that you might pick up on in an appointment (these can also be typical aspects of grief).
> 1. Excessive worry or fear about the situation.
> 2. Depression signs, such as, changes in their sleep patterns, appetite or movement, loss of concentration, energy, thoughts of guilt, suicidal ideation.
> 3. Confusion or problems paying attention
> 4. Strong feelings of anger (remember, this can be a normal part of grief)
> 5. Difficulties relating to people (either other people in the family or you)
> 6. Additional warning signs require longer-term observation—such as avoiding friends or social situations, extreme mood changes, difficulty perceiving reality, substance abuse, and physical ailments (always has a headache, or stomachache, for example.)
> 7. If you notice some of these signs, get a mental health expert involved in continued care (NAMI Staff, 2018).

Suicidal owners—When confronted with a suicidal owner, there are many steps a veterinarian can take. Suicide ideation is complex; they may tell you they are planning to commit suicide, they may not. The people who do not verbalize their desire to die will be challenging to help. There may be clues that make you concerned that they may harm themselves. Calling in a mental health professional post death of their beloved pet could be significant to furthering their grief process and help them through suicidal thinking.

Possible signs to watch for:

1. There may be statements made by a client, such as, "when my pet dies, I want to die," or "can you kill me too?"
2. Any statements that may indicate if they have a plan. It is ok to ask if they have a plan directly.
3. Use of drugs or alcohol (noting some impairment while at the house does not mean they will commit suicide, but taking note of it and documenting it in the medical record).
4. If they or other family members have mentioned, a family member has a mental illness. Mental illness can include anxiety and depression, which may not be apparent at the house call, though if you are concerned, follow up with a trusted family member, and if the client or family member mentions it, ask if they have a counselor available to them that you can follow up with.
5. They may mention their plan. It is ok to ask if the client has a weapon. Though if it might compromise your safety, do not.
6. Many of the other signs listed on suicide websites may not pertain to a one-time visit. Know that people who have complicated grief may be more prone to considering or committing suicide (Mayo Clinic Staff, 2018).

> **National Suicide Hotline 1-800-273-8255 (US)** (NSPL Staff, 2018)
> **UK Suicide Hotlines—Hotline: +44 (0) 8457 90 90 90 (UK—local rate)**
> **Hotline: +44 (0) 8457 90 91 92 (UK minicom)**
> **Hotline: 1850 60 90 90 (ROI—local rate)**
> **Hotline: 1850 60 90 91 (ROI minicom)** (Suicide.org, 2018)
> **Australia Hotline 13 11 14 and website:** https://www.lifeline.org.au/get-help/get-help-home (Lifeline Staff, 2018)

What can you do for those who you are concerned might be considering suicide?

1. If you are concerned, give them information. A suicide hotline or a crisis hotline, in addition to counselors trained in pet loss support. Leaving grief information at the first palliative or hospice appointment includes a suicide or crisis hotline and mental health information.
2. If mental health or family support is coming to the appointment, sitting with the client while you are waiting, talking to them, or sitting in silence until they have support. Just your physical presence may show a person, they are cared for.
3. Be empathetic and respectful of their feelings.
4. If they do not have support at the appointment, ask if they have a friend or family member who can be with them after you leave.
5. If they have mentioned mental illness, find out who their counselor is and get the counselor's information if they are willing to give it. Get the person's permission to contact them and let them know what is going on.
6. Get additional training in pet loss and suicide or crisis support (Mayo Clinic Staff, 2018).

A word on self-defense

Self-defense training is a fantastic way to help you plan for difficult, potentially dangerous situations. One class, however, may not be enough to get you out of a physically threatening situation. You will need ongoing training for years before you will have the muscle memory to help you not freeze in fear when you need to act. Because women (in particular) have been socially trained to go along and be helpful, having a change in mindset to be able to harm another even in the face of danger also takes time.

Mindfulness workshops or classes may also help with calming your body and mind during stressful situations. Yoga, exercise may also be great stress relievers.

Start creating plans

Before you start seeing house calls, think about things that might concern you. Write them down, and then plan for each item on your list. Put the plan in writing. For those things that will require you to be physical, get into training, and keep training. Do not stop training because it is in the muscle memory of doing the self-defense work that it will make it come naturally when you are put in a stressful situation.

One class may not help you in a stressful situation. It might give you some good tools, to begin with, but they may be forgotten if someone is trying to choke you or harm you in another way.

If you choose to carry a weapon, get training, and keep training. Police officers do not take one-gun class; they practice and they practice frequently. They continually train in stressful situations to hopefully not make a mistake when put in an actual stressful situation. Find a local gun range and find a teacher that you feel comfortable with and start training if you are going to carry a weapon.

If you choose pepper spray or mace, take training to use it. The last thing you want is to spray yourself in the face in the moment of a dangerous situation. Know that you can be overpowered and that any weapon may be used against you.

Planning begins when you enter a home; making a mental map of the layout of the house, escape routes, doors that have been locked. Many people automatically lock their front door, so knowing that you will have to unlock it if something comes up should be in your mental plan. When you go into a house, be aware of your surroundings, what might block you from getting out. Note locks, doors, windows, other rooms you can get into. Note chairs or other things to climb on, and consider carrying a tool to break a window if you must. Make a mental plan quickly on your ability to get out. Call the police as soon as you are safe. The first person who calls is the first person who documents a dangerous situation.

Above all, if you are in a stressful situation, permit yourself to get out of it. Get out of the house, give an excuse to go to the car, you forgot equipment, you need a medication for them, anything to get you out. You can regroup there or drive away and call the police. If you are attacked, fight back, even without training. Fighting back may get you an opening to escape. Do not allow anyone to remove you from a location to a secondary location if you can prevent it.

Another option would be to take a second person. A technician, a husband, or an adult child can help keep things safer. Having a dog in the car that you could let out might be another option.

We do not like to think about this scenario, it is scary and possibly triggering to think about. However, we prepare for other aspects of a house call, what meds we are bringing, what equipment, etc.; why not be prepared for your safety?

Other difficult home visits

People you do not connect with

While this chapter has been chiefly about personal safety, you will occasionally meet people with whom you do not connect with emotionally. You may also run into people who need your attention all of the time. You do not have to help every client that crosses your path. Maybe they do not trust you, or you do not trust them, you get a weird vibe, they are drug seekers, they want a different type of practice than you provide. Many reasons can be possible that you are not a good fit for them or vice versa. It is ok to give them options, send them to another veterinarian, say you are not a good fit. Not taking on an appointment may be hard to do when you are beginning a business. However, in the long run, "choose discomfort over resentment," quoting Brene Brown. If you do take on a client like this, you need to establish early boundaries, especially if they have poor boundaries themselves.

Cancellations

Cancellations happen, even with long-term businesses. Planning for cancellations can be a way to set a boundary and encourage early cancellation. Clients are human. Things in life happen, family emergencies, death of a pet. Sometimes clients cancel at the last minute or even as you show up at the house. These can be frustrating, as you have made an effort to be there, and it costs your business if you could have scheduled another appointment at that time. Build a cancellation policy into your boundary list. Setting up your cancellation policy can establish payment for your time and decrease late cancelations.

You can make a cancellation policy as you think would work for your practice. Consider the following questions:

1. What is the timeline you think would be fair to you and your business? What would be fair to the client, considering that many of our patients are dying?
2. Do you want to be headed their way and have them cancel; do they need to do it 24 h in advance? Do you want to allow them up to an hour or two before the appointment? Are there going to be tiers for cancellation?
3. How much are you going to charge if you show up at their door and no one is home, or they already euthanized the dog without informing you?
4. Do you have a prepaid deposit?
5. How are you going to collect if you do not get a prepaid nonrefundable deposit?
6. Under what circumstances would you be ok not charging for you showing up?
7. Will it be different for current palliative clients or euthanasia-only appointments?
8. What if you have associates? How are you going to pay them for their time?

Firing clients

No one wants to have to fire a client. And, there are many reasons not to establish a client/patient/veterinary relationship. Once established as a client, there can be reasons to discontinue your relationship. You will have boundaries that you will not allow to be crossed. Once crossed, it may be time to stop seeing a client. When a client is repeatedly late, rude to you or the staff, verbally, emotionally, or physically abusive, firing a client is a way to set a permanent boundary.

Reasons to fire a client:

1. Verbal, emotional, sexual, or physical abuse to you or your team.
2. Abuse of the animal.
3. Dangerous animals.
4. The client is not concerned about your safety.
5. Consistently noncompliant clients.
6. Failure to Pay—this is less common with house calls than at a brick-and-mortar practice.
7. Clients who are threatening lawsuits, professional reputation.
8. Drug Seeking clients (Corp-Minamiji, 2013).

Firing a client letter

1. There are many templates online from various business websites.
2. The letter should be short and may include the following things:
3. Concern that the client is no longer satisfied with the service.
4. Their latest transgression, or perhaps a thorough list of all the documented transgressions (This may make a situation with them worse, and could be left out).
5. As stated, we can no longer provide service for you and perhaps include reasons, but as number 3, stating reasons may cause additional problems.
6. A statement about records either to be sent, have the next veterinarian call for records, or records are provided with this letter. All documentation of transgressions should be in the medical record. And just the facts, not the emotions of the situation.
7. Concern again for their well-being, happiness, future endeavors (Fig. 14.4) (Opperman, 2006).

The euthanasia that has gone poorly

Euthanasias that have not gone well can be one of the more challenging home visits. More is covered in the euthanasia chapter on what to do when you have a challenging euthanasia visit.

BUSINESS NAME HERE

Here is a generic sample letter written by Dr. Eve Harrison and used with her permission.

The key with a firing letter is to be direct, be kind, and follow-through. There is a saying in parenting, never threaten what you can't carry out.

Start with the behavior that you want to address:
Dear John,
"I wanted to reach out and touch base about your experience today. I'm so sorry to hear that you were unhappy with the way things went earlier in the day."

You can give them a warning shot here:

"Sadly (warning shot), after careful consideration, I think you may be right that this is not a good match after all. Veterinarians and clients need to be able to trust and that needs to be mutual."

State the reason you are removing them from your practice:

"Without trust and an assumption of my best intentions, it seems my practice will not be able to meet your needs for veterinary care."

Follow with a positive:

"You deserve to work with a team you trust. I would never want to force a rapport when there is a distrustful feeling towards my best efforts to help [companion animal]. I'm really sorry for an experience that didn't work for you."

FIGURE 14.4

Generic firing letter sample.

Written by Lynn Hendrix, Eve Harrison ©2021 Harrison, E. H. (2021). Generic firing letter. (Los Angeles, CA, USA).

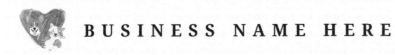

BUSINESS NAME HERE

Add in your follow-through, this tells people you mean what you say:

"I will be happy to provide the veterinarian of your choice with copies of all medical records at no charge to you. If your new veterinary practice would like information beyond what is in the medical record, I will be happy to provide them with additional information over the phone to facilitate the transition.

I wish all the best for you, and [companion animal]."

And sign it, date it to make it official:

"Take care,
Dr. Eve Harrison
8/9/2020"

And then send it certified mail and have them sign for it so that you know you they have received it. And follow through with sending records to the next veterinarian.

FIGURE 14.4 cont'd.

Conclusion

Thinking about all the dreadful things that can happen when going to a stranger's house during a very emotional time can be overwhelming. The author wants you to know, most people you will see in their home are lovely and the likelihood of something going wrong is rare. Planning for concerns can help you arrive and help each family you see to be the best person you can be for each situation you come to find yourself in. Planning and training are the keys to success, as much as it is with your veterinary training. Terrible things can come up, and this is an emotional time for people, be prepared before you get into a situation that can go bad. And know that the incidence of running into challenging people is much less common than in a brick and mortar. Screening people over the phone, planning as you walk in the door, and follow up can be vital to having a successful home palliative or hospice or in-home euthanasia practice, as can setting boundaries early, and in writing and having a plan and a crisis kit to empower your clients.

References

Addictionblog.org Staff. (2018). *How to tell if someone has drug seeking behavior*. Retrieved from Addictionblog.org http://addictionblog.org/FAQ/identifying-addiction/how-to-identify-drug-seeking-behavior/.

Corp-Minamiji, C. (September 23, 2013). *VINZ insights*. Retrieved from VIN.com https://www.vin.com/vetzinsight/default.aspx?pid=756&catId=5874&id=5959405.

DEA Staff. (1999). *Don't be scammed by a drug abuser (from 1999 brochure)*. Retrieved from DEA Diversion Control Division https://www.deadiversion.usdoj.gov/pubs/brochures/drugabuser.htm.

Harrison, E. H. (2021). *Generic firing letter* (Los Angeles, CA, USA).

Lifeline Staff. (2018). *Get help*. Retrieved from Lifeline.org https://www.lifeline.org.au/get-help/get-help-home.

Martin, R. (2018). *5 ways to deal with angry people*. Retrieved from Psychology Today https://www.psychologytoday.com/us/blog/all-the-rage/201506/5-ways-deal-angry-people.

Mayo Clinic Staff. (2018). *Suicide: What to do when someone is suicidal*. Retrieved from Mayo Clinic https://www.mayoclinic.org/diseases-conditions/suicide/in-depth/suicide/art-20044707.

NAMI Staff. (2018). *Know the warning signs*. Retrieved from NAMI- National Alliance on Mental Illness https://www.nami.org/Learn-More/Know-the-Warning-Signs.

NSPL Staff. (2018). *National suicide prevention lifeline*. Retrieved from National Suicide Prevention Lifeline https://suicidepreventionlifeline.org/.

Opperman, M. (May 1, 2006). *Show bad clients the door*. Retrieved from DVM 360 veterinarybusiness.dvm360.com/sample-client-termination-letter.

Shear, K. S.-F. (2011). Complicated grief and related bereavement issues for DSM-5. *Depression and Anxiety*, 103—117.

Suicide.org. (2018). *United Kingdom suicide hotlines*. Retrieved from Suicide.org http://www.suicide.org/hotlines/international/united-kingdom-suicide-hotlines.html.

US DOL Staff. (2018). *DOL workplace violence program - appendices*. Retrieved from United States Department of Labor https://www.dol.gov/oasam/hrc/policies/dol-workplace-violence-program-appendices.htm.

Further reading

Barbour, L. (2021). *Professional-patient boundaries in palliative care*. Retrieved from Palliative Care Network of Wisconsin https://www.mypcnow.org/fast-fact/professional-patient-boundaries-in-palliative-care/.

Expanding access to palliative medicine education and organization

Lynn Hendrix, AA, BA, DVM, CHPV [1,2,3,4]

[1]*Owner, Veterinarian, Beloved Pet Mobile Vet, Davis, CA, United States;* [2]*Former Board of Directors, IAAHPC, Chicago, IL, United States;* [3]*Consultant, Hospice, Palliative Medicine, End of Life, VIN, Davis, CA, United States;* [4]*President, Founder, World Veterinary Palliative Medicine Organization, Davis, CA, United States*

In the past 10 years, the animal hospice movement has become a hot topic in veterinary medicine. The early adoptors looked to expand education, public awareness, and eventually build a specialty in palliative medicine. Additional training in palliative medicine and hospice techniques may be found with different organizations, and there are increasing lecture topics at the major conferences. With more veterinarians adopting hospice or palliative medicine into their practice, the public and colleagial awareness has increased.

Hospice or palliative medicine?

The International Association for Animal Hospice and Palliative Care recruited six authors in 2012 to work on comprehensive guidelines for best practices in hospice and palliative care. The authors discussed topics from terminology to definitions in writing these landmark veterinary guidelines. One of the topics of discussion was what to call this field. The guideline authors decided to focus on the term hospice and settled on animal hospice. The guidelines were published on the IAAHPC website in 2013 and revised in 2017. In 2016, AAHA and the IAAHPC cowrote 3-page guidelines changing the terminology to end-of-life care (Bishop, 2016). In 2017, the AVMA revised their hospice guidelines, removed the word hospice and replaced it with end-of-life care, and are utilizing the cowritten guidelines. So why are terminology changes happening?

A possible explanation could be the term hospice, in human medicine, has a negative connotation (Rogers, 2009). In the traditional human end of life model, doctors perform with the standard of curative care (Diehl, 2021) up to the point in the illness where curative medicine is no longer working and then send the terminally ill to hospice care. That model was endorsed early by Medicare in the United

States (Medicare Staff, 2018) and has continued to be the traditional standard of care until the Temel study in 2010 (Temel, 2010). People also avoid going into hospice until the very end of their disease for a number of reasons, such as fear, or the medical community has not suggested it to them. The ability to have difficult discussions and the death denial culture also play a role in the late enrollment into hospice (Zimmermann, 2007). At what point do we change our focus from curative to palliative (Gawande, 2010)? As mentioned, Temel's landmark study began to change the paradigm. The Temel study shifted how MDs and their teams promoted palliative care, medicine (Cruz-Oliver, 2017, pp. 110—115; Temel, 2010). Palliative medicine provides comfort and support at the end-of-life, and while it is most frequently used in end-of-life care, it can also be utilized with many advanced, progressive, chronic diseases.

With the changes in the AVMA, the AAHA guidelines, and the shift in human medicine, the author believes veterinary palliative medicine is the future of end-of-life care. More veterinarians may be interested in palliative medicine and could incorporate it into their practice, even if they choose not to do hospice care. General practitioners could advance their palliative skills for end-of-life, advanced, progressive chronic patients, expand their communication skills, add to their education and support for the family, or caregivers. Broadening education to include veterinary palliative medicine and patient/client-centered care will expand upon current skills and advance the veterinary field.

Current organizations

Starting with the organizations that are currently available and adding the other areas where you can find additional information on either Animal Hospice or Palliative Medicine is the starting place in changing the paradigm of end-of-life care in veterinary medicine. While there are only a few at this time, the future will build upon the present.

IAAHPC

The IAAHPC founded in 2009 by Dr. Amir Shanan, et. al., provides education for veterinarians, veterinary technicians and mental health professionals. The organization has an annual conference that focuses on topics in animal hospice, palliative care, oncology, business and marketing of animal hospice practices, social media, hospice in veterinary technology, and mental health for animal hospice providers and their clients. The organization also has a business circle group that provides education and support for veterinarians wanting to establish their own hospice or palliative practice. They have developed certification programs on animal hospice and palliative care for veterinarians and licensed veterinary technicians. https://www.iaahpc.org

IVAPM

The International Veterinary Academy of Pain Management (IVAPM) is dedicated to pain management for all pets: surgical, acute, and chronic. The IVAPM provides course work, lectures from certified pain specialists at continuing education around the world, and a certification program on pain management for both veterinarians and veterinary technicians. They are a wonderful resource for increasing your pain management skills. https://ivapm.org/

The future of veterinary palliative medicine organizations

As human hospice developed, so did the organizations of professionals to support the work that they were doing. As veterinarians develop additional skills and education, there will be specialized organizations that will be formed. There is a recent Veterinarian Palliative Medicine organization, and as the medicine grows and becomes more mainstream, the author suspects there will be organizing for Veterinary Technicians and Veterinary Social Work or other mental health organization, and the development of local chapters.

WVPMO

In 2018, the World Veterinary Palliative Medicine Organization (WVPMO) was developed by Drs. Lynn Hendrix and Caroline Ficker. Dr. Hendrix and Dr. Ficker studied human palliative medicine separately before they met in 2012 at an IAAHPC conference. They became board members of the IAAHPC in 2016 and 2017, respectively, and saw a need for expansion in the education and research. They began a Facebook group for veterinarians interested in veterinary palliative medicine that grew exponentially with veterinarians from 60+ countries as of this writing. They saw a need for an international organization for veterinarians interested in veterinary palliative medicine, and WVPMO was born.

They are currently recruiting experts in various fields in veterinary medicine to provide high-quality education in oncology, internal medicine, behavior, emergency medicine, communication, and others, for small intimate workshops around the world in diverse topics pertaining to end-of-life care for animals. They plan to bring the high quality of human palliative medicine and translate it to veterinary medicine to bring a gold standard of care for veterinary palliative medicine. They also plan on helping start-up organizations around the world for local chapters interested in pursuing veterinary palliative medicine. And, they will be involved in developing a specialty in Veterinary Palliative Medicine. https://www.wvpmo.org/

Local organizations around the world

Currently, there are not many hospice or veterinary palliative care or medicine organizations that are specific to veterinary palliative care. The next step is to design more local chapters for additional areas to bring palliative medicine or hospice education. Hopefully, other veterinarians are inspired to develop their own local chapter as palliative medicine grows.

The Australian Veterinary Palliative Care Advisory Council

The Australian Veterinary Palliative Care Advisory Council was established in 2017 to harness expertise from a range of specialties across veterinary and allied health fields in Australia.

"It aims to develop and support best end-of-life care practices within veterinary medicine, encourage cross-discipline interaction between veterinarians and allied health practitioners to improve patient outcomes, and be a source of practical advice for veterinary practitioners looking to increase their clinical skills in this area. It also endeavors to openly encourage conversations about death and bereavement within the veterinary and animal health field."

Campbell (2017).

Other conferences

AVMA, CVC, Western States, NAVC—now VMX, and local VMAs are all discussing Animal Hospice. The London Vet Show had information on Animal Hospice in 2016 (Ficker, 2016). There was recently a holistic European Conference that included Animal Hospice. Australia just had its first conference in 2018 on Animal Hospice and Palliative Care. They need to start having speakers discussing veterinary palliative medicine.

Veterinary palliative medicine is expanding into the mainstream veterinary field, and hospice, which has been the hot topic word, is an aspect of veterinary palliative medicine. The challenge for the future is to provide veterinary palliative medicine education at the veterinary school level, to establish a residency program, to provide training in communication, in multimodal and targeted chronic and cancer pain management that we can use while treating the disease and beyond where the traditional curative medicine stops, in multimodal and targeted symptom management, and training and educating clients on end-of-life caregiving.

Online education

Webinars and other online education on Animal Hospice and Palliative care can be found in just a few places and the detail, the quality may vary, and the author has included to give you options. VIN has occasional webinars on hospice or palliative care (IAAHPC staff, 2018; VIN staff, 2018). AAHA has a short CE course on Animal Hospice (Cooney, 2018).

HSVMA has some end-of-life webinars in their archived continuing education (HSVMA staff, 2018).

Online education on Veterinary Palliative Medicine is harder to find, nearly impossible. Most of the education in palliative medicine is available in the human field, and NHPCO (the National Hospice and Palliative Care Organization) list of end-of-life care resources is a good place to start looking for educational opportunities (NHPCO staff, 2018). https://www.nhpco.org/resources/end-life-care-resources

The IVAPM has monthly webinars on assorted topics in pain management (IVAPM staff, 2018) and a Facebook group.

And on the Facebook group, Veterinarian Palliative Medicine, has files of studies, and the WVPMO will have online educational opportunities. The WVPMO looks to expand the veterinary palliative medicine education for veterinarians.

VIN folder

Started in October of 2015, the Veterinary Information Network added a folder for veterinarians to meet, ask questions, and find support in doing hospice, end-of-life care, and euthanasia. The consultant is the author of this book, and there is an associate editor chosen for their commitment to the education and support of veterinarians. The current consultant and editor have provided rounds on hospice, communication, and some palliative medicine as well, as have other veterinarians in various fields. From 2018-2021, there have been over 21,000 unique views of the topics in the VIN folder.

Facebook group—Veterinarian Palliative Medicine Group

The founders of the WVPMO started a Facebook group called the Veterinarian Palliative Medicine Group in 2017. It has grown from about 50 core people, in 2017 to 2700 veterinarians, in 2021 from around the world (https://www.facebook.com/groups/worldvetpalliativemedicine). They have basic information on veterinary palliative medicine, with Question-and-Answer FB live events, support from the members, and the leaders in the field are members and can provide answers to questions that arise and can help people starting out or wanting to find out more about palliative medicine in the veterinary field. There are two sister sites for veterinary techicians and veterinary students https://www.facebook.com/groups/VeterinaryPCNurses, https://www.facebook.com/groups/StudentVPM.

Conclusion

Veterinary palliative medicine has become hot topic in veterinary medicine. Being able to improve upon the current research, the support of the veterinarian, the client, and the pet is appealing to GPs, specialists, and veterinarians interested in specializing in palliative medicine. Veterinarians are looking for ways to improve end-of-life care, and future education and research in palliative medicine is key. There has been momentum forward in veterinary palliative medicine, and it will benefit the end-of-life patients, their families, and future veterinarians around the world.

References

Bishop, G. C. (2016). *2016 AAHA/IAAHPC end-of-life care guidelines*. Retrieved from AAHA.org https://www.aaha.org/professional/resources/end_of_life_care_guidelines.aspx.

Campbell, J. (2017). *About AVPCAC*. Retrieved from avpcac.com https://www.avpcac.com/about-avpcac/.

Cooney, K. (2018). *Animal hospice & palliative care certificate program*. Retrieved from AAHA.org https://www.aaha.org/professional/education/animal_hospice_palliative_care_certificate_program.aspx.

Cruz-Oliver, D. (2017). *Palliative care: An update. Missouri medicine*.

Diehl, S. (2021). *Palliative conversations with Dr Diehl. (L. Hendrix, interviewer)*.

Ficker, C. (2016). *Informal discussion . (L. Hendrix, interviewer)*.

Gawande, A. (2010, 8 2). *Letting go*. Retrieved from The New Yorker.com https://www.newyorker.com/magazine/2010/08/02/letting-go-2.

HSVMA staff. (2018). *Continuing education webinars - archived webinars*. Retrieved from HSVMA.org http://www.hsvma.org/archivedwebinars.

IAAHPC staff. (2018). *Professional webinars*. Retrieved from IAAHPC.org https://www.iaahpc.org/education/products/professionals.html.

IVAPM staff. (2018). *Veterinary CE webinars*. Retrieved from International Veterinary Academy of Pain Management https://ivapm.org/professionals/veterinary-ce-webinars/.

Medicare staff. (2018). *Your Medicare coverage- hospice and respite care*. Retrieved from Medicare.gov https://www.medicare.gov/coverage/hospice-and-respite-care.html.

NHPCO staff. (2018). *End-of-Life care resources*. Retrieved from NHPCO.org https://www.nhpco.org/resources/end-life-care–resources.

Rogers, T. (2009). Hospice myths: What is hospice really about? *Pennsylvania Nurse*, 4—8.

Temel, J. E. (2010). Early palliative care for patients with metastatic non-small cell lung cancer. *The New England Journal of Medicine*, 733—742.

VIN staff. (2018). *Home page*. Retrieved from Veterinary Information Network https://www.vin.com/vin/.

Zimmermann, C. (2007). Death denial: Obstacle or instrument for palliative care? An analysis of clinical literature. *Sociology of Health and Illness*, 297—314.

Further reading

Wagner, T. (2017). *Animal hospice from the perspective of*. Retrieved from Pet Loss Grief Counseling Certification.com http://pet-loss-grief-counseling-certification.com/class-animal-hospice/.

Redefining veterinary medicine: The future of veterinary palliative medicine and animal hospice

16

Lynn Hendrix, AA, BA, DVM, CHPV [1,2,3,4]

[1]*Owner, Veterinarian, Beloved Pet Mobile Vet, Davis, CA, United States;* [2]*Former Board of Directors, IAAHPC, Chicago, IL, United States;* [3]*Consultant, Hospice, Palliative Medicine, End of Life, VIN, Davis, CA, United States;* [4]*President, Founder, World Veterinary Palliative Medicine Organization, Davis, CA, United States*

Where do we need to go?

Veterinary Palliative Medicine is the future of end-of-life care and foreseeably will become a specialty. Veterinarians providing veterinary palliative medicine can bridge the possible gap in care between terminal diagnosis and euthanasia or death. Veterinary medicine needs to build a more extensive evidence base with additional research in palliative medicine and euthanasia. Veterinary students need expanded education in palliative medicine and hospice, as well as euthanasia, psychology, business, and communication. Palliative medicine can evolve, utilizing more targeted therapies and multimodal approaches for pain and other symptom management.

Getting veterinary palliative care to more people and their pets

Human beings around the world do not often have access to palliative care with their end of life process. Increasing access to care for pets may prove to be even more challenging. A big challenge in veterinary medicine is cost of care. This has been a challenge in the past in human medicine. In human hospice, the insurance companies decided to pay for palliative care/hospice in the United States in 1982 via the Tax Equity and Fiscal Responsibility Act of 1982 whcih helped with their access to care (NHPCO staff, 2016). Yet they still have challenges getting care to everyone. This is more a problem in low income areas of the US and other areas of the world. Cost is still a concern for providing quality care for end-of-life patients. How could we help more folks pay for veterinary palliative care?

Animal Hospice and Palliative Medicine for the House Call Veterinarian
https://doi.org/10.1016/B978-0-323-56798-5.00007-2

Veterinarians have proposed helping clients with cost of care in many different ways. Clients may use pet insurance to help cover costs associated with hospice and palliative care. Veterinarians can start an "Angel fund" and have it crowdfunded or placing a small amount aside each month to help defray costs for a low-income client. Clients can Find a rescue to help fund or sometimes individual crowdfunding can also help. Adding education in palliative care for SPCA and animal shelters may be another way to provide palliative care to low-income families and their pets. Financial aid for animals also exists in the US. This webpage, https://bestfriends.org/resources/financial-aid-pets, has a comprehensive list of financial assistance by state (Financial Aid for Pets, 2018).

The AVMA has a program called the American Veterinary Medical Foundation that can support veterinarians to help clients who face financial struggles. The website is https://avmf.org/ for more information.

Increasing the public awareness of veterinary palliative medicine will also assist more animals to receive care. House call veterinarians can utilize their advertising, marketing dollars to reach more people. Social media, newspaper articles, getting on TV and radio can also increase the reach for housce call veterinarians. Adding to those strategies, educating colleagues and students will be another way to take precedence of the future of palliative medicine.

Increasing the number of universities educating students in the end-of-life care, and adding to the research being completed in veterinary palliative care will upgrade the level of care and increase the number of veterinarians practicing this important medicine focus.

Certification to specialization

In 2014, the IAAHPC started developing the first certification program on hospice and palliative care for veterinarians and veterinary technicians. The first group of veterinarians and a few veterinary technicians began a journey through 110 hours of four modules, developing case studies, and finished in 2017 with a comprehensive test. The IAAHPC have recently launched their certificate program for social workers.

In 2013, an organizing committee formed and put together the first step in paperwork with the AVMB to start the veterinarian specialization process. Specialization is a 10-year process, and we have made slow but steady work to become a specialty service in veterinary medicine. Like other specialties, there will be internships, residencies, and a board exam to be a diplomate in Animal Hospice and Veterinary Palliative Medicine. The specialty is still in the early stages of development.

What more could we do?

A goal for future growth in veterinary palliative medicine in the United States and then internationally will be developing a program at every veterinary school. The author has found there is interest all over the world in veterinary palliative medicine. Developing programs in veterinary palliative medicine will increase the number of veterinarians who can provide care to clients and their beloved pets. There is more work to do, to develop training in veterinary schools. In 2015, an informal phone call survey of universities and colleges that have veterinary programs in the United States found while about $\frac{1}{3}$ of them mentioned the word hospice in their programs, most have a class on euthanasia (States, 2015). The University of Michigan did have a hospice program in 2013, but it is no longer in service. Colorado State University does have the Argus Institute that incorporates hospice for animals. Cornell University has an end-of-life program (States, 2015). UC Davis has a communications course as does Colorado that discusses euthanasia and difficult client situations.

Involving more veterinary technicians and mental health

Human hospice originally began in England in 1967 because Cecily Saunders saw a need to make the end of life better for people (Cecily Saunders International, 2018). Nurses are heavily involved in the care of dying humans all over the world. A nurses association formed in 1987, about 20 years after Cecily Saunders developed the first concepts (O'Rawe, 2001). Developing education and then organization for veterinary techinicians can support veterinarians who are interested in this type of care. Adding a specialty for veterinary technicians in animal hospice would further support their education. Veterinary Technical schools could provide additional training in animal hospice and palliative care, and this would give students an opportunity to expand their abilities and knowledge and increase the job market.

Increasing the mental health field in veterinary palliative care should be another goal. The University of Tennessee has a veterinary social work program. The Colorado State University has the Argus institute, and they do have volunteers and mental health workers practicing animal hospice and palliative care. Those with advanced degrees in mental health can find additional training with APLB (the Association for Pet Loss and Bereavement), American Institute of Health Care Professionals, Inc., The Animal Loss, and Grief Support Institute (AIHCP staff, 2018; APLB staff, 2018; Wagner, 2017).

Research

While there is research in human hospice and palliative medicine, research is lacking in animal hospice and veterinary palliative medicine. Evidence-based palliative medicine will need to be established with research. The IAAHPC, and a new organization for veterinarians, the World Veterinary Palliative Medicine Organization, are dedicated to adding more new research in animal hospice and palliative medicine. These organizations can collaborate with universities and may be able to obtain further funding for research in veterinary palliative medicine.

Building other interdisciplinary organizations

Veterinary-guided animal hospice will need further training in palliative medicine for veterinarians, veterinary technicians, mental health professionals, and other team members to provide improved palliative care for the animals with advanced, progressive, chronic and terminal diseases. There are organizations for MDs, Nurses, Mental health professionals, and broader scope organizations on the human side. The author would encourage the reader to join a human organization, and these are a few from parts of the world:

1. *In the United States*, National Hospice and Palliative Care Organization
2. National Hospice Foundation
3. American Academy of Hospice and Palliative Medicine
4. American Board of Hospice and Palliative Medicine
5. Center to Advance Palliative Care
6. Hospice and Palliative Nurses Association
7. *In Canada*, The Canadian Hospice Palliative Care Association
8. *In the United Kingdom*, The Association of Palliative Medicine
9. Hospice United Kingdom
10. Irish Association for Palliative Care
11. Irish Hospice Foundation
12. National Association for Hospice at Home
13. The National Care Forum
14. Rapid Effective Assistance for Children with Potentially Terminal Illness
15. *In Europe*, European Association for Palliative Care
16. European Organization for Research and Treatment of Cancer
17. *In Australia*, Palliative Care Australia
18. Australian and New Zealand Society of Palliative Medicine

(NPCRC, 2013; NCPC, 2015; IAHPC, 2018)

The IAAHPC is a good umbrella organization for veterinarians, veterinary technicians, and mental health professionals looking to find more animal hospice information. Veterinarians, veterinary technicians, and mental health professionals will also need profession-specific organizations to increase the funding for research, education, and specificity for each field of study which need to be developed.

Technology for veterinary palliative medicine

With the world pandemic of Covid-19 in 2020, telemedicine, telehealth, and other ways to connect to clients became a more significant part of veterinary medicine. Telehealth has continued to grow assisting veterinarians in seeing their clients and patients with video calls, texting, and other technologies. Ultrasound probes are now available for phones, adding to the at-home procedures we can provide for the care of our patients. Placing indwelling catheters for epidurals, chest tubes in the home could happen with newer, more portable technology. Artificial intelligence, and phone applications may assist us in our abilities to diagnose and prognose patients in the future. Newer technologies like immunotherapies, monoclonal antibodies, m-RNA technology may expand our ability to care for our end-of-life patients.

Integration of early palliative care into practice

The easiest and most important aspect of increasing palliative care is instituting it early. As studies have shown since Dr. Temel et al. had their landmark study in 2010, early integration of palliative care can make an impact on the life of the terminally ill patient. Dr. Temel's group examined early integration in a large cohort of patients and found less depression and higher quality of life over a 24-week study for patients with lung cancer and GI cancer (Temel, 2017).

As the future of veterinary palliative medicine and animal hospice continues to develop and grow, more services will provide higher standards of care, round-the-clock service with additional team members, and added mental health and grief support from mental health professionals. Increasing our level of education in palliative medicine, drawing on our human counterparts information will increase the current level of care provided to animals and their caregiver families. Educating both clients and students will help raise public awareness of this service and provide a better foundation for delivering quality care for animals at the end of life. The standard of palliative care will increase with new organizations, new education, new technology, such as telemedicine, and adding to the research that we currently have to improve our evidence base (Diehl, 2021). Here is to looking forward to the future of veterinary palliative medicine.

References

AIHCP staff. (2018). *Pet loss grief recovery certification.* Retrieved from American Institue of Health Care Professionals https://aihcp.net/pet-loss-grief-recovery-certification/.

APLB staff. (2018). *Counselor training.* Retrieved from APLB.org https://aplb.org/training-courses/counselor-training/.

Cecily Saunders International. (2018). *Dame Cecily Saunders biography.* Retrieved from Cecily Saunders International https://cicelysaundersinternational.org/dame-cicely-saunders/.

Diehl, S. (2021). *Palliative conversations with Dr Diehl. (L. Hendrix, interviewer).*

Financial Aid for Pets. (2018). *Retrieved from best friends animal society.* https://bestfriends.org/resources/financial-aid-pets.

IAHPC. (June 14, 2018). *Global directory of palliative care services and organizations.* Retrieved from International Association for Hospice And Palliative Care https://hospicecare.com/global-directory-of-providers-organizations/search/?idregion=5.

NCPC. (2015). *UK palliative care organisations.* Retrieved from The National Council for Palliative Care http://www.ncpc.org.uk/uk-palliative-care-organisations.

NHPCO staff. (March 28, 2016). *History of hospice care*. Retrieved from National Hospice and Palliative Care Organization https://www.nhpco.org/history-hospice-care.

NPCRC. (2013). *Palliative care organizations*. Retrieved from National Palliative Care Research Center http://www.npcrc.org/content/26/Palliative-Care-Organizations.aspx.

O'Rawe, A. (2001). History of the hospice nurses association, 1986-1996. *Journal of Hospice and Palliative Nursing*, 128–136.

States, V. S. (2015). *Topic- do you have a hospice program? (D. L. Hendrix, interviewer)*.

Temel, J. S.-J. (2017). Effects of early integrated palliative care in patients with lung and GI cancer: A randomized clinical trial. *Journal of Clinical Oncology*, 834–841.

Wagner, T. (2017). *Training and certification program*. Retrieved from The Animal Loss and Grief Support Institute https://pet-loss-grief-counseling-certification.com/.

Appendix

Sample Checklists for Clients and Practitioners in Palliative Medicine

Sample Nursing care checklist

- ☐ Assessment of the client
  - ☐ Do they have new worries or concerns?
  - ☐ How are medications going?
  - ☐ What are they currently giving? (does it match with what was prescribed?)
  - ☐ How do they feel about continuing care?
- ☐ Assessment of the patient
  - ☐ Physical exam
  - ☐ Validated pain score assessment
  - ☐ Any major changes with the animal
  - ☐ Contact veterinarian
- ☐ Patient needs
  - ☐ Any changes needed to be made?
  - ☐ Are their needs being met?
  - ☐ Quality of Life assessment
    - ▪ Emotional
    - ▪ Physical
    - ▪ Will to live still present.
- ☐ Adjust Plan/Goals
  - ☐ Contact veterinarian for changes in plan, medication
- ☐ Application of plan
- ☐ Re-evaluation/Check-in appointment made
  - ☐ Phone check-in
  - ☐ In-person check in with veterinary nurse
  - ☐ In-person check in with veterinarian
  - ☐ Need for Social Worker/Counselor
  - ☐ Additional support

FIGURE 1

Sample nursing checklist.

389

Created by Dr. Lynn Hendrix ©2021.

Sample Checklist for the Veterinarian and Team

Basic Needs of the client/caregiver

Establish the goals of the owner/caregiver

- ☐ What are their concerns, worries, fears?
- ☐ What do they understand about their animal's disease?
  - ☐ Give education materials regarding the end of life of their animal's disease
- ☐ Death due to illness- Palliated
- ☐ Death due to Euthanasia
- ☐ Establish DNR status
  - ☐ Do they want rescue status?
  - ☐ Do they want a do not resuscitate status if the animal ends up in an emergency room?
- ☐ Establish where they would like the death to happen- usually at home
- ☐ Create a timetable for their disease
  - ☐ Stable disease- likely has at least a year to live
  - ☐ Unstable disease- likely has six months or less to live
  - ☐ Deteriorating disease- likely has two months or less to live
  - ☐ Final Days- likely have two weeks or less to live.
- ☐ Check in's (times can vary depending on the situation)
  - ☐ For stable patients, at least every six months
  - ☐ For unstable patients, at least once a month
  - ☐ For deteriorating patients, at least weekly
  - ☐ For final days patients-daily
- ☐ Educate and create a plan for the client on common clinical signs to monitor for the disease.
  - ☐ Signs with stable disease
  - ☐ Signs with unstable disease
  - ☐ Signs with deteriorating disease
  - ☐ Signs of final days
  - ☐ Imminent death signs
- ☐ Create an Advanced Directive for both the patient and the client
- ☐ Give written educational information
  - ☐ Quality of Life
  - ☐ Chronic pain information
  - ☐ Another symptom management
- ☐ Crisis information
  - ☐ Where to call if there is a crisis-ER, your practice, RDVM

FIGURE 2
___
Sample palliative care checklist with team building.

Created by Dr. Lynn Hendrix© 2021.

- ☐ Assess the need for other support
    - ☐ Nursing support
- ☐ Mental Health support
    - ☐ Assess coping skills of family
    - ☐ Address for possible unfinished issues with family
    - ☐ Assess need for increase social worker intervention through visits, telephone calls
    - ☐ Bereavement risk

- ☐ Grooming support
    - ☐ Local groomers who are knowledgeable in caring for elderly patients
        - ☐ Animals can lay down while being bathed
        - ☐ They recognize the signs of pain
- ☐ Respite support
    - ☐ Pet sitting support
        - ☐ Local pet sitters who understand the needs of an elderly, frail patient
    - ☐ Family Respite support
    - ☐ Housesitting/pet sitting
- ☐ Spiritual support
    - ☐ Assess for cultural beliefs & values, beliefs about death and dying
    - ☐ Establish resource list
    - ☐ Education for staff to improve sensitivity for the spiritual needs of all clients
- ☐ Aftercare support
    - ☐ Review Cremation services
    - ☐ Review other body care options
    - ☐ Review memorial items
    - ☐ Review Grief services
        - ☐ Pet Loss Support Hotlines
        - ☐ Online support
        - ☐ In-Person Local support

Patient Needs

- ☐ Create a personalized plan for the patient
    - ☐ Consider pain management
        - ☐ Mild, moderate, or severe chronic pain, or unrelenting pain
            - ☐ Use pain scales to assess pain with clients
        - ☐ Acute pain
        - ☐ Acute pain flare-up on top of chronic pain

FIGURE 2 cont'd.

- ☐ Review pain management at each point of contact
  - ☐ Review current dosing- what is the owner giving, how often, at what dose?
  - ☐ Review need for additional medication
  - ☐ Review need for refills
- ☐ Consider other symptom management
  - ☐ Bleeding
    - ☐ Where are they bleeding from?
    - ☐ Skin
    - ☐ Spleen
    - ☐ Liver
    - ☐ Kidney/Urinary tract
    - ☐ GI
    - ☐ Pulmonary
    - ☐ Head/Neck
    - ☐ Third space- abdomen, pericardium, pleural space
  - ☐ Breathlessness/dyspnea
  - ☐ Constipation
    - ☐ Straining
    - ☐ Frank Blood in stool
    - ☐ Dark stool
  - ☐ Carcinomatosis/Metastasis
  - ☐ Chronic Renal Disease
  - ☐ Delirium
  - ☐ Dementia
  - ☐ Diarrhea
  - ☐ Dysphagia
  - ☐ Dysrexia
    - ☐ Anorexic
    - ☐ Hyporexic
  - ☐ Fever/Chill
  - ☐ Frailty
  - ☐ Hydration
  - ☐ Hypercalcemia

FIGURE 2 cont'd.

- ☐ Lethargy
- ☐ Liver disease, end-stage
- ☐ Lymphatic disease
- ☐ Neuromuscular disease
  - ☐ Degenerative Myelopathy
  - ☐ GOLPP
- ☐ Nutrition
- ☐ Osteoarthritis
- ☐ Pancreatic disease
- ☐ Seizures
  - ☐ How long are the seizures lasting?
  - ☐ How often do they have them?
  - ☐ When did they have the last seizure?
  - ☐ Medications prescribed_____
- ☐ Sleep/wake disturbances
- ☐ Urination
  - ☐ Are they incontinent?
  - ☐ Are they urinating frequently?
  - ☐ Are they not urinating? Or Oliguric?
  - ☐ Straining to urinate.
  - ☐ Blood in urine
- ☐ Vomiting/ Nausea
- ☐ Skin health
  - ☐ Monitor for redness, irritation, licking at pressure points
  - ☐ Monitor for ulcerations, "bedsores"
  - ☐ Monitor for insects, fleas, flies, maggots
  - ☐ Monitor for petechiae, ecchymosis

FIGURE 2 cont'd.

- Eyes, Nose, Throat, Oral hygiene
  - Keeping the ENT moist
  - Checking for ulcers on eyes, oral mucosa
- Anxiety/Terminal Delirium
- Interventional therapies/Client declines/approves
  - Feeding Tubes
  - Epidural pain management
  - IV infusions
  - Joint infusions
  - SQ port placement
  - TENS unit
  - Urinary Catheters
- Review Symptom management at each point of contact
- Establish a Crisis kit
  - Address the concerns of the client- what are they worried about, concerned about, what are they most scared about happening
  - Address what you are, the veterinarian, concerned about happening with this particular disease as it progresses towards death
  - Establish medications that will address those concerns if you are not available
  - Have specific instructions for each medication
    - when to use
    - what it is used for
    - how to give
    - how long it will last before they may have to re-dose
    - possible side effects of each medication
  - Decide what you are comfortable giving and what your client is comfortable giving, oral, transmucosal, transdermal, injections. (recognize that not all clients will be able to give injections or want to)
- Equipment needs
  - Animal Wheelchair (does the client need education?)
  - Splint
  - Orthotic device
  - Harness/sling
  - Stroller/wagon

FIGURE 2 cont'd.

- □ Raised Dishes
- □ Rugs
- □ Foot covers/toe grips
- □ Diapers/Pee Pads
- □ Syringes for feeding, water
- □ As they approach imminent death
  - □ Educate owners on the imminent death
  - □ Monitor for pre-active dying signs (possibly hours to a week or two before death- often the time when nursing care increases, owners may elect euthanasia at this time)
    - □ Weakness and fatigue
    - □ Disorientation
    - □ Withdrawal from family
    - □ Dyspnea, especially with heart failure patients
    - □ Increased respiratory rate due to pain
    - □ Increased risk of decubitus ulcers
    - □ Decreasing urine output
    - □ Decreasing food and water intake (can go weeks without eating, can go many days without water)
    - □ May have difficulties swallowing
  - □ Monitor for Active dying signs (sometimes minutes to a day or so before death)
    - □ Decreasing mentation
    - □ "Death Rattle"- thickening of secretions in the pharynx
    - □ Dyspnea in heart failure patients
    - □ Brain stem breathing to include Cheyne- Stokes breathing,
    - □ Pads, ears, nose (if pink) may become dusky, mottled, or blue
    - □ Limbs and ears are cold to touch
    - □ Decreased to Absent urine output
    - □ Terminal delirium – vocalizations
    - □ Tachycardia, hypotension

Team Support

- □ Create team plan of care for patient and caregiver(s)
  - □ Review the best plan of support for the client
  - □ Review updated plans/timetable
  - □ Triage
- □ Check-in with team daily
  - □ How did the caseload go?
  - □ Medication check

FIGURE 2 cont'd.

- ☐ Follow up drug logs
- ☐ Are files complete?
- ☐ Any challenges? What could we do to improve?
- ☐ Any wins? How did we support a family well?
- ☐ Check-in with team weekly
  - ☐ Assess client interactions
  - ☐ Difficulties that have come up with clients/patients
  - ☐ Challenges with team efforts
    - ☐ What could we do better?
    - ☐ How could we support each other in this situation?
  - ☐ Wins- what went right?
  - ☐ Shout outs-
    - ☐ Who felt good about a case? Tell us about it!
    - ☐ Recognition of fellow team member
  - ☐ Working together shout-outs- who felt great about team effort?
- ☐ Check-in with team monthly
  - ☐ How has the month has gone for each individual?
  - ☐ Challenges we have not addressed?
  - ☐ What could we do better?
  - ☐ Ideas to improve care?
  - ☐ Best experience this month?
- ☐ Referral letters- summary of palliative visits, should mimimally include, current physical problem list, assessment, plan.
- ☐ Check-in timetables with client list.

FIGURE 2 cont'd.

Client centered planning sample checklist- what can the client plan for?

<u>Family support</u>
- ☐ Spiritual support
- ☐ Friends
- ☐ Family members

<u>Anticipatory Grief support</u>
- ☐ Online support
- ☐ In-person support

<u>Setting for euthanasia</u>
- ☐ Outdoor
- ☐ Indoor
- ☐ Candles
- ☐ Music
- ☐ Bed present/not present
- ☐ Blanket

<u>Children</u>
- ☐ Broaching topic of death
- ☐ Discussing if they would like to participate
- ☐ Giving them Resources - age specific, books, coloring books, videos to watch
- ☐ Have a plan if they need to go to a sitter, grandparent's house, parent takes for a walk…

<u>Rituals and Ceremony</u>

<u>Crisis Kit</u>

<u>Planning</u>
- ☐ Day/Time
- ☐ Scheduling appointment with veterinarian
    - ☐ First Choice_____
    - ☐ Second Choice_____
    - ☐ Third Choice/Emergency_____
- ☐ People to contact who may want to be there or would like the chance to say goodbye.
- ☐ Arranging for childcare if needed.
- ☐ Time off for grieving.
- ☐ Consider Aftercare
    - ☐ Private Cremation (You receive your pet's ashes back)
    - ☐ Communal Cremation (Your pet's ashes are scattered)
    - ☐ Burial- you will comply with the rules and regulations in your city or county. It is your responsibility to check with your local municipality.
- ☐ Grief Resources
    - ☐ Online support
    - ☐ In-person support
    - ☐ Pet Loss Hotlines available

FIGURE 3

Sample client centered planning checklist.

Created by Dr. Lynn Hendrix ©2021.

Crisis- Make sure you have a crisis kit from your veterinarian

<u>Respiratory distress</u>- working hard at breathing
- ☐ abdominal effort
- ☐ nostril flare
- ☐ open mouth breathing in cats
- ☐ resting respiratory rates higher than 60 breaths in a minute (normal is 20-30).
- ☐ coughing (frequent or increasing frequency).
- ☐ blood from nose, rapid, repeated sneezing.

<u>Brain distress</u>
- ☐ Seizures
- ☐ vestibular disease (head tilt, eyes bouncing back and forth, falling over, and circling)
- ☐ howling (especially in a kitty, although not always distress)
- ☐ head pressing, getting stuck in corners, seeming confused (last 3 are often signs of headache.)

<u>GI distress</u>
- ☐ Vomiting
- ☐ Diarrhea, especially if there is blood in it.
- ☐ Constipation (straining to defecate and producing very little or no feces).
- ☐ Bloated abdomen with retching.
- ☐ Painful abdomen.

<u>Urinary stress</u>
- ☐ straining to urinate
- ☐ blood in urine
- ☐ urinating more frequently
- ☐ drops of urine, or no urine production (sometimes they are holding it or can't get up and seem distressed)
- ☐ crying when they urinate.
- ☐ Urinating on self, unable to get up or away from urine.

<u>Cardiac distress</u>
- ☐ Clot going to other body parts- back legs in cats (become paralyzed, very painful), to the lungs (trouble breathing suddenly), to the heart (often sudden death), to the brain (stroke),
- ☐ Sudden death
- ☐ Rapid heart rate (often manifesting in rapid breathing.)>120 in dogs, >180 in cats.

<u>Musculoskeletal distress</u>
- ☐ Pain, difficulty getting up, falling over.
- ☐ Bone pain (can happen with cancer.)
- ☐ Not wanting to eat (can be pain in teeth or jaw).
- ☐ Significant muscle loss that weakens them, keeps them from being mobile.

<u>Skin distress</u>
- ☐ Bed sores
- ☐ Ulcerated tumors/Weeping tumors
- ☐ Hot spots
- ☐ Severe itching (can be pain related)
- ☐ Constant licking one spot (can be pain related).
- ☐ Urine scald (Irritated skin from laying on urine)

<u>Emotional distress</u>
- ☐ Cannot get up
- ☐ Urinating or defecating on self

FIGURE 4

Sample basic daily/weekly palliative checklist.

Created by Dr. Lynn Hendrix ©2021.

- ☐ Struggling to get up
- ☐ Frustration
- ☐ Confusion
- ☐ Depression
- ☐ Avoidance behavior, withdrawing from family.
- ☐ Sighing.
- ☐ Moaning/Groaning
- ☐ Cannot do things they want to do. (Different than apathy- does not care to do anymore)

Lynn Hendrix DVM, CHPV© 2021

FIGURE 4 cont'd.

BASIC PALLIATIVE CHECKLIST

☐ **Short term Palliative Goals for Pet**

☐ What are the families short term goals.?

☐ Have we met those goals?
- ☐ Today
- ☐ This week
- ☐ This month

☐ Have there been any changes we need to address?
- ☐ Today
- ☐ This week
- ☐ This month

☐ What tools are we using to measure progress or regress?
- ☐ Canine Brief Pain Inventory
- ☐ Liverpool Osteoarthritis in Dogs
- ☐ Helsinki Chronic Pain Index
- ☐ Feline Grimace Scale
- ☐ Scale of your choice

☐ Review Current interventions

☐ Discuss with Family members and re-evaluate short term goals
- ☐ Make changes to medical palliative plan

☐ **Short-term Caregiver needs**

☐ Have there been changes in their lives that need to be addressed?

☐ Create a plan for next 24 hours, 48 hours, 1 week, 1 month

☐ Re-evaluate as needed

☐ Next Check-in Time

NOTES

FIGURE 4 cont'd.

BEGINING PALLIATIVE CHECKLIST

- ☐ Goals of Care for Caregivers
  - ☐ Their Understanding of the disease process
  - ☐ Psychosocial Needs
  - ☐ Spiritual Needs
  - ☐ Review of disease progression and trajectory
  - ☐ Review plan for death-Euthanasia vs Palliated death
  - ☐ Review of Imminent Death Signs
- ☐ Medications needed
  - ☐ Pain Management
  - ☐ Symptom management
- ☐ Equipment/Environmental needs
  - ☐ Wheelchair/Orthotic
  - ☐ Mobility Aids
  - ☐ Changes to flooring
  - ☐ Enviromental changes
  - ☐ Other needs, such as grooming supplies,
- ☐ Educational Materials left with caregivers
  - ☐ Chronic pain information
  - ☐ Quality of Life information
  - ☐ Disease specific information
  - ☐ Symptom specific information
- ☐ Grief Support
  - ☐ Local In-Person Grief Group Support
  - ☐ Anticipatory Loss Support
  - ☐ Online Grief Support
- ☐ Crisis kit medications
  - ☐ For euthanasia preparation
  - ☐ For specific clinical signs
    - ☐ Acute Pain
    - ☐ Seizures
    - ☐ Breathlessness
    - ☐ Bleeding
    - ☐ Anxiety
    - ☐ Night Waking
    - ☐ Excess saliva
    - ☐ Skin issues (disease specific)

NOTES

FIGURE 5

Sample first appointment palliative checklist.

Created by Dr. Lynn Hendrix© 2021.

Index

'*Note*: Page numbers followed by "f" indicate figures, "t" indicate tables and "b" indicate boxes.'

Printed and bound by CPI Group (UK) Ltd, Croydon, CR0 4YY

03/10/2024

01040300-0014